STRUCTURAL FETAL ABNORMALITIES
THE TOTAL PICTURE

STRUCTURAL FETAL ABNORMALITIES

THE TOTAL PICTURE

EDITOR

ROGER C. SANDERS, M.D.
Medical Director
Ultrasound Institute of Baltimore, Lutherville, Maryland

Clinical Professor, Radiology, Obstetrics, and Gynecology
University of Maryland School of Medicine, Baltimore, Maryland

ASSISTANT EDITORS

LILLIAN R. BLACKMON, M.D.
Associate Professor of Pediatrics
University of Maryland School of Medicine, Baltimore, Maryland

W. ALLEN HOGGE, M.D.
Associate Professor, Obstetrics, Gynecology and Reproductive Sciences
University of Pittsburgh School of Medicine
Medical Director, Department of Genetics
Magee-Womens Hospital, Pittsburgh, Pennsylvania

ERIC A. WULFSBERG, M.D.
Associate Professor of Pediatrics
Division of Human Genetics
University of Maryland School of Medicine, Baltimore, Maryland

with 206 illustrations

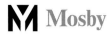

St. Louis Baltimore Boston Carlsbad Chicago Naples New York Philadelphia Portland
London Madrid Mexico City Singapore Sydney Tokyo Toronto Wiesbaden

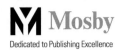

Mosby
Dedicated to Publishing Excellence

A Times Mirror
Company

Editor-in-Chief: Susan Gay
Managing Editor: Elizabeth Corra
Project Manager: Linda Clarke
Production Editor: Veda King
Designer: Nancy McDonald
Cover Design: Carolyn O'Brien
Electronic Production Coordinator: Pamela Merritt
Manufacturing Manager: Betty Richmond

Printed in the United States of America
Composition by Mosby Electronic Production, Philadelphia
Printing/binding by Maple Vail—York

Mosby–Year Book, Inc.
11830 Westline Industrial Drive
St. Louis, Missouri 63146

Library of Congress Cataloging-in-Publication Data
Structural fetal abnormalities: the total picture/editor, Roger C. Sanders;
    assistant editors, Lillian R. Blackmon, W. Allen Hogge, Eric A. Wulfsberg.
        p.   cm.
    Includes bibliographical references and index.
    ISBN 0-8151-7838-7
    1. Fetus—Abnormalities. 2. Fetus—Ultrasonic imaging.
I. Sanders, Roger C., 1936-   .
    [DNLM: 1. Abnormalities—ultrasonography—atlases.
2. Ultrasonography, Prenatal—atlases.   WQ 17 S927 1996]
RG626.S78   1996
618.3'2—dc20
DNLM/DLC
for Library of Congress   95-23082
                                                            CIP

97 98 99 00 / 9 8 7 6 5 4 3

Contributors

LILLIAN R. BLACKMON, M.D.
Associate Professor of Pediatrics
University of Maryland School of Medicine
Baltimore, Maryland

DUKE CAMERON, M.D.
Associate Professor of Cardiac Surgery
The Johns Hopkins School of Medicine
Director of Pediatric Cardiac Surgery
The Johns Hopkins Hospital
Baltimore, Maryland

CRAIG R. DUFRESNE, M.D., F.A.C.S.
Co-Director, Center for Facial Rehabilitation
Fairfax Hospital, Inova Medical Institution
Fairfax, Virginia
Clinical Assistant Professor, Departments of Neurosurgery
and Plastic Surgery
The Johns Hopkins University
Baltimore, Maryland
Clinical Assistant Professor of Plastic Surgery
Georgetown University
Washington, D.C.

DAVID L. DUDGEON, M.D.
Professor of Surgery and Pediatrics
Case Western Reserve University of Medicine
Director of Pediatric Surgery and Surgeon,
Division Chief of Pediatric Surgery
Rainbow Babies and Childrens Hospital
Cleveland, Ohio

JOHN P. GEARHART, M.D., F.A.C.S., F.A.A.P.
Director of Pediatric Urology
The Johns Hopkins Hospital
Baltimore, Maryland

JOHN E. HERZENBERG, M.D., F.R.C.S.C.
Associate Professor of Orthopaedic Surgery and Pediatrics
University of Maryland School of Medicine
Co-Director, Maryland Center for Limb Lengthening
Kernan Hospital
Baltimore, Maryland

W. ALLEN HOGGE, M.D.
Associate Professor, Obstetrics, Gynecology and
Reproductive Sciences
University of Pittsburgh School of Medicine
Medical Director, Department of Genetics
Magee-Womens Hospital
Pittsburgh, Pennsylvania

CHARLES N. PAIDAS, M.D.
Assistant Professor of Surgery, Pediatrics,
Oncology, Anesthesia, and Critical Care Medicine
Director, Pediatric Trauma
The Johns Hopkins University School of Medicine
Baltimore, Maryland

DROR PALEY, M.D., F.R.C.S.C.
Co-Director, Maryland Center for Limb Lengthening and
Reconstruction
Associate Professor of Orthopaedic Surgery
Chief, Pediatric Orthopaedics
University of Maryland School of Medicine and Kernan
Hospital
Baltimore, Maryland

JOHN RAGHEB, M.D.
Clinical Instructor, Pediatric Neurosurgery
University of Maryland Medical System
Baltimore, Maryland

ROGER C. SANDERS, M.D.
Medical Director
Ultrasound Institute of Baltimore
Lutherville, Maryland
Clinical Professor, Radiology, Obstetrics, and Gynecology
University of Maryland School of Medicine
Baltimore, Maryland

JANET N. SCHEEL, M.D.
Assistant Professor
Division of Cardiology
Department of Pediatrics
University of Maryland Medical System
Baltimore, Maryland

ERIC A. WULFSBERG, M.D.
Associate Professor of Pediatrics
Division of Human Genetics
University of Maryland School of Medicine
Baltimore, Maryland

Preface

Most fetal abnormalities discovered in utero are found in the course of a diagnostic ultrasound examination. On occasion, sonograms are performed in a specific effort to find an abnormality because of family history or a positive screening test, such as an abnormal alpha-fetoprotein. More often, ultrasound examinations that uncover abnormalities are performed for unrelated reasons. For instance, many sonograms are requested when there is a date versus examination discrepancy or vaginal bleeding is present. This book is designed to provide a comprehensive picture of the genetic, epidemiologic, and ultrasonographic features; the obstetrical, neonatal, and surgical management; and the prognosis of the more common abnormalities discovered by ultrasound examination. Many conditions that may be discovered with invasive prenatal testing, but which do not have ultrasonographic features, such as Tay-Sachs disease and Fragile X syndrome, are not considered.

When a fetus with an unusual ultrasound appearance is seen, many questions arise. Parents may experience varying levels of grief, guilt, and worry. Often there is no correlation between the level of concern and the ultrasonographic findings. However, these concerns stimulate spoken and unspoken questions about the pregnancy and neonatal consequences. The obstetrician who encounters fetal malformations infrequently is faced with unfamiliar dilemmas concerning the pregnancy management such as delivery timing, route, and site. Whoever discovers the abnormality, whether it be a sonographer, radiologist, or obstetrician, encounters some unplanned worrying responsibilities. Is the finding real or merely an artifact? Is the diagnosis specific, or is there a wide differential? Is it lethal? Is it correctable? Is it hereditary? This book attempts to answer many of these questions.

Prenatal care of both mother and fetus is a joint effort. Today, most prenatal centers have established fetal abnormality management groups. These groups meet at regular intervals to coordinate care. Depending on the nature and severity of the finding, responsibility for care is shared between the obstetrician, perinatologist, neonatologist, and surgeon. In practice, clinical staff such as sonographers, nurses, and genetic counselors play a very significant role in both diagnosis and care. In addition, consultations with specialty experts, such as those in pediatric cardiology, dysmorphology, or maxillofacial surgery,

may be required. The patient, in this way, is assured a more caring, comprehensive care plan. Each care provider must have some knowledge of the other specialties involved and of the long-term prognosis. This volume includes sections written by experts in each area. Sonologist Roger C. Sanders provides the ultrasonographic findings of each abnormality followed by the perspective of each involved expert. Eric A. Wulfsberg— pediatric geneticist and dysmorphologist; W. Allen Hogge— perinatologist; Lillian Blackmon— neonatologist; Janet Scheel— pediatric cardiologist, John Gearhart—pediatric urologist, and several surgeons (David Dudgeon, Dror Paley, Charles Paidas, Craig Dufresne, John Herzenberg, John Ragheb, and Duke Cameron) have joined forces to complete this comprehensive picture of diagnosis and management of the more common structural fetal abnormalities detected by obstetrical ultrasound.

There are thousands of conditions and syndromes that cause fetal deformities. Conditions presented here were chosen either because they are frequently recognized with ultrasound, or because a distinct ultrasonographic feature exists that allows definitive diagnosis and prognosis (the "hitchhiker" thumb of diastrophic dwarfism distinguishes this syndrome from other dwarfisms). Some of the more common sonographic dilemmas that sometimes indicate underlying fetal problems, such as amniotic bands or cord masses, are also included. Many rare malformations or syndromes are mentioned in the discussion of differential diagnosis.

Each abnormality is considered in a similar manner. The template for each entity has been designed to facilitate location of a specific feature of any condition whether it be the recurrence rate, ultrasonographic differential diagnosis, or surgical complications. In the first appendix there is a list of the differential diagnosis of fetal ultrasonographic findings. Included in the second appendix is a brief description of the ultrasonographic appearance of many of the more rare syndromes or abnormalities. The authors hope that the book will be used during pregnancy in the same fashion as *Smith's Recognizable Patterns of Human Malformation* is used postdelivery, as an easy reference when an abnormality is found. There is a sizable bibliography following the section on each abnormality to afford the reader greater detail for each condition.

Acknowledgment

This book would not have been possible without the organization, skill, and agreeable coercion of Billie J. Fish. Billie is the perfectionist who made sure that the contributions from so many diverse sites and individuals were melded together into the finished product.

Contents

1. Chromosomes
1.1 Triploidy, 1
1.2 Trisomy 13, 3
1.3 Trisomy 18, 6
1.4 Trisomy 21 (Down Syndrome), 9
1.5 Turner's Syndrome, 12

2. The Central Nervous Sytem
2.1 Agenesis of the Corpus Callosum, 14
2.2 Anencephaly, 17
2.3 Aqueductal Stenosis, 20
2.4 Arachnoid Cyst, 23
2.5 Caudal Aplasia/Dysplasia (Regression) Sequence, 25
2.6 Dandy-Walker Malformations, 27
2.7 Encephalocele, 30
2.8 Holoprosencephaly (Alobar, Lobar, Semilobar), 34
2.9 Hydranencephaly, 37
2.10 Iniencephaly, 39
2.11 Intracranial Hemorrhage, 41
2.12 Intracranial Teratoma, 43
2.13 Microcephaly, 45
2.14 Spinal Dysraphism (Myelomeningocele, Myeloschisis, Meningocele), 47
2.15 Vein of Galen Malformation, 51

3. Cardiac
3.1 Bradycardias, 54
3.2 Cardiac Rhabdomyoma, 57
3.3 Coarctation of the Aorta, 59
3.4 Double-Outlet Right Ventricle, 62
3.5 Ebstein's Anomaly, 65
3.6 Ectopia Cordis (Pentalogy of Cantrell), 68
3.7 Endocardial Cushion Defect (Atrioventricular Canal), 71
3.8 Hypoplastic Left Heart Syndrome, 73
3.9 Premature Atrial Contractions ("Dropped Beats"), 76
3.10 Tachycardias, 78
3.11 Tetralogy of Fallot, 81
3.12 Transposition of the Great Arteries (D-Transposition of Simple Transposition), 84
3.13 Ventricular Septal Defect, 87

4. The Genitourinary Tract
4.1 Adrenal Hematoma, 89
4.2 Exstrophy of the Bladder, 91
4.3 Hydronephrosis (Ureteropelvic Junction Obstruction and Reflux), 93
4.4 Infantile Polycystic Kidney Disease, 97
4.5 Multicystic Dysplastic Kidney, 100
4.6 Ovarian Cysts, 103
4.7 Posterior Urethral Valves, 106
4.8 Renal Agenesis, 109
4.9 Sacrococcygeal Teratoma, 112
4.10 Ureterocele, 116

5. The Chest
5.1 Cystic Adenomatoid Malformation of the Lung, 118
5.2 Diaphragmatic Hernia, 122
5.3 Esophageal Atresia (Tracheal Atresia, Tracheoesophageal Fistula), 126
5.4 Pleural Effusion, 130

6. The Gastrointestinal System
6.1 Anal Atresia (Imperforate Anus), 132
6.2 Duodenal Atresia, 134
6.3 Gastrointestinal Atresia or Stenosis, 137
6.4 Gastroschisis, 140
6.5 Meconium Cyst (Peritonitis), 144
6.6 Meconium Ileus, 147
6.7 Omphalocele, 149

7. The Neck and Face
7.1 Cleft Lip and Palate, 153
7.2 Cystic Hygroma, 158
7.3 Thyroid Enlargement/Goiter, 161

8. The Limbs

8.1 Achondrogenesis, 163
8.2 Achondroplasia, 166
8.3 Amniotic Band Syndrome, 169
8.4 Arthrogryposis, 172
8.5 Camptomelic Dysplasia, 174
8.6 Club and Rocker-Bottom Feet (Vertical Talus), 176
8.7 Diastrophic Dysplasia, 179
8.8 Focal Femoral Hypoplasia, 182
8.9 Klippel-Trenaunay-Weber Syndrome, 185
8.10 Limb-Body Wall Complex (Body Stalk Complex, Cyllosomas), 188
8.11 Multiple Pterygium Syndrome, 191
8.12 Osteogenesis Imperfecta, 193
8.13 Polydactyly, 197
8.14 Radial Ray Problems (Radial Ray Aplasia/Hypoplasia), 199
8.15 Thanatophoric Dwarfism (Dysplasia), 201

9. Infections

9.1 Cytomegalic Inclusion Disease, 203
9.2 Parvovirus (Fifth Disease), 206
9.3 Congenital Syphilis, 208
9.4 Toxoplasmosis, 210
9.5 Varicella Infection (Varicella-Zoster Virus), 213

10. Drugs

10.1 Fetal Alcohol Syndrome, 215
10.2 Antiseizure Drugs (Phenytoin, Carbamazepine, Valproic Acid, and Phenobarbital), 217
10.3 Illegal Drugs (Cocaine, Heroin), 219

11. Twins

11.1 Acardiac Twin (Acardiac Monster) Holoacardius (Twin Reversed Arterial Perfusion Sequence), 221
11.2 Conjoined Twins, 223
11.3 Stuck Twin, 228
11.4 Twins: Intrauterine Growth Retardation, 230
11.5 Twin-Twin Transfusion, 232

12. Miscellaneous Abnormalities

12.1 Chorioangioma, 235
12.2 Nonimmune Hydrops Fetalis, 237
12.3 Rhesus Incompatibility, 240
12.4 VACTERL Association, 242

13. Abnormal Sonographic Findings

13.1 Amniotic Membranes, 244
13.2 Cord Cyst, 246
13.3 Intrauterine Growth Retardation, 248
13.4 Macrosomia, 250
13.5 Oligohydramnios, 252
13.6 Polyhydramnios, 254

Appendix I   Differential Diagnoses of Abnormal in utero Sonographic Findings, 255
Appendix II   Sonographic Features of Less Common Fetal Abnormalities, 269

STRUCTURAL FETAL ABNORMALITIES

THE TOTAL PICTURE

1 Chromosomes

1.1 TRIPLOIDY

EPIDEMIOLOGY/GENETICS

Definition   Rare, lethal chromosomal abnormality. An entire extra haploid set of chromosomes resulting in 69 chromosomes instead of the usual 46. Severe growth retardation affects the skeleton more than the head.

Epidemiology   One to two percent of human conceptions are triploid, but most end in spontaneous miscarriage. Very rare at birth (M1.5:F1).

Embryology   A complete extra set of chromosomes results in 69 XXX or XYY. Sixty percent result from fertilization with two sperm, 40% result from fertilization of a diploid egg. Central nervous system malformations include hydrocephalus, holoprosencephaly, and neural tube defects. Hypertelorism, cleft lip/cleft palate, syndactyly of fingers three and four and congenital heart defects are typical features.

Inheritance Patterns   Sporadic.

Teratogens   None.

Screening   Serum alpha-fetoprotein (AFP) levels may be markedly elevated (e.g., 8 multiples of the median [MOM]).

Prognosis   Lethal antenatally or in the newborn period. Rare mosaic cases survive with moderate to severe mental retardation.

SONOGRAPHY

Findings
1. **Fetus:** The sonographic findings include:
   a. Severe early onset of intrauterine growth retardation.
   b. Isolated ventriculomegaly. Arnold Chiari malformation, holoprosencephaly, or agenesis of the corpus callosum.
   c. Cystic hygroma may be present, but is unusual.
   d. Facial clefts.
   e. Limb abnormalities, such as club foot or syndactyly.
   f. Congenital heart disease.
   g. Renal anomalies such as hydronephrosis.
   h. Omphalocele.
   i. Meningocele.
2. **Amniotic Fluid:** Oligohydramnios is often seen.
3. **Placenta:** The placenta is often abnormal. Either there is an enlarged placenta with normal texture or an enlarged placenta with cystic spaces, similar to a molar pregnancy (partial mole).
4. **Measurement Data:** Severe early onset of intrauterine growth retardation (IUGR) is usually seen. Intrauterine growth retardation may develop as early as 12 to 14 weeks.
5. **When Detectable:** Placental changes and some of the more severe structural changes may be seen as early as 12 to 14 weeks.

Pitfalls   Structural changes are highly variable and the placenta may be tiny and senescent.

Differential Diagnosis   Trisomy 13 and 18.

Where Else to Look   The lead finding (placentomegaly or IUGR) mandates a careful look at the rest of the fetus.

PREGNANCY MANAGEMENT

Investigations and Consultations Required   Amniocentesis, chorionic villi sampling (CVS), or umbilical blood sampling establish the diagnosis. Once a cytogenetic diagnosis has been established, no further investigations or consultations are necessary.

Monitoring   If pregnancy termination is not an option, monitor for preeclampsia or hyperthyroidism.

Pregnancy Course   Molar changes in the placenta predispose to hyperemesis gravidarum, early preeclampsia, theca lutein cysts, and, on occasion, hyperthyroidism.

Pregnancy Termination Issues   Suction dilatation and evacuation is appropriate once a cytogenetic diagnosis has been established.

Delivery   Fetal monitoring and cesarean section are both contraindicated for the pregnancy complicated by a triploid gestation.

NEONATOLOGY

Resuscitation   Contraindicated if the diagnosis is definite because of the established lethal prognosis.

Transport   Only indicated if diagnostic confirmation, counselling, and long-term care planning is not available locally.

Testing and Confirmation   Lymphocyte karyotype can confirm the chromosome abnormality.

Nursery Management   Provision of basic supportive care—warmth, hygiene, nourishment, and comfort only—until prognosis for protracted survival is defined and long-term care decisions can be addressed by family.

BIBLIOGRAPHY

Crane JP, Beaver HA, Cheung SW: Antenatal ultrasound findings in fetal triploidy syndrome. *J Ultrasound Med* 1985; 4:519-524.

Edwards MT, Smith WL, Hanson J et al: Prenatal sonographic diagnosis of triploidy. *J Ultrasound Med* 1986; 5:279-281.

Gorlin RJ, et al (eds): In: *Syndromes of the head and neck*, 3rd edition. Oxford University Press, New York. 1990. pp. 64-65.

Jones KL (ed): In: *Smith's recognizable patterns of human malformations*. WB Saunders, Philadelphia. 1988. pp. 10-15.

Lockwood C, Scioscia A, Stiller R et al: Sonographic features of the triploid fetus. *Am J Obstet Gynecol* 1987; 157:285-287.

Pircon RA, Porto M, Towers CV et al: Ultrasound findings in pregnancies complicated by fetal triploidy. *J Ultrasound Med* 1989; 8:507-511.

Shepard TH, Fantel AG: Embryonic and early fetal loss. *Clin Perinatol* 1979; 6:219-243.

Wertecki W, Graham JM Jr, Sergovich GP: The clinical syndrome of triploidy. Obstet Gynecol 1976; 47:69.

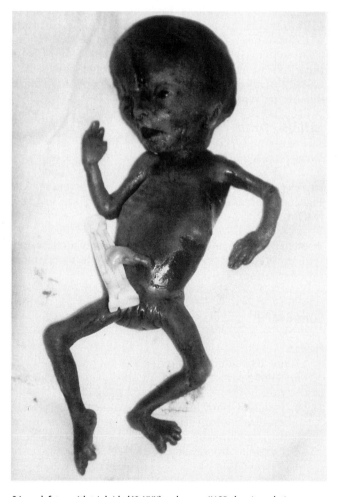

24-week fetus with triploidy (69, XXX) and severe IUGR showing relative macrocephaly and 3–4 finger syndactyly.

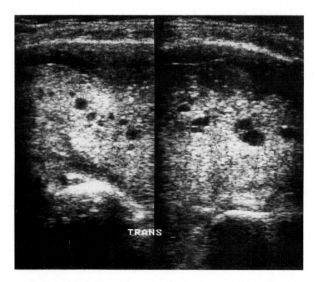

Triploidy. Composite view of the placenta. The placenta is enlarged and there are numerous cystic areas within. On other views, a small, but otherwise normal-appearing fetus. In other examples of triploidy the placenta may be large, but without cysts.

1.2 TRISOMY 13

EPIDEMIOLOGY/GENETICS

Definition   Trisomy 13 is the third most common multiple malformation, autosomal trisomy syndrome recognized at birth. Infants have a characteristic phenotype that includes major cardiac, brain, gastrointestinal, and limb malformations.

Epidemiology   1 out of every 5,000 to 10,000 births.

Embryology   The phenotype is due to full trisomy 13. Increased maternal age has been documented in this disorder. Rare mosaic, partial trisomy 13 syndromes (with varying phenotypes) and translocation patients have been reported. Microcephaly, holoprosencephaly, microphthalmia, polydactyly, facial clefts, and abnormal helices are found in greater than 50% of patients. Eighty percent of patients have congenital heart defects with atrial septal defects (ASDs) and ventricular septal defects (VSDs) being the most common, but many patients have complex heart lesions. Other distinctive abnormalities include polycystic kidneys (30% of patients) and omphalocele (less than 20% of patients).

Inheritance Patterns   Most cases are sporadic with a 1 out of 100 risk of recurrence in future pregnancies. Rare familial translocations have a higher recurrence risk depending on the specific translocation.

Teratogens   None.

Screening   Maternal serum biochemical marker screening (*triple screen*) is not helpful in detecting trisomy 13 fetuses.

Prognosis   This condition is lethal or has a very poor prognosis in all cases. Seventy percent of affected infants are stillborn or die by age 6 months and 85% die in the first year. All survivors with full trisomy 13 have profound mental retardation. In infancy, severe failure to thrive, feeding difficulties, seizures, apneic attacks, and visual and hearing deficits occur in the majority of infants, secondary to the orofacial and central nervous system (CNS) defects.

SONOGRAPHY

Findings
1. **Fetus**
   a. Holoprosencephaly (see Chapter 2.8) (40%).
   b. Central cleft lip and palate of all types (see Chapter 7) (45%).
   c. Enlarged cisterna magna (15%).
   d. Eyes—Close-set eyes with many variations, for example, hypotelorism, single orbit with two globes, cyclops, or micropthalmia.
   e. Cystic hygroma (21%).
   f. Nose—The nose may have a single nostril or be absent and replaced by a proboscis.
   g. Hand and feet problems—Polydactyly, club and rocker-bottom feet, club hands, and overlapping fingers may occur.
   h. Congenital heart disease—Numerous different abnormalities are seen, principally hypoplastic left heart and VSD.
   i. Cystic kidneys—The kidneys may be more echogenic, not enlarged, and may contain a few small cysts. Occasionally, hydronephrosis may be seen.
   j. Omphalocele (see Chapter 6.7) (18%).
   k. Neural tube defects (see Chapter 2.14).
   l. Echogenic chordae tendinae (35%). All fetuses had other sonographic findings.
2. **Amniotic Fluid:** Polyhydramnios was seen in 15%, oligohydramnios in 10%.
3. **Placenta:** Normal.
4. **Measurement Data:** IUGR is often present. Microcephaly is frequent (12%).
5. **When Detectable:** With vaginal probe at about 12 weeks.

Differential Diagnosis   This is a very distinct entity. Holoprosencephaly without trisomy 13 may occur.

Where Else to Look   A detailed look at all organs is required when this karyotype abnormality is suspected.

PREGNANCY MANAGEMENT

Investigations and Consultations Required   Amniocentesis, CVS, or umbilical blood sampling establish the diagnosis. For patients in whom the diagnosis is made beyond the point of legal pregnancy termination or those who decide to continue the pregnancy, a neonatologist should consult with the family about appropriate perinatal and neonatal management.

Monitoring   Only routine prenatal care should be performed. The family should be offered supportive psychological care throughout the pregnancy.

Pregnancy Course   Intrauterine growth retardation is common, and aggressive management such as monitoring or early delivery is inappropriate.

Pregnancy Termination Issues   Suction dilatation and evacuation is appropriate once a cytogenetic diagnosis has been established.

Delivery   Electronic fetal monitoring and cesarean section should be avoided unless requested by the family after a thorough discussion of the prognosis for infants with trisomy 13.

NEONATOLOGY

Resuscitation   A decision whether or not to give life support should be considered prior to delivery when the diagnosis is established. If unknown prior to birth, providing life support is appropriate until diagnosis can be established.

Transport   Only indicated if diagnostic confirmation, counselling, and long-term care planning is not available locally.

Testing and Confirmation   Birth weight is frequently normal. Lymphocyte karyotype can confirm the chromosome abnormality.

Nursery Management   Full life support is appropriate until the diagnosis is confirmed and the family has time for weighing options for duration and intensity of support. Care requirements will be contingent upon associated organ involvement and the long-term goals of the family. Central nervous system, cardiac, and orofacial defects are usually the major problems. Feeding mode and respiratory drive are most commonly the key issues for interim care.

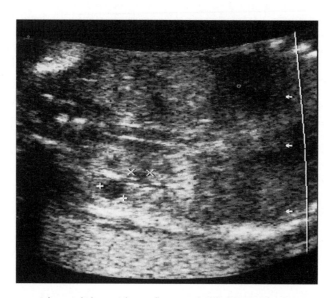

Echogenic kidneys with cysts (between the x's) due to trisomy 13.

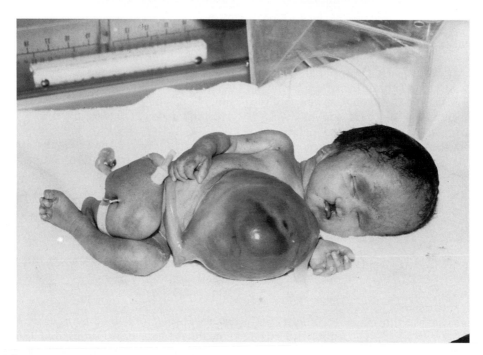

19-week fetus with trisomy 13 (47,XX, + 13) exhibiting the classical features including midline facial cleft, omphalocele, and polydactyly.

BIBLIOGRAPHY

Benacerraf BR, Frigoletto FD Jr et al: Abnormal facial features and extremities in human trisomy syndromes: prenatal US appearance. *Radiology* 1986; 159:243-246.

Benacerraf BR, Miller WA, Frigoletto FD Jr: Sonographic detection of fetuses with trisomy 13 and 18: accuracy and limitations. *Am J Obstet Gynecol* 1988; 158:404-409.

Carey JC: Health supervision and anticipatory guidance for infants with congenital defects. In Ballard RA (ed): *Pediatric care of the ICN graduate*. Philadelphia, WB Saunders, 1988.

Gorlin RJ et al (eds): *Syndromes of the Head and Neck*, 3rd edition. New York, Oxford University Press. 1990. pp. 40-43.

Greene MF, Benacerraf BR, Frigoletto FD Jr: Reliable criteria for the prenatal sonographic diagnosis of alobar holoprosencephaly. *Am J Obstet Gynecol* 1987; 156:687-689.

Hodes ME, Cole J, Palmer et al: Clinical experience with trisomies 18 and 13. *J Med Genet* 1978; 15:48-60.

Jones KL (ed): In: *Smith's recognizable patterns of human malformations*. Philadelphia, WB Saunders Company. 1988. pp. 20-21.

Lehman CD, Nyberg DA, Winter TC III et al: Trisomy 13 syndrome: prenatal US findings in a review of 33 cases. Radiology 1995; 194:217-222.

Taylor AI: Autosomal trisomy syndromes: a detailed study of 27 cases of Edwards' syndrome and 27 cases of Patau's syndrome. *J Med Genet* 1968; 5:227-252.

Warkany J, Passarge E, Smith LB: Congenital malformations in autosomal trisomy syndromes. *Am J Dis Child* 1966; 112:502-517.

1.3 TRISOMY 18

EPIDEMIOLOGY/GENETICS

Definition Trisomy 18 is the second most common multiple malformation, autosomal trisomy syndrome and presents with IUGR, microcephaly, and congenital heart defects (80%).

Epidemiology 1 out of every 3,000 to 5,000 (M1:F3).

Embryology Most infants have full trisomy 18. Rare patients with mosaic karyotypes, partial trisomy 18 syndromes (with varying phenotypes), and translocation cases have been reported. Infants with trisomy 18 present with severe IUGR, microdolichocephaly with a prominent occiput, malformed ears, micrognathia, clenched hands, and congenital heart defects (80%) that are characterized by complex polyvalvular abnormalities with VSDs. Malformations that occur in less than 50% of cases include cleft lip and palate, limb defects, omphalocele, and diaphragmatic hernias.

Inheritance Patterns Most cases are sporadic with a 1 out of 100 risk of recurrence in future pregnancies. Rare familial translocations have a higher recurrence risk depending on the specific translocation.

Teratogens None.

Screening Maternal serum biochemical marker screening (the *triple screen*) may detect as many as 80% of trisomy 18 fetuses.

Prognosis Trisomy 18 is lethal, or has a very poor prognosis in all cases. Fifty percent of affected infants will die in the first 2 months of life and 90% will die in the first year. All survivors with full trisomy 18 have profound mental retardation. Associated cardiac and gastrointestinal anomalies are usually life threatening and definitely life limiting, if not corrected or palliated by surgery. Failure to thrive and feeding difficulties occur in all who survive the immediate neonatal period.

SONOGRAPHY

Findings
1. **Fetus**
   a. Limbs—abnormal with persistently clenched hands and overlapping of the fourth digit. Club and rocker-bottom feet are typical. Unusually positioned or absent thumb or radial agenesis occur. Persistently extended legs may be seen.
   b. Face—Micrognathia is common (a good quality profile view is desirable); unilateral or bilateral cleft lip and/or palate may occur.
   c. Congenital heart disease—VSD is most common; tetralogy of Fallot, transposition, and coarctation of the aorta are less frequent.
   d. Omphalocele—usually containing only bowel is seen in about 25% of cases.
   e. Diaphragmatic hernia (about 10%).
   f. Neural tube defects (20%).
   g. Choroid plexus cysts (25%)—Between 2% and 9% of choroid plexus cysts are associated with trisomy 18. A choroid plexus cyst as the sole feature of trisomy 18 is very rare. The number of cysts does not influence the likelihood of trisomy 18. Larger cysts are thought by some to be more likely due to trisomy 18.
   h. Single umbilical artery.
   i. Cystic hygroma (15%).
   j. Enlarged (greater than 10 mm) cisterna magna.
   k. Lemon-like head shape with or without spinal dysraphism. A strawberry-shaped head may also be seen.
2. **Amniotic Fluid:** Twenty-five percent have polyhydramnios with IUGR. Oligohydramnios may occur.
3. **Placenta:** Normal.
4. **Measurement Data:** Early onset of IUGR is seen in over 50% of cases (prior to 18 weeks).
5. **When Detectable:** Fifteen to 16 weeks—earlier if congenital heart disease or omphalocele is present.

Pitfalls A medial indentation on the border of the choroid plexus may be mistaken for a choroid plexus cyst.

Differential Diagnosis
1. Pena Shokeir syndrome.
2. Arthrogryposis.

Where Else to Look May affect any organ.

PREGNANCY MANAGEMENT

Investigations and Consultations Required A karyotype should be obtained by amniocentesis or percutaneous umbilical blood sampling (PUBS). Once a cytogenetic diagnosis has been established, consultation should be obtained from a neonatologist to discuss a plan for management of the newborn with the family. An isolated choroid plexus cyst with a normal *triple screen* is considered by many as so unlikely to be due to trisomy 18 that karyotyping is not essential.

Monitoring Maternal status should be monitored in standard fashion. Fetal evaluation is not appropriate because emergency intervention is not warranted. The family should be offered supportive psychological care.

Pregnancy Course   Fetuses with trisomy 18 are likely to develop severe IUGR and, if monitored, evidence of fetal distress in labor.

Pregnancy Termination Issues   Suction dilatation and evacuation techniques are appropriate once a cytogenetic diagnosis has been established.

Delivery   Electronic fetal monitoring and cesarean section should be avoided unless requested by the family after a thorough discussion of the prognosis for infants with trisomy 18.

NEONATOLOGY

Resuscitation   A decision of whether or not to give life support should be considered prior to delivery when the diagnosis is definite. If unknown prior to birth, providing life support is appropriate until the diagnosis can be established.

Transport   Only indicated if diagnostic confirmation, counselling, and long-term care planning is not available locally.

Testing and Confirmation   Lymphocyte karyotype can confirm the abnormality.

Nursery Management   Decisions regarding surgical intervention for cardiac and gastrointestinal defects are the primary concerns in the postnatal period. If no surgical intervention is desired by the family, care requirements are determined primarily by feeding difficulties.

BIBLIOGRAPHY:

Benacerraf BR, Miller WA, Frigoletto FD Jr: Sonographic detection of fetuses with trisomies 13 and 18: accuracy and limitations. *Am J Obstet Gynecol* 1988; 158:404-409.

Bundy AL, Saltzman DH, Pober B et al: Antenatal sonographic findings in trisomy 18. *J Ultrasound Med* 1986; 5:361-364.

Carey JC: Health supervision and anticipatory guidance for infants with congenital defects. In Ballard RA (ed): *Pediatric care of the ICN graduate.* Philadelphia, WB Saunders, 1988.

Gorlin RJ et al (eds): *Syndromes of the head and neck,* 3rd edition. New York, Oxford University Press. 1990. pp. 43-46.

Hepper PG, Shahidullah S: Trisomy 18: behavioral and structural abnormalities. An ultrasonographic case study. *Ultrasound Obstet Gynecol* 1992; 2:48-50.

Hodes ME, Cole J, Palmer CG et al: Clinical experience with trisomies 18 and 13. *J Med Genet* 1978; 15:48-60.

Jones KL (ed): *Smith's recognizable patterns of human malformations.* Philadelphia. WB Saunders, 1988. pp. 16-17.

Nadel AS, Bromely BS, Frigoletto FD Jr et al: Isolated choroid plexus cysts in the second trimester fetus: is amniocentesis really indicated? *Radiology* 1992; 185:545-548.

Nyberg DA, Kramer D, Resta RG et al: Prenatal sonographic findings of trisomy 18: review of 47 cases. *J Ultrasound Med* 1993; 2:103-113.

Palomaki GE, Knight GJ, Haddow JE et al: Prospective intervention trial of a screening protocol to identify fetal trisomy 18 using maternal serum alpha-fetoprotein, unconjugated oestriol, and human chorionic gonadotropin. *Prenat Diagn* 1992; 12:925-930.

Swan TJ, Rouse GA, DeLange M: Sonographic findings in trisomy 18: a pictorial essay. *JDMS* 1991; 7:255-263.

Taylor AI: Autosomal trisomy syndromes: a detailed study of 27 cases of Edwards' syndrome and 27 cases of Patau's syndrome. *J Med Genet* 1968; 5:227-252.

Thurmond AS, Nelson DW, Lowensohn RI et al: Enlarged cisterna magna in trisomy 18: prenatal ultrasonographic diagnosis. *Am J Obstet Gynecol* 1989; 161:83-85.

Warkany J, Passarge D, Smith LB: Congenital malformations in autosomal trisomy syndromes. *Am J Dis Child* 1966; 112:502-517.

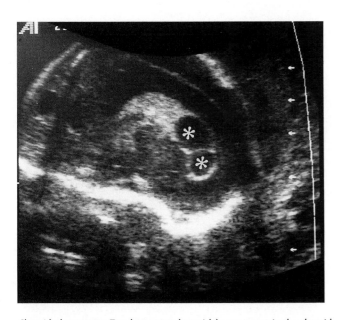

Choroid plexus cysts. Two large cysts (*asterisks*) are present in the choroid plexus. This finding, if isolated, has a slight but statistically significant association with trisomy 18.

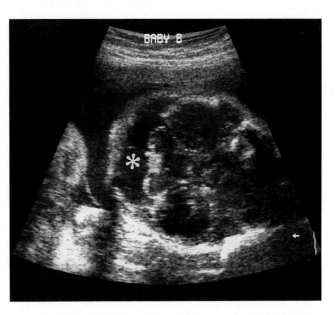

Large cisterna magna over 10 mm wide (*asterisk*). Although associated with trisomy 18, this finding has not so far been the only abnormality seen in a trisomy 18 case.

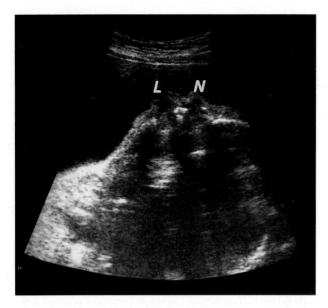

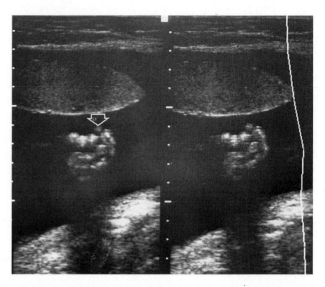

Micrognathia. The chin is unduly small and recessed posterior to the forehead. This is a frequent finding in trisomy 18. *L*, lips, *N*, nose.

Abnormal hand in trisomy 18. The hand is clenched and the fingers are crowded with the third finger overriding (*arrow*).

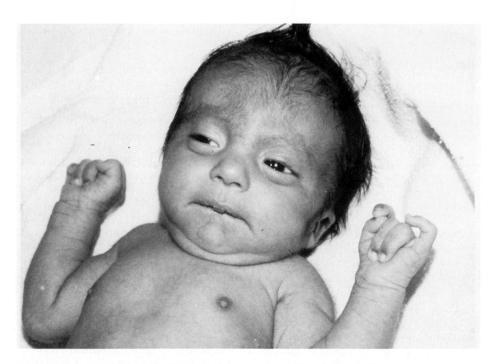

Newborn with trisomy 18 (47, XY, + 18) exhibiting the classic features including round face with short nose and clenched fists.

1.4 TRISOMY 21
DOWN SYNDROME

EPIDEMIOLOGY/GENETICS

Definition   Trisomy 21 (Down syndrome) is the most common multiple-malformation, chromosome abnormality in newborns and results in a characteristic phenotype with major malformations, including congenital heart disease and duodenal atresia.

Epidemiology   Occurs in 1 out of 800 live births (M1:F1). No racial differences have been noted, but there is a significant increase in incidence with increasing maternal age.

Embryology   The phenotype is due to trisomy for all or part (21q22) of chromosome 21. Ninety-five percent of cases are due to full trisomy 21, 3% are translocation and 2% are mosaic. Infants with trisomy 21 have a characteristic craniofacial appearance that includes microbrachycephaly, midface hypoplasia, excess nuchal skin, and small overfolded ears. There is generalized shortening of the limbs with small hands, clinodactyly of the fifth fingers (60%), single palmar creases (45%) and wide spacing between the first and second toes. Approximately 50% of patients have congenital heart disease with endocardial cushion defects and VSDs being the most common lesions. Two thirds of cases of endocardial cushion defects have trisomy 21. Alimentary tract defects—duodenal atresia, tracheoesophageal fistula, imperforate anus, Hirschsprung's disease—occur in approximately 10% of infants with trisomy 21.

Inheritance Patterns   Most cases are sporadic with a 1 out of 100 risk of recurrence in future pregnancies. Rare familial translocations have a higher recurrence risk depending on the specific translocation.

Teratogens   None.

Screening   Assuming all women would elect to have CVS or amniocentesis, the use of advanced maternal age would detect approximately 25% of trisomy 21 fetuses. Combining maternal age with maternal serum biochemical markers raises the detection rate to 60%. It is uncertain how many additional cases are identified with sonographic markers.

Prognosis   Cardiac abnormalities are the major cause of increased mortality in infancy. Mortality between infancy and age 40 years is not much increased over the general population, but then increases because of premature aging. Intelligence quotients (IQs) range from 25-50 in childhood, but fall in adulthood. Alimentary tract defects present major life limitations and therefore, ethical issues, following birth. Survival without surgical correction in the immediate neonatal period is not possible.

SONOGRAPHY

Findings
1. **Fetus**
   a. Thickened nuchal fold—At least 40% of Down syndrome fetuses have *nuchal translucency* (nuchal edema) at 13 weeks. There is an echopenic area extending from the back of the skull to the sacrum. By 18 weeks the nuchal fold has regressed into *nuchal thickening*. A standard *cerebellar* view will show nuchal thickening of greater than 6 mm. About one in seven fetuses with nuchal thickening of this type will have Down syndrome. Although Down syndrome is typically associated with nuchal edema, cystic hygroma may also be seen.
   b. Congenital heart disease—Fetuses with Down syndrome often have congenital heart disease (about 50%). Endocardial cushion defect with extensive ASD and VSD and abnormal mitral and tricuspid valve is typical of Down syndrome. Ventricular septal defect alone is also common. Hypoplastic left-heart syndrome and tetralogy of Fallot occur.
   c. Duodenal atresia—The stomach and duodenal bulb are dilated. Appropriate transducer angulation shows the pyloric connection. The small and large bowel are empty. Other gut atresias such as tracheoesophageal atresia may occur.
   d. Omphalocele—Although more typical of trisomy 13 and 18, omphalocele may be seen.
   e. Short humerus and femur—Both femur and humerus are mildly shortened to 0.91 of the biparietal diameter value. This sign has about a 1 in 10 likelihood of being Down syndrome.
   f. Mild renal pelvic dilatation—Renal pelvic dilatation to greater than 3 mm has a weak, but convincing, association with Down syndrome.
   g. Short middle phalanx of fifth finger—This structure is difficult to measure, but there is an association with Down syndrome.
   h. Flattened facial profile—The nose is small and recessed.
   i. Posterior urethral valve (PUV) syndrome—Particularly when the onset of PUV occurs very early, e.g. 12 weeks, Down syndrome may be responsible.
   j. Isolated pleural effusion and isolated fetal ascites with retained lymph fluid have an approximately 5% association with Down syndrome.
   k. Non immune hydrops—One of the numerous causes is trisomy 21.
   l. Echogenic bowel—A group of adjacent small bowel loops with an echogenicity as great as bone increases the risk of Down syndrome.

m. The big toe may be separated from the remaining toes.

n. Choroid plexus cysts have been reported with Down syndrome.

o. Mild lateral ventriculomegaly.

2. **Amniotic Fluid:** Normal.

3. **Placenta:** Normal.

4. **Measurement Data:** Growth is usually normal. Intra-uterine growth retardation only occurs occasionally. Brachycephaly may be seen with decreased frontothalamic distance.

5. **When Detectable:** Some manifestations, such as nuchal edema and posterior urethral valves, are detectable at 11 weeks; cushion defects have been detected at 13 weeks with endovaginal echocardiography. Duodenal atresia is usually detected after 24 weeks.

Pitfalls

1. Nuchal folds at 18 weeks are difficult to measure accurately and can easily be over-measured. Make sure that the cerebellum and cortical brain structures are satisfactorily visualized at the same time.

2. Duodenal atresia usually presents late (after 24 weeks).

3. An unfused amniotic membrane may be confused with nuchal edema if the fetus is lying on its back.

Differential Diagnosis   Other chromosomal anomalies (e.g., Turner's syndrome) can have some of the same findings (e.g., cystic hygroma).

Where Else to Look   Any component of the fetus can be affected by Down syndrome.

PREGNANCY MANAGEMENT

Investigations and Consultations Required   A precise diagnosis depends on chromosome studies by amniocentesis, chorionic villus sampling or percutaneous umbilical blood sampling. The high incidence of cardiac defects requires fetal echocardiography, which also may be helpful in assessing prognosis.

Monitoring   No alterations in prenatal care are necessary.

Pregnancy Course   Duodenal atresia results in severe polyhydramnios and resultant pre-term labor.

Pregnancy Termination Issues   Suction dilatation and evacuation techniques are appropriate once a cytogenetic diagnosis has been established.

Delivery   The fetus with Down syndrome should be managed like a fetus with normal chromosomes. Cesarean section should be performed if there are obstetric indications. If structural malformations are present, delivery should be in a tertiary center.

NEONATOLOGY

Resuscitation   Rarely contraindicated unless multiple complex associated anomalies have been confirmed antenatally and a prior decision has been made by family not to begin life support measures. If diagnosis not known prior to birth, providing life support is appropriate initially.

Transport   Indicated if cardiac or alimentary tract anomalies are suspected or if diagnostic confirmation, counselling, and long-term care planning are not available locally.

Testing and Confirmation   Children with trisomy 21 present in the newborn period with hypotonia and a characteristic craniofacial appearance. Lymphocyte karyotype can confirm the chromosome abnormality.

Nursery Management   The major objectives of care are comprehensive evaluation to identify all associated problems and the development of a postnursery plan of care to facilitate parental adaptation. The initial priorities are to determine the presence and type of cardiac and alimentary defects and plan surgical interventions. Short-term issues include polycythemia in 25%, feeding difficulties (particularly if preterm or with concurrent cardiac or alimentary anomalies), and neutrophil abnormalities, which are uncommon and usually transient.

BIBLIOGRAPHY

Baird PA, Sadovnick AD: Life expectancy in Down syndrome. *J Pediatr* 1987; 110:849-854.

Benacerraf BR, Barss VA, Laboda LA: A sonographic sign for the detection in the second trimester of the fetus with Down's syndrome. *Am J Obstet Gynecol* 1985; 151:1078-1079.

Benacerraf BR, Cnaan A, Gelman R et al: Can sonographers reliably identify anatomic features associated with Down syndrome? *Radiology* 1989; 173:377-380.

Benacerraf BR, Neuberg D, Bromley B et al: Sonographic scoring index for prenatal detection of chromosomal abnormalities. *J Ultrasound Med* 1992; 11:449-458.

Bronshtein M, Bar-Hava I, Blumenfeld I et al: The difference between septated and nonseptated nuchal cystic hygroma in the early second trimester. *Obstet Gynecol* 1993; 81:683-687.

Brumfield CG, Hauth JC, Cloud GA et al: Sonographic measurements and ratios in fetuses with Down syndrome. *Obstet Gynecol* 1989; 73:644-646.

Carey JC: Health supervision and anticipatory guidance for infants with congenital defects. In: Ballard RA (ed): *Pediatric care of the ICN graduate.* Philadelphia. WB Saunders, 1988.

Gorlin RJ et al (eds): In: *Syndromes of the head and neck*, 3rd edition. New York. Oxford University Press, 1990. pp. 33-40.

Jones KL: *Smith's recognizable patterns of human malformations*, 4th edition. Philadelphia. WB Saunders Company, 1988.

Lynch L, Berkowitz GS, Chitkara U, et al: Ultrasound detection of Down syndrome: is it really possible? *Obstet Gynecol* 1989; 73:267-270.

Miller M, Cosgriff JM: Hematological abnormalities in newborn infants with Down syndrome. *Am J Med Genet* 1983; 16:173-177.

1990; 76:370-377.

Nicolaides KH, Azar G, Snijders RJ et al: Fetal nuchal oedema: Associated malformations and chromosomal defects. *Fetal Diagn Ther* 1992; 7:123-131.

Warkany J, Passarge E, Smith LB: Congenital malformations in autosomal trisomy syndromes. *Am J Dis Child* 1966; 112:502-517.

Nyberg DA, Resta RG, Luthy DA et al: Prenatal sonographic findings of Down syndrome: review of 94 cases. *Obstet Gynecol*

Wilkins I: Separation of the great toe in fetuses with down syndrome. *J Ultrasound Med* 199; 13:229-231.

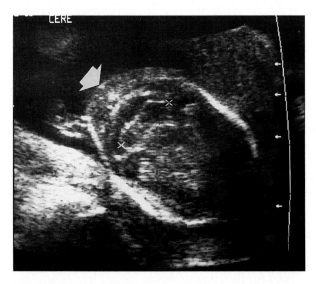

Nuchal thickening. At the level of an intracranial view, which shows the cerebellum (*between the x's*), thickened skin is seen at the back of the neck (*arrow*).

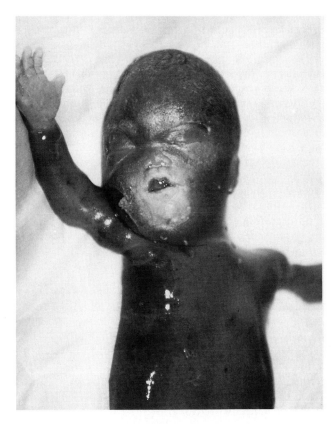

23-week fetus with Down syndrome. Note midface hypoplasia with short nose and small hand.

1.5 Turner's Syndrome

EPIDEMIOLOGY/GENETICS

Definition Turner's syndrome is a rare sex chromosome abnormality characterized by a complete or partial monosomy for one X chromosome.

Epidemiology Occurs in 1 out of every 5,000 to 10,000 births (M0:F1).

Embryology Turner's syndrome is due in most cases to a 45,X karyotype that results from chromosomal nondisjunction. No maternal age effect has been noted. Forty percent of newborns with Turner's syndrome are mosaic or have variant chromosome patterns whereas only seven percent of those spontaneously aborted. Over 95% of 45,X conceptions are spontaneously aborted. Characteristic cardiac abnormalities (20%) include a bicuspid aortic valve and coarctation of the aorta. Horseshoe kidney and other renal structural abnormalities occur in 60% of patients. A nuchal cystic hygroma with or without hydrops is the most common antenatal presentation.

Inheritance Patterns Sporadic.

Teratogens None.

Screening Maternal serum AFP is elevated only in cases of cystic hygroma and hydrops.

Prognosis If hydrops is present, death will almost always occur during pregnancy. Isolated cystic hygroma, without hydrops, regress during pregnancy. Early death in infancy results from associated cardiac defects and is infrequent with current surgical and postoperative intensive care. The potential life span is uncertain, but those who survive early infancy usually reach adulthood. Skeletal growth retardation occurs in all and perceptive hearing impairment in 50%. Absence of secondary sexual characteristics and infertility are uniformly present. Hormone replacement therapy will be necessary for maturational changes in adolescence. Most have normal or near normal intelligence.

SONOGRAPHY

Findings
1. Fetus
   a. Cystic hygromas (see Chapter 7.2) develop in the late first to early second trimester. Skin thickening with cystic spaces separated by septum are seen in the skin starting in the upper torso. Hydrops often develops.
   b. Lymph collections may occur in other sites such as isolated fetal ascites, pleural effusion, or lymphangiomata.
   c. Congenital heart disease most likely involving the left side of the heart, such as coarctation of the aorta is often seen; the aortic narrowing with coarctation is almost never visible in utero. Secondary right-heart enlargement may occur.
   d. Renal anomalies: renal agenesis, horseshoe kidney, and pelvic kidney are seen.
2. **Amniotic Fluid:** There may be oligohydramnios.
3. **Placenta:** Normal.
4. **Measurement Data:** Usually not affected.
5. **When Detectable:** Cystic hygroma are detectable from 10 weeks on.

Pitfalls Cystic hygroma may be seen in fetuses that are eventually normal (20% to 30%).

Differential Diagnosis Other causes of cystic hygroma include: 1. Noonan's syndrome (male or female often with hypoplastic pulmonary valves); 2. Multiple pterygium syndrome (see Chapter 8.11); 3. Down syndrome (see Chapter 1.4); and 4. Roberts' syndrome.

Where Else to Look
1. Look for flexed arms and extended legs—features of multiple pterygium syndrome
2. Look at the gender—Turner's syndrome fetuses have female genitalia, but Noonan's fetuses can be either male or female.

PREGNANCY MANAGEMENT

Investigations and Consultations Required Amniocentesis, CVS, or umbilical blood sampling establish the diagnosis. Once a cytogenetic diagnosis has been established, fetal echocardiography should be performed because of the high incidence of congenital heart disease. Consultations with surgical specialists will be dependent on the types of structural malformations seen.

Monitoring No change in standard obstetric care is needed.

Pregnancy Course Whereas cystic hygroma with hydrops is virtually always fatal, cystic hygroma without hydrops slowly regresses and leaves a webbed neck.

Pregnancy Termination Issues Should a family choose pregnancy termination, suction dilatation and evacuation techniques are appropriate once a cytogenetic diagnosis has been established.

Delivery If congenital heart disease is present, delivery should occur in a tertiary center. In other cases the site of delivery can be the family's and physician's choice.

NEONATOLOGY

Resuscitation   There is no contraindication to full resuscitation. As coarctation of the aorta is the most frequently occurring cardiac defect, peripheral perfusion may be dependent upon flow through the ductus arteriosus. Prolonged exposure to high oxygen concentrations is not advisable until the cardiac anatomy is known.

Transport   Indicated if a cardiac malformation is suspected, and counselling and long-term care planning are not available locally. If asymptomatic and no cardiac involvement is suspected, outpatient evaluation in early infancy is appropriate.

Testing and Confirmation   Newborns present with a short webbed neck (50%) with a low hairline (80%), lymphedema of hands and feet, prominent ears (80%), and cardiac abnormalities. Patients not detected in infancy are detected in childhood with short stature and delayed puberty due to ovarian dysgenesis. Lymphocyte karyotype with special attention to possible mosaicism confirms the diagnosis.

Nursery Management   Diagnostic evaluation should include an echocardiogram and renal sonogram irrespective of symptomatology. No intervention is usually required for lymphedema. Peripheral invasive procedures should be minimized to decrease the potential for systemic infection.

BIBLIOGRAPHY

Brown BSJ, Thompson DL: Ultrasonographic features of the fetal Turner syndrome. *J Can Assoc Radiol* 1984; 35:40-46.

Carey JC: Health supervision and anticipatory guidance for infants with congenital defects. In: Ballard RA (ed): *Pediatric care of the ICN graduate*. Philadelphia. WB Saunders, 1988.

Chervenak FA, Isaacson G, Blakemore KJ et al: Fetal cystic hygroma: cause and natural history. *N Engl J Med* 1983; 309:822-825.

Gorlin RJ et al (eds): In: *Syndromes of the head and neck*, 3rd edition. New York. Oxford University Press, 1990. pp. 54-58.

Haddad HM, Wilkins L: Congenital anomalies associated with gonadal aplasia: review of 55 cases. *Pediatrics* 1959; 23:885.

Jones KL (ed): *Smith's recognizable patterns of human malformations*. Philadelphia. WB Saunders, 1988. pp. 10-15.

Litvak AS, Rousseau TG, Wrede LD et al: The association of significant renal anomalies with Turner's syndrome. *J Urol* 1978; 120:671-672.

Robinow M, Spisso K, Buschi AJ et al: Turner syndrome: sonography showing fetal hydrops simulating hydramnios. *Am J Roentgenol* 1980; 135:846-848.

Sculerati N, Ledesma-Medina J, Finegold DN et al: Otitis media and hearing loss in Turner syndrome. *Arch Otolaryngol Head Neck Surg* 1990; 116:704-707.

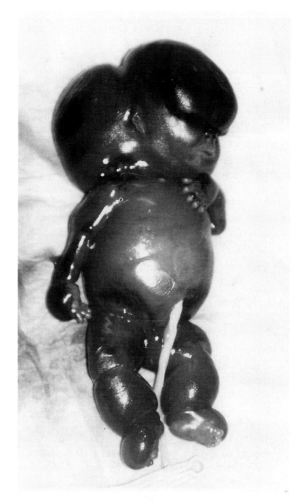

18-week fetus with massive cystic hygroma and lymphedema as a result of Turner's syndrome (45,X).

2 The Central Nervous System

2.1 Agenesis Of The Corpus Callosum

EPIDEMIOLOGY/GENETICS

Definition   Complete or partial failure of the callosal commissural fibers to cross in the midline and form the corpus callosum between the two cerebral hemispheres.

Epidemiology   Incidence may be as high as 1% with many asymptomatic individuals.

Embryology   The corpus callosum develops between the 12th and the 22nd week of gestation. Vascular disruption or failure of formation may cause complete or partial agenesis. Associated abnormalities include hydrocephalus, microcephaly, pachygyria, and lissencephaly. Over 80 sporadic, genetic, and chromosomal syndromes have been described with agenesis of the corpus callosum including trisomies 13 and 18.

Inheritance Patterns   Most isolated defects are sporadic. Autosomal dominant, recessive, and X-linked syndromes have been described.

Teratogens   None known.

Prognosis   Isolated agenesis of the corpus callosum (ACC) may be asymptomatic although seizures occur in some patients. The prognosis of some syndromes such as the Dandy-Walker syndrome is worsened when there is concomitant ACC.

SONOGRAPHY

Findings
1. Fetus
   a. Because the corpus callosum is absent, the third ventricle lies high between widely separated lateral ventricles. The lateral ventricles are more parallel to the midline than usual, so the medial wall is well seen at a more superior level.
   b. There may be a cyst arising from the superior aspect of the third ventricle, which communicates with the lateral ventricles. It usually has a more or less round shape with multiple projections. A mass—the bundles of Probst—causes an impression on the lateral aspects of the cystic area.
   c. The gyri are normally horizontally aligned. They assume a vertical orientation with agenesis. A

sagittal view through the midline (difficult to obtain) will show absence of the normal corpus callosum and the radiating gyri.
   d. The occipital horns of the lateral ventricle are locally dilated (colpocephaly) forming an appearance on axial views similar to *bulls horns*.
2. **Amniotic Fluid:** Normal, unless there is an associated anomaly.
3. **Placenta:** Normal, unless there is an associated anomaly.
4. **Measurement Data:** Normal.
5. **When Detectable:** At about 20 weeks—The corpus callosum forms by this time.

Pitfalls   The sonographic findings are technically difficult to detect. A coronal view is the best for seeing the relationship to the lateral ventricles. A sagittal view, if obtainable, will show gyri radiating from the lateral ventricle. The cavum pellucidum and cavum verga can be mistaken for ACC, but there will be a third ventricle in normal position.

Differential Diagnosis
1. Lobar holoprosencephaly—The lateral ventricles and apparent third ventricle are joined. There is no midline falx and the lateral ventricles are squared off.
2. Arachnoid cyst—Irregular shape and unlikely to be exactly midline. There is usually no ventricular dilation.
3. Mild lateral ventriculomegaly—The entire ventricle is dilated and the third ventricle will be mildly dilated and in a normal position.

Where Else to Look
1. Dandy-Walker syndrome is the most common association. The vermis of the cerebellum will be small and will be surrounded by a fourth ventricular cyst.
2. Encephalocele or myelomeningocele—There will be no visible cisterna magna and the cerebellum will be banana shaped.
3. Aicardi syndrome—males only. There are also vertebral anomalies.
4. Chromosomal anomalies (trisomy 8, 13, and 18)—Look for the stigmata.
5. Diaphragmatic hernia (see Chapter 5.2).
6. Cardiac malformations.

7. Lung agenesis or dysplasia.
8. Absent or dysplastic kidneys are more frequent with ACC.

PREGNANCY MANAGEMENT

Investigations and Consultations Required Chromosome studies of the fetus are essential. Evaluation of the parents for signs of autosomal dominant conditions, such as basal cell nevus syndrome and tuberous sclerosis, should be performed by a dysmorphologist. Fetal echocardiography should be done to detect congenital heart disease. Maternal serum toxoplasmosis, rubella, cytomegalovirus, and herpes simplex virus (TORCH) titers should be drawn. Additional consultations will depend on the associated abnormalities found.

Monitoring No change in standard obstetric practice is indicated for isolated ACC. The aggressiveness of fetal intervention must be based on the underlying etiology, if that can be determined. Isolated ACC should not progress, but if associated with a cyst, a third trimester examination is desirable to make sure the cyst has not enlarged and that other processes have not been missed.

Pregnancy Course Obstetric complications are not expected on the basis of ACC alone.

Pregnancy Termination Issues Because many conditions have ACC as a component, an intact fetus should be delivered in an institution with expertise in dysmorphology and fetal pathology.

Delivery Because of the high association with other non–central nervous system (CNS) abnormalities, delivery should occur in a tertiary center with full capabilities for diagnosis and management of infants with multiple malformations.

NEONATOLOGY

Resuscitation No specific issues except in those infants with additional CNS defects, in which case the associated defect will be the dominant factor in decisions regarding intervention.

Transport Referral to a tertiary center after birth is not indicated with an isolated lesion and asymptomatic course. If any neurologic symptoms or associated CNS lesions are present, the infant should be referred promptly to a tertiary perinatal center with pediatric neurology capabilities for definitive evaluation.

Testing and Confirmation Postnatal confirmation of the defect and evaluation for other associated lesions is best achieved with magnetic resonance imaging (MRI). Screening for inherited metabolic disorders is indicated with isolated lesions of the corpus callosum.

Nursery Management Subsequent course and management are dictated by the associated lesion(s).

BIBLIOGRAPHY

Bamforth F, Bamforth S, Poskitt K et al: Abnormalities of corpus callosum in patients with inherited metabolic diseases. *Lancet* 1988; 2:451.

Bertino RE, Nyberg DA, Cyr DR et al: Prenatal diagnosis of agenesis of the corpus callosum. *J Ultrasound Med* 1988; 7:251-260.

Cohen MM Jr, Kreiborg S: Agenesis of the corpus callosum: its associated anomalies and syndromes with special reference to the Apert syndrome. *Neurosurg Clin N Am* 1991; 2:565-568.

Comstock CH, Culp D, Gonzalez J et al: Agenesis of the corpus callosum in the fetus: its evolution and significance. *J Ultrasound Med* 1985; 4:613-616.

Dobryns WB: Agenesis of the corpus callosum and gyral malformations are frequent manifestations of nonketotic hyperglycinemia. *Neurology* 1989; 39:817.

Franco I, Kogan S, Fisher J et al: Genitourinary malformations associated with agenesis of the corpus callosum. *J Urol* 1993; 149:1119-1121.

Malinger G, Zakut H: The corpus callosum: normal fetal development as shown by transvaginal sonography. *Am J Roentgenol* 1993; 161:1041-1043.

Pilu G, Sandri F, Perolo A et al: Sonography of fetal agenesis of the corpus callosum: a survey of 35 cases. *Ultrasound Obstet Gynecol* 1993; 3:318-329.

Vergani P, Ghidini A, Mariani S et al: Antenatal sonographic findings of agenesis of corpus callosum. *Am J Perinatol* 1988; 5:105-108.

Vergani P, Ghidini A, Strobelt N et al: Prognostic indicators in the prenatal diagnosis of agenesis of corpus callosum. *Am J Obstet Gynecol* 1994; 170:753-758.

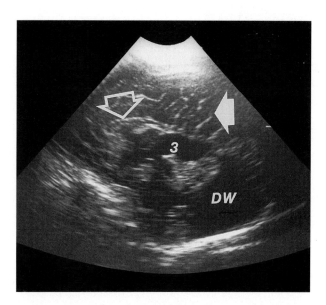

Partial agenesis of the corpus callosum. Midline sagittal view. The anterior portion of the corpus callosum is present (*open arrow*). Posteriorly where the corpus callosum is absent, the gyri are aligned vertically (*solid arrow*). The patient also had Dandy-Walker syndrome with an enlarged third ventricle (*3*) and a posterior fossa cyst (*DW*).

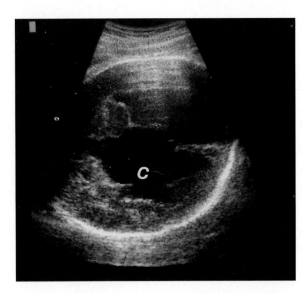

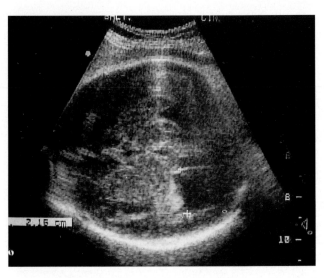

Axial view. A centrally placed cyst (*C*) communicates with both lateral ventricles. Such a centrally placed cyst is not uncommon with agenesis of the corpus callosum.

Axial view showing marked colpocephaly. Not the large size of the occipital horn (between the x's) whereas the anterior horn (arrow) is very narrow.

2.2 ANENCEPHALY

EPIDEMIOLOGY/GENETICS

Definition Anencephaly is a defect in closure of the anterior neural tube characterized by complete or partial absence of the forebrain, overlying meninges, skull, and skin.

Epidemiology The incidence is geographic and population dependent and ranges from about 1 out of 1000 births in the United States to 1 out of 100 in parts of the British Isles (M1:F3.7).

Embryology Neural tube closure occurs between 20 and 28 days of pregnancy with abnormalities of cephalic closure, which occurs late, resulting in anencephaly. Anencephaly is characterized by the absence of the cranial vault with exposed neural tissue and is associated with spina bifida, facial and nasal clefts, and omphalocele. Amniotic band disruptions are also a common cause of anencephaly.

Inheritance Patterns Multifactorial inheritance with both genetic and environmental factors is implicated. Recurrence risk after one affected pregnancy is two to three percent for any open neural tube defect. Rare families have been reported with X-linked inheritance.

Teratogens Valproic acid, folic acid antagonists (such as methotrexate and aminopterin), maternal diabetes, hyperthermia, and folic acid deficiency are associated with an increased risk for neural-tube defects.

Screening Maternal serum alpha-fetoprotein screening will detect most cases of anencephaly.

Prognosis Anencephaly is invariably lethal, with about 50% of cases being stillborn, and the remainder dying in the newborn period.

SONOGRAPHY

Findings
1. Fetus
   a. Skull development, usually completed by 10 weeks, never occurs. The exposed brain is gradually eliminated after exposure to the amniotic fluid. When diagnosed between 10 and 14 weeks, the brain is still present to a variable extent. The remaining brain has an irregular outline. By about 17 weeks the brain has been eliminated, but intracranial vessels remain as a superior bulge.
   b. Facial and brainstem structures persist, so there is a typical frog-like appearance to the fetal face.
   c. Myelomeningoceles in the lumbosacral or cervical region are quite frequent.
2. **Amniotic Fluid:** Polyhydramnios is common, but not invariable (about 75%). Because of the polyhydramnios, there can be increased fetal movement.
3. **Placenta:** Normal.
4. **Measurement Data:** Appropriate for dates.
5. **When Detectable:** First detectable at 11 weeks when all of the brain will be present. The brain will have an irregular, *floppy* outline because the skull is absent.

Pitfalls
1. An irregular fetal head outline at 10 to 12 weeks can easily be overlooked.
2. If the head is deep in the pelvis and no endovaginal probe study is done, the defect may be overlooked and the absence of the skull thought to be a technical problem.

Differential Diagnosis
1. Large encephalocele—The skull will be visible on close inspection.
2. Microcephaly—A small skull will be present.
3. Iniencephaly is often seen with anencephaly. Because of the delivery complications that may be associated with iniencephaly, this condition must be ruled out before deciding on an appropriate management plan.

Where Else to Look
1. Look at the cervical spine for shortening and rachischisis. Iniencephaly is commonly associated with anencephaly.
2. Myelomeningocele may also be present in the lumbosacral region.
3. Diaphragmatic hernia, hydronephrosis, cleft lip, and cardiac malformations have been reported with anencephaly. Because the condition is lethal, an extensive search for additional malformations seems futile.
4. Occasional cases of anencephaly are due to the amniotic band syndrome. The amniotic bands may be visible on careful ultrasonic inspection.

PREGNANCY MANAGEMENT

Investigations and Consultations Required No specific antenatal evaluations or consultations are necessary.

Monitoring In pregnancies that are continued, clinical assessment for the presence of polyhydramnios is indicated. The most important component of the prenatal care is emotional support for the family.

Pregnancy Course Always lethal at or shortly after birth.

Pregnancy Termination Issues   Suction dilatation and evacuation techniqes are appropriate. Karyotyping abortus material is worthwhile to detect the rare case caused by chromosome anomaly, such as trisomy 18.

Delivery   There are no special conditions regarding delivery. The majority of anencephalic infants will deliver in the breech presentation.

NEONATOLOGY

Resuscitation   Given the lethal prognosis neonatal resuscitation is never indicated. Prenatal diagnosis and counseling should focus on preparing family for nonintervention.

Transport   Not an issue.

Testing and Confirmation   The abnormality is obvious at birth. Evidence of amniotic band disruptions should be sought.

Nursery Management   Provision of warmth, hygiene, and facilitation of parental grief are the principal elements of care. Some infants may survive for several days with intermittent periods of stable cardiorespiratory function that parents and staff may find disturbing.

BIBLIOGRAPHY

Bronshtein M, Ornoy A: Acrania: anencephaly resulting from secondary degeneration of a closed neural tube: two cases in the same family. *J Clin Ultrasound* 1991; 19:230-234.

Goldstein RB, Filly RA: Prenatal diagnosis of anencephaly: spectrum of sonographic appearances and distinction from the amniotic band syndrome. *Am J Roentgenol* 1988; 151:547-550.

Hendricks SK, Cyr DR, Nyberg DA et al: Exencephaly—clinical and ultrasonic correlation to anencephaly. *Obstet Gynecol* 1988; 72:898-900.

Melnick M, Myrianthopoulos NC: Studies in neural tube defects. II. Pathologic findings in a prospectively collected series of anencephalics. *Am J Med Genet* 1987; 26:797-810.

Salamanca A, Gonzalez-Gomez F, Padilla MC et al: Prenatal ultrasound semiography of anencephaly: sonographic-pathological correlations. *Ultrasound Obstet Gynecol* 1992; 2:95-100.

Van Allen MI, Kalousek DK, Chernoff GF et al: Evidence for multisite closure of the neural tube in humans. *Am J Med Genet* 1993; 47:723-743.

Vergani P, Ghidini A, Sirtori M et al: Antenatal diagnosis of fetal acrania. *J Ultrasound Med* 1987; 6:715-717.

Wilkins-Haug L, Freedman W: Progression of exencephaly to anencephaly in the human fetus—an ultrasound perspective. *Prenat Diagn* 1991; 11:227-233.

Worthen NJ, Lawrence D, Bustillo M: Amniotic band syndrome: antepartum ultrasonic diagnosis of discordant anencephaly. *J Clin Ultrasound* 1980; 8:453-455.

Yang YC, Wu CH, Chang FM et al: Early prenatal diagnosis of acrania by transvaginal ultrasonography. *J Clin Ultrasound* 1992; 20:343-345.

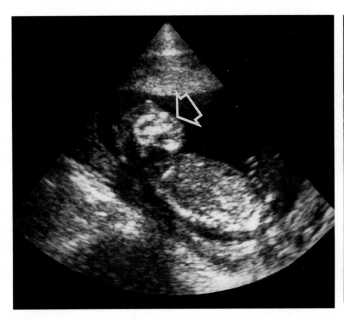

Anencephaly at 16 weeks. Little brain and no skull is present superior to the orbits (*arrow*).

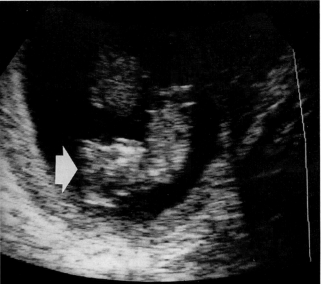

Acrania at 11 weeks. Although the brain is present (*arrow*), the skull is absent. If this fetus is followed, by approximately 16 weeks the brain tissue will no longer be visible.

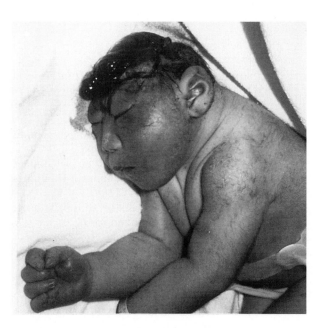

Newborn with isolated anencephaly.

2.3 Aqueductal Stenosis

EPIDEMIOLOGY/GENETICS

Definition   Aqueductal stenosis is an obstruction or maldevelopment of the aqueduct of Sylvius resulting in congenital hydrocephalus.

Epidemiology   1 out of 2000 (M1.8:F1). Ninety percent of cases of congenital hydrocephalus are the result of Arnold-Chiari malformations, whereas 3% to 5% have aqueductal stenosis.

Embryology   The aqueduct of Sylvius is the connection between the third and fourth ventricles in the brain. It develops at about 6 weeks gestation. Histologic evidence of gliosis is found in approximately 50% of cases of aqueductal stenosis, suggesting inflammatory or infectious causes. The etiology is heterogenous and includes congenital tumors, hemorrhage, infections, and genetic syndromes. Flexion and adduction deformities of the thumbs are seen in 20% of boys with X-linked aqueductal stenosis.

Inheritance Patterns   Most cases are sporadic. Estimates suggest that 2% to 5% of cases of hydrocephalus, not associated with neural tube defects, have X-linked recessive inheritance.

Teratogens   Congenital infections including cytomegalovirus (CMV), rubella, and toxoplasmosis.

Prognosis   There is a 10% to 30% neonatal mortality, partly dependent upon associated abnormalities. The prognosis for aqueductal stenosis discovered in utero is very poor. Approximately 10% of survivors will have an IQ greater than 70. The X-linked recessive form is associated with profound mental retardation and a poor prognosis.

SONOGRAPHY

Findings
1. **Fetus**
    a. With aqueductal stenosis there is enlargement of the lateral and third ventricles, but not of the fourth ventricle. A dilated proximal aqueduct of Sylvius may occasionally be visible. Unless the ventriculomegaly is very severe, the cisterna magna and cerebellum are normal. With very severe lateral ventricular enlargement, the cisterna magna may not be seen and the cerebellum may be technically difficult to find.
    b. Mild asymmetry of the lateral ventricular dilatation is possible. Facial structures remain of a size appropriate for gestational age.
    c. Mild lateral ventricular dilation (10 to 15 mm) may not progress and may indicate a chromosomal anomaly (trisomy 21) rather than early

aqueductal stenosis. The *hanging choroid* sign is a helpful indication that a mild lateral ventricle measurement increase indicates hydrocephalus.
    d. Measurement of the remaining cortical mantle has some relationship to prognosis. It is customarily measured at the occipital, parietal, and frontal areas. The occipital mantle thickness is usually the smallest.
    e. Flexion and adduction of the thumb is seen in some boys with the X-linked form.
2. **Amniotic Fluid:** Usually normal.
3. **Placenta:** Normal.
4. **Measurement Data:** The head size is larger than predicted for gestational age. If the head size is not increased, other etiologies such as cerebral atrophy need to be considered. Intrauterine growth retardation (IUGR) may be seen.
5. **When Detectable:** Usually detectable by 17 weeks, but may develop later.

Pitfalls
1. Ventriculomegaly is present in many different entities. When ventriculomegaly is very severe, aqueductal stenosis can be confused with Arnold-Chiari malformation or holoprosencephaly.
2. If there is ventriculomegaly, but a head circumference measurement that is decreased or appropriate for gestational age, consider cerebral atrophy or Arnold-Chiari malformation with myelomeningocele.
3. Do not mistake the echogenic blush superior to the lateral ventricle, previously termed the lateral border of the lateral ventricle, for the true lateral ventricles. The choroid plexus should be visible within the lateral ventricle.
4. Mantle thickness measurement looks much more severe in utero. Once a shunt is in place the cortical mantle regains thickness. Mantle thickness is especially thin posteriorly.

Differential Diagnosis
1. Arnold-Chiari malformation—Look for absence of cisterna magna and cerebellar deformity.
2. Holoprosencephaly—Look for a fused thalamus and absent third ventricle.

Where Else to Look
1. Up to 16% of aqueductal stenosis cases have other anomalies elsewhere, but up to 80% of ventriculomegaly cases have associated abnormalities. There is a moderate, but definite association with karyotypic abnormalities.
2. Look for the gender of the fetus considering that there is an X-linked form of aqueductal stenosis.
3. Look for stigmata of CMV, a known cause of mild hydrocephalus. Calcification in the lateral aspect of the lateral ventricle border is characteristic.

PREGNANCY MANAGEMENT

Investigations and Consultations Required Chromosome evaluation and viral studies (both maternal serum and amniotic fluid) should be performed. Pediatric neurosurgical consultation should be obtained to plan management.

Fetal Intervention Theoretically, aqueductal stenosis should be the perfect situation for in utero shunt placement. However, the experience to date has been quite disappointing. There are many reasons for the relatively poor outcomes that have been seen. Misdiagnosis has been a common finding in all series, as has been failure to detect associated abnormalities. Morbidity has been high, reflecting the difficulties of exact shunt placement in the fetus. For these reasons, and the lack of data to support a clear benefit of fetal surgical intervention, in utero ventriculoamniotic shunts are not indicated in the management of fetal ventriculomegaly.

Monitoring
1. Ventriculomegaly, due to aqueductal stenosis may abruptly increase in severity over a few weeks, therefore ultrasonic monitoring every 2 or 3 weeks is desirable.
2. Spontaneous resolution of mild to moderate hydrocephalus has been reported.
3. Aqueductal stenosis is a condition that should have few complications given a carefully managed pregnancy with early intervention, if necessary.

Pregnancy Termination Issues The method should be a nondestructive one and at a site with special expertise in neuropathology.

Delivery In theory, early delivery followed by shunt placement could improve outcome. However, the centers using this approach have limited data to support the benefits of this approach over the risks of prematurity from delivery at 32 to 37 weeks gestation. Further study is needed before clear recommendations can be made. Mode of delivery can be vaginal, if the head is relatively normal size and the fetus is in a vertex presentation. Occasionally excessive head growth and fetal position may necessitate cesarean section. Delivery should occur where appropriate neonatal and neurological support services are available.

NEONATOLOGY

Resuscitation The decision regarding support of the onset of respiration should be discussed with the family prior to delivery. Except in circumstances of extreme enlargement of the head or presence of other severe CNS abnormalities, initial resuscitation is indicated. Delay in spontaneous onset of respiration secondary to fetal distress from dystocia from macrocephaly occurs frequently. Prematurity (if early delivery is chosen

because of rapidly advancing hydrocephalus) may also cause respiratory distress.

Transport Immediate referral to a tertiary perinatal center with pediatric neurology and neurosurgery capabilities is always indicated. Precautions during transport are dictated by the maturity of the infant, presence of respiratory distress, and other associated abnormalities.

Testing and Confirmation Both cranial computerized tomography (CT) and magnetic resonance imaging (MRI) are useful to establish a definite anatomic diagnosis. Further imaging studies to be considered are echocardiography and abdominal sonography if physical examination findings suggest other abnormalities and studies were not obtained prenatally.

Nursery Management The first priority is to determine the severity of the increased intracranial pressure as immediate reduction may be needed to achieve clinical stability.

SURGERY

Preoperative Assessment Issues of importance with respect to the surgical management of aqueductal stenosis are as follow.
1. The presence of other anomalies (i.e., cardiac, renal, spinal, or limb deformities) are associated with a poor overall prognosis.
2. The presence of posterior fossa mass or compressive lesion such as congenital tumor or tectal mass.
3. Rate of ventricular enlargement and head growth.

Operative Indications Evidence of progressive ventricular enlargement or accelerated head growth are indications for surgical intervention.

Types of Procedures Standard surgical therapy for aqueductal stenosis has been ventricular shunting with either a ventriculoperitoneal or a ventriculoatrial shunt using a pressure-regulated valve system. Ventricular shunts have been associated with a high failure rate. Nearly 80% will require revision within 5 years. Alternative therapy available since the resurgence of ventriculoscopy is the fenestration of the floor of the third ventricle opening an alternative cerebrospinal fluid (CSF) pathway into the basal cisterns. This procedure, called a third ventriculostomy, is typically performed within the first year of life in children with proven aqueductal stenosis. The procedure has a better than 50% success rate in avoiding the need for a shunt, with potential for improvement as techniques improve.

Surgical Results/Prognosis In the absence of associated CNS or non-CNS abnormalities or shunt complications, these children have a good overall prognosis.

BIBLIOGRAPHY

Benacerraf BR, Birnholz JC: The diagnosis of fetal hydrocephalus prior to 22 weeks. *J Clin Ultrasound* 1987; 15:531-536.

Bowerman RA, DiPietro MA: Erroneous sonographic identification of fetal lateral ventricles: relationship to the echogenic periventricular "blush". *AJNR* 1987; 8:661-664.

Callen PW, Hashimoto BE, Newton TH: Sonographic evaluation of cerebral cortical mantle thickness in the fetus and neonate with hydrocephalus. *J Ultrasound Med* 1986; 5:251-255.

Cardoza JD, Filly RA, Podrasky AE: The dangling choroid plexus: a sonographic observation of value in excluding ventriculomegaly. *Am J Roentgenol* 1988; 151:767-770.

Cochrane DD, Myles ST, Nimrod C et al: Intrauterine hydrocephalus and ventriculomegaly: associated anomalies and fetal outcome. *Can J Neurol Sci* 1985; 12:51-59.

Holmes LB, Nash A, ZuRhein GM et al: X-linked aqueductal stenosis: clinical and neuropathological findings in two families. *Pediatrics* 1973; 51:697-704.

Levitsky DB, Mack LA, Nyberg DA et al: Fetal aqueductal stenosis diagnosed sonographically: How grave is the prognosis? *Am J Roentgenol* 164:725-730, 1995.

McClone DSG, Naidich TP, Cunningham T: Posterior fossa cysts: management and outcome. *Conc Ped Neurosurg* 1987; 7:134.

McCullough DC, Balzer-Martin LA: Current prognosis in overt neonatal hydrocephalus. *J Neurosurg* 1982; 57:378-383.

Pretorius DH, Davis K, Manco-Johnson ML et al: Clinical course of fetal hydrocephalus: 40 cases. *Am J Roentgenol* 1985; 144:827-831.

Vintzileos AM, Campbell WA, Weinbaum PJ et al: Perinatal management and outcome of fetal ventriculomegaly. *Obstet Gynecol* 1987; 68:5-11.

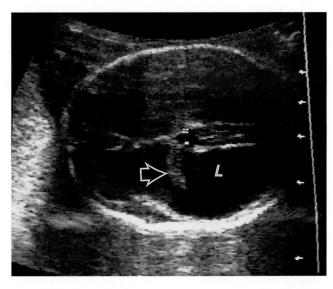

Aqueductal stenosis. There is a dilated lateral ventricle (*L*) showing the *hanging choroid* sign of ventriculomegaly (*arrow*). The third ventricle is dilated (*small x's*).

2.4 ARACHNOID CYST

EPIDEMIOLOGY/GENETICS

Definition Arachnoid cysts are membrane-lined fluid-filled cavities that may occur anywhere within the brain or spinal cord in association with the arachnoid or ventricular lining.

Epidemiology Very rare (M>F).

Embryology Arachnoid cysts can occur anywhere in the lining of the brain or spinal cord. Many arise postnatally and are associated with trauma or infection. The etiology of congenital cysts is unclear. They may represent maldevelopment of the leptomeninges or acquired destructive events.

Inheritance Patterns Rare autosomal recessive families with isolated arachnoid cysts have been described.

Teratogens Congenital infections.

Prognosis Because these cysts generally compress normal brain structures, the outcome is usually favorable unless it is associated with other congenital abnormalities or there are significant complications related to treatment.

SONOGRAPHY

Findings
1. **Fetus:** Intrabrain cystic collections of random shape and size that abut the meninges. One type, centrally located, may expand and compress brain substance.
2. **Amniotic Fluid:** Should be unaffected unless the cystic area involves swallowing control.
3. **Placenta:** Normal.
4. **Measurement Data:** Head size may be small or normal.
5. **When Detectable:** Arachnoid cysts have been seen as early as 23 weeks.

Pitfalls If the cyst is in the dependent part of the skull and the nondependent portion of the brain can never be seen due to acoustic shadowing, arachnoid cysts can be confused with bilateral processes such as holoprosencephaly. They may be missed altogether if they lie in the portion of the brain closest to the transducer.

Differential Diagnosis
1. Porencephalic cyst—The cystic area will border on the ventricle.
2. Vein of Galen aneurysm—There will be blood flow in a centrally placed cyst.
3. Intracranial bleed—There will be internal echoes in the apparent cyst if the gain is increased.
4. Schizencephaly—disorganized cystic area extending across the midline involving both hemispheres.

Depending on the location of the cyst, obstructive hydrocephalus may develop. An attempt should be made to exclude conditions not associated with a risk of significant in utero ventriculomegaly.

Where Else to Look Usually this is an isolated finding.

PREGNANCY MANAGEMENT

Investigations and Consultations Required Despite the low reported incidence of chromosome abnormalities, cytogenic studies should be performed. No other diagnostic evaluations are indicated. Consultation with a pediatric neurosurgeon should be arranged.

Fetal Intervention Invasive fetal intervention is not indicated because of the relatively benign course of the malformation.

Monitoring Serial ultrasound examinations should be performed every 3 to 4 weeks to detect or follow ventriculomegaly.

Pregnancy Course Obstetric complications are not to be expected.

Pregnancy Termination Issues The method should be a nondestructive procedure at a site with expertise in neuropathology.

Delivery The site of delivery should be at a location with expertise in the management of neonates with CNS malformations.

NEONATOLOGY

Resuscitation The most likely intrapartum risk is for distress secondary to head compression or hemorrhage into the cyst. Prematurity (from early delivery because of rapidly developing hydrocephalus) may also impact on early adaptation.

Transport Referral to a tertiary center with pediatric neurology and neurosurgery capabilities is always indicated.

Testing and Confirmation: Presentations at birth include macrocephaly or a bulging fontanelle with widened stutures. The cysts cause their symptoms through pressure and mass effect. Small to moderate cysts are frequently asymptomatic. Postnatal CT or MRI will accurately define these abnormalities. Determination of the degree of increased intracranial pressure governs the urgency of surgical intervention.

Nursery Management   Hemorrhage into the cyst may complicate the course at any point and should be suspected if an abrupt clinical deterioration occurs. Preoperative and postoperative course is determined by the location of the cyst and the neurologic dysfunction that results.

SURGERY

Preoperative Assessment   Location of the arachnoid cysts with respect to the ventricular system, the basal cisterns, and the structures of the posterior fossa is important for surgical planning. Computed tomographic scan or MRI scanning, with the occasional addition of intravenous contrast, are used to rule out a cystic neoplasm.

Operative Indications   Small, asymptomatic arachnoid cysts warrant observation only, with periodic CT or MRI follow-up. If stable over time, then no intervention is needed. Larger cysts, those that present with hydrocephalus, a progressive increase in cyst size, the presence of a neurologic deficit, or poorly controlled seizures require surgical intervention.

Types of Procedures
1. Shunting of the cyst to the peritoneal cavity or the right atrium.

2. Marsupialization of the cyst into the basal cisterns or surrounding subarachnoid space. This technique is useful only for arachnoid cysts that present at the skull base adjacent to basal cisterns.
3. Fenestration of the cyst into an adjacent ventricle. This technique can be done endoscopically using a ventriculoscope.

Surgical Results/Prognosis   Arachnoid cysts in general have an excellent outcome and are not typically associated with neurologic or cognitive impairment. Children who present with poorly controlled epilepsy respond well to cyst decompression. Controversy exists as to the best surgical approach, though most surgeons will choose to avoid shunt placement if at all possible. In some situations, fenestration or marsupialization may fail, ultimately requiring placement of a shunt.

BIBLIOGRAPHY
Diakoumakis EE, Weinberg B, Mollin J: Prenatal sonographic diagnosis of a suprasellar arachnoid cyst. *J Ultrasound Med* 1986; 5:529-530.

Meizner I, Barki Y, Tadmor R et al: In utero ultrasonic detection of fetal arachnoid cyst. *J Clin Ultrasound* 1988; 16:506-509.

Wilson WG, Deponte KA, McIlhenny J et al: Arachnoid cysts in a brother and sister. *J Med Genet* 1988; 25:714-715.

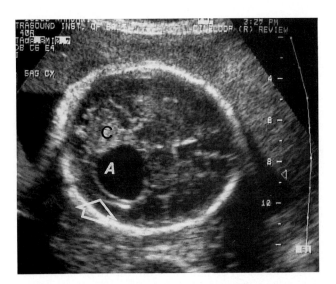

Arachnoid cyst. A cyst (*A*) lies alongside the tentorium, displacing the lateral ventricle (*arrow*) laterally. The cyst arises in a cistern and displaces but does not destroy brain tissue.

2.5 CAUDAL APLASIA/DYSPLASIA (REGRESSION) SEQUENCE

EPIDEMIOLOGY/GENETICS

Definition   Caudal aplasia/dysplasia sequence is the total or partial agenesis of the distal neural tube resulting in sacral agenesis/dysgenesis with associated abnormalities of the lower extremities, gastrointestinal, or genitourinary tracts.

Epidemiology   Occurs in about 1 to 5 out of 100,000 births (M1:F1).

Embryology   Differentiation of the lower spine is usually complete before the seventh week of pregnancy. The term caudal "regression" is probably inaccurate as the caudal defects in this condition are primary malformations rather than the result of "regression" of structures. Sirenomelia may represent one end of the spectrum of this condition or may be etiologically separate. Heart defects are common associated malformations.

Inheritance Patterns   Most often sporadic. Rare families showing autosomal and X-linked dominant inheritance have been reported.

Teratogens   Approximately 16% of cases are seen in infants of diabetic mothers.

Prognosis   Dependent on the severity of the defect and presence of associated abnormalities. Bowel and urinary complications are common and may not be compatible with life.

SONOGRAPHY

Findings
1. **Fetus:** Shortened spine with missing sacral and lower lumbar vertebrae. Normally the superior aspect of the iliac crest lies at the level of L5; in this condition, no vertebrae are seen at this level.
2. **Amniotic Fluid:** Normal.
3. **Placenta:** Normal.
4. **Measurement Data:** Normal.
5. **When Detectable:** About 18 weeks.

Pitfalls   Because the sacrum does not calcify until 22 weeks, the syndrome may be difficult to identify before that time.

Differential Diagnosis
1. Myelomeningocele with cord tethering.
2. Sirenomelia is a related condition in which both legs are fused. In sirenomelia, there is oligohydramnios or absent fluid and the kidneys may appear to be absent, obstructed, or dysplastic.

There may be a single lower extremity or both legs may be fused and lie alongside each other.

Where Else to Look
1. Look at the cranium for hydrocephalus.
2. Look at the kidneys for hydronephrosis and multicystic kidney.
3. Look at the legs for movement and club feet. (In sirenomelia, both legs are close together and straight). Both legs may be crossed and positioned over the abdomen.
4. Look at the spine for hemivertebrae and cord tethering.

PREGNANCY MANAGEMENT

Investigations and Consultations Required   Evaluation of the mother for diabetes should be performed. Fetal echocardiography should be performed to evaluate for associated cardiac defects. Pediatric surgical consultations should be obtained to plan with the family for neonatal management.

Monitoring   No specific alterations in obstetric care are necessary. The diagnosis is difficult, therefore a repeat ultrasound in the third trimester is worthwhile.

Pregnancy Termination Issues   In the patient with known diabetes no special autopsy requirements are necessary. In the absence of maternal diabetes, full autopsy of an intact fetus should be performed to establish the diagnosis.

Delivery   The high likelihood of neonatal complications requires delivery at a tertiary site. Breech presentation may warrant cesarean section because of the marked body/head discrepancy that may be present.

NEONATOLOGY

Resuscitation   Beyond the issues of prematurity and of infants of diabetic mothers, there are no special concerns in planning for resuscitation. In a small number of cases there may be other serious anomalies (CNS or cardiac) that could govern approach. If there are other life-threatening and potentially uncorrectable defects known to be present, prenatal discussion with the parents regarding nonintervention is appropriate.

Transport   Referral to a tertiary center with multiple pediatric subspecialty capabilities is indicated.

Testing and Confirmation   The physical findings are apparent at birth. Echocardiography, to exclude concomitant cardiac anomalies, and cranial CT scan or MRI, for CNS defects, should be obtained prior to invasive interventions.

Nursery Management   Approach and management are governed by both the suspected etiology (i.e., maternal diabetes, associated anomalies) and the location of the defect. In general, with the exception of hydrocephalus, the long-term issues of ambulation and bowel and bladder function are very similar to those of a high to mid-lumbar myelomeningocoele.

BIBLIOGRAPHY

Andrish J, Kalamchi A, MacEwen GD: Sacral agenesis: a clinical evaluation of its management, heredity and associated anomalies. *Clin Orthop* 1979; 139:52-57.

Loewy JA, Richards DG, Toi A: In-utero diagnosis of the caudal regression syndrome: report of three cases. *J Clin Ultrasound* 1987; 15:469-474.

Mills JL: Malformations in infants of diabetic mothers. *Teratology* 1982; 25:385-394.

Price DL, Dooling EC, Richardson EP Jr: Caudal dysplasia (caudal regression syndrome). *Arch Neurol* 1970; 23:212-220.

Rusnak SL, Driscoll SG: Congenital spinal anomalies in infants of diabetic mothers. *Pediatrics* 1965; 35:989.

Twickler D, Budorick N, Pretorius D et al: Caudal regression versus sirenomelia: Sonographic clues. *J Ultrasound Med* 1993; 12:323-330.

Welch JP, Aterman K: The syndrome of caudal dysplasia: a review, including etiologic considerations and evidence of heterogeneity. *Pediatr Pathol* 1984; 2:313-327.

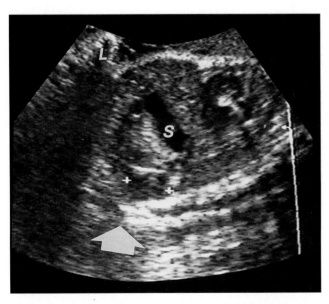

Caudal regression. The lumbar spine ends at about L2 (*arrow*). Note how close the stomach (*S*) is to the lower end of the spine. The legs (*L*) are crossed over the anterior aspect of the abdomen.

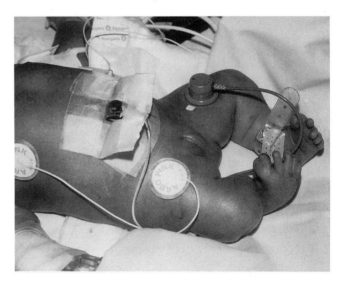

Newborn infant of a diabetic mother with caudal agenesis/dysgenesis and tetralogy of Fallot. Note the short, twisted lower extremities with bifid toes.

2.6 DANDY-WALKER MALFORMATIONS

EPIDEMIOLOGY/GENETICS

Definition Dandy-Walker malformations (DWM) are characterized by: 1. a posterior fossa cyst; 2. a defect in the cerebellar vermis that provides a communication between the cyst and the fourth ventricle; and 3. variable hydrocephalus.

Epidemiology 1 out of 25,000 to 35,000. Occurs in approximately 4% of cases of hydrocephalus.

Embryology The Dandy-Walker malformation is an abnormality in the development of the CNS that probably occurs before the sixth to seventh week of gestation. Associated intracranial abnormalities occur in about 50% of cases and associated extracranial abnormalities in 35% of cases. Common associated defects are agenesis of the corpus callosum, ventricular septal defect, and facial clefts. Chromosomal abnormalities are seen in approximately 15% to 30% of cases including trisomies 13, 18, and 21.

Inheritance Patterns The Dandy-Walker malformation can be a feature of mendelian genetic syndromes including the Meckel-Gruber syndrome (autosomal recessive [AR]), Walker-Warburg syndrome (AR), and the Aicardi syndrome (X-linked dominant).

Teratogens Congenital infections.

Prognosis Postnatal mortality is approximately 35% and is dependent on the associated abnormalities. One third of survivors, with isolated abnormalities, have IQ's above 80. Shunting is usually required for associated hydrocephalus.

SONOGRAPHY

Findings
1. Fetus
   a. A Dandy-Walker cyst is seen as a fluid collection separating the lobes of the cerebellum. It represents an intracerebellar cyst connected to the fourth ventricle. Visualization is enhanced by using an exaggerated cerebellar view.
   b. The vermis of the cerebellum is usually hypoplastic and may be difficult to see with large Dandy-Walker cysts. The remainder of the cerebellum may also be partially or completely absent.
   c. With larger cysts there is secondary dilatation of the third and lateral ventricles.
2. **Amniotic Fluid:** Normal, unless the Dandy-Walker cyst is secondary to a chromosomal abnormality when oligohydramnios or polyhydramnios may occur.

3. **Placenta:** Normal.
4. **Measurement Data:** Biparietal diameter and head circumference are usually increased in size. There can be IUGR if associated syndromes are present.
5. **When Detectable:** The syndrome has been detected as early as 13 weeks by endovaginal probe use.

Pitfalls
1. An enlarged cisterna magna of greater than 1 cm diameter, but with a normally formed cerebellum is called a Dandy-Walker variant by some, although it does not carry the same generally gloomy prognosis.
2. A small cyst inferior to the cerebellum is frequently seen. This is an unimportant normal variant if small.

Differential Diagnosis
1. When an infracerebellar cyst becomes very large it is known as an extraaxial cyst. Such arachnoid cysts can be distinguished from Dandy-Walker cysts by the size and appearance of the cerebellum. Although compressed, a normal cerebellum is still present.
2. Enlarged cisterna magna. The cerebellum has a normal appearance.
3. If the posterior fossa is difficult to examine, the secondary findings of bilateral, lateral, and third ventricular dilatation may be confused with aqueduct stenosis.

Where Else to Look
1. Agenesis of the corpus callosum is commonly associated and markedly worsens the prognosis. The corpus callosum is best seen on midline sagittal views, but such views are difficult to obtain in utero. Transverse coronal views or endovaginal views may be helpful (see Chapter 2.1).
2. Look for stigmata of trisomy 13 and 18, which are associated with Dandy-Walker cysts in about 15% to 30% of cases.
3. Encephaloceles (including Meckel-Gruber and Walker-Warburg) often have Dandy-Walker cysts in addition.
4. Neural tube defects are associated with Dandy-Walker cysts.

PREGNANCY MANAGEMENT

Investigations and Consultations Required Chromosome studies should be performed at any gestational age at which the initial diagnosis is made. The high association with trisomy 18 and the dismal prognosis of this chromosome abnormality would preclude any aggressive obstetric management. Fetal echocardiography should be performed to detect the commonly associated cardiac lesions. A pediatric neurosurgeon should be consulted to discuss prenatal and neonatal management.

Fetal Intervention   Despite the reports of "successful" in utero placement of shunts for the DWM, fetal intervention is contraindicated because of the poor prognosis and high incidence of associated abnormalities in this disorder.

Monitoring   Serial ultrasound examinations should be performed every 3 to 4 weeks to assess for the presence and degree of ventriculomegaly.

Pregnancy Course   Many of the syndromes of which the DWM is a component may be associated with IUGR and decisions regarding management of this complication will be highly dependent on the prognosis of the underlying condition.

Pregnancy Termination Issues   As with other CNS malformations, special expertise in neuropathology is essential for a precise diagnosis and the resultant counseling that will be necessary following this diagnosis.

Delivery   Early delivery after 32 weeks may be considered when there is progressive and severe ventriculomegaly. However, this approach is controversial because of the inherent poor prognosis for normal neurologic development in the infant with DWM.

NEONATOLOGY

Resuscitation   The major issues relate to: 1) fetal distress secondary to dystocia from macrocephaly; and 2) prematurity, if early delivery is chosen because of rapidly advancing hydrocephalus. Given the very poor prognosis, if there are associated CNS or other organ system anomalies, a prenatal discussion with the family regarding intervention to initiate respirations is appropriate. No special techniques are required.

Transport   Referral to a tertiary center with pediatric neurosurgery capabilities is indicated.

Testing and Confirmation   The priority issue is the identification of associated CNS abnormalities by cranial CT and MRI. In the majority of infants, hydrocephalus develops by 2 months of age if not present prenatally.

If karyotyping was not performed on the fetus, it should be obtained after birth before invasive interventions are undertaken, especially if there are other dysmorphic features.

Nursery Management   Hemorrhage into the cyst can occur at any point and should be suspected with an abrupt clinical deterioration.

SURGERY

Preoperative Assessment   Magnetic resonance imaging scan and CT scan of the head, and a careful search for associated extracranial anomalies.

Operative Indications   The DWM without hydrocephalus does not necessarily require treatment in asymptomatic infants. In infants who have hydrocephalus or who are symptomatic (i.e., with poor feeding, recurrent aspiration, hoarse or weak cry, or a poor suck), the treatment is initially directed at the DWM. Subsequent treatment of the hydrocephalus is occasionally necessary.

Types of Procedures   Treatment of DWM in the absence of hydrocephalus usually involves shunting the cyst to the peritoneal cavity. In the presence of hydrocephalus, controversy exists about the management. Some advocate simultaneously shunting the ventricular system and the Dandy-Walker cyst, whereas others advocate shunting the Dandy-Walker cyst only with the hope that the hydrocephalus will resolve once the posterior fossa cyst is decompressed. Should the child remain symptomatic or the ventricular size remain enlarged, ventriculoperitoneal shunting is performed.

Surgical Results/Prognosis   Outcome in children with DWM in isolation is reasonably good. These children can have normal cognitive development though the risk of shunt malfunction and the need for revision is significantly greater with the presence of dual shunt systems in many of these children. The DWM with the presence of associated anomalies generally has a poor prognosis with less than 25% of children demonstrating a normal IQ.

BIBLIOGRAPHY

Cornford E, Twining P: The Dandy-Walker syndrome: the value of antenatal diagnosis. *Clin Radiol* 1992; 45:172-174.

Estroff JA, Scott MR, Benacerraf BR: Dandy-Walker variant: prenatal sonographic features and clinical outcome. *Radiology* 1992; 185:755-758.

Hart MN, Malamud N, Ellis WG: The Dandy-Walker syndrome: a clinicopathological study based on 28 cases. *Neurology* 1972; 22:771-780.

Hill LM, Martin JG, Fries J et al: The role of the transcerebellar view in the detection of fetal central nervous system anomaly. *Am J Obstet Gynecol* 1991; 164:1220-1224.

Hirsch JF, Pierre-Kahn A, Renier D et al: The Dandy-Walker malformation: a review of 40 cases. *J Neurosurg* 1984; 61:515-522.

Kollias SS, Ball Jr WS, Prenger EC: Cystic malformations of the posterior fossa: differential diagnosis clarified through embryologic analysis. *Radiographics* 1993; 13:1211-1231.

Hudgins R, Edwards MSB: Management of hydrocephalus detected in utero. In: Scott M (ed): *Concepts of neurosurgery: hydrocephalus.* Williams & Wilkins, 1990; p. 99-108.

McCullough DC, Balzer-Martin LA: Current prognosis in overt neonatal hydrocephalus. *J Neurosurg* 1982; 57:378-383.

Murray JC, Johnson JA, Bird TD: Dandy-Walker malformation: etiologic heterogeneity and empiric recurrence risks. *Clin Genet* 1985; 28:272-283.

Nyberg DA: The Dandy-Walker malformation: prenatal sonographic diagnosis and its clinical significance. *J Ultrasound Med* 1988; 7:65-72.

Nyberg DA, Cyr DR, Mack LA et al: The Dandy-Walker malformation prenatal sonographic diagnosis and its clinical significance. *J Ultrasound Med* 1988; 7:65-71.

Nyberg DA, Mahony BA, Hegge FN et al: Enlarged cisterna magna and the Dandy-Walker malformation: factors associated with chromosome abnormalities. *Obstet Gynecol* 1991; 77:436-442.

Nyberg DA, Pretorius DH: Cerebral malformations. In: Nyberg DA, Mahony BS, Pretorius DH (eds): *Diagnostic ultrasound of fetal anomalies.* Chicago. Mosby–Year Book, 1990; pp. 83-145.

Pilu G, Goldstein I, Reece EA et al: Sonography of fetal Dandy-Walker malformation: a reappraisal. *Ultrasound Obstet Gynecol* 1992; 2:151-157.

Raman S, Rachagan SP, Lim CT: Prenatal diagnosis of a posterior fossa cyst. *J Clin Ultrasound* 1991; 19:434-437.

Russ PD, Pretorius DH, Johnson MJ: Dandy-Walker syndrome: a review of fifteen cases evaluated by prenatal sonography. *Am J Obstet Gynecol* 1989; 161:401-406.

Tal Y, Freigang B, Dunn HG et al: Dandy-Walker syndrome: analysis of 21 cases. *Dev Med Child Neurol* 1980; 22:189-201.

Rekate H: Treatment of hydrocephalus. In: Cheek W (ed): *Pediatric Neurosurgery*, 3rd edition, chapter 13, pp. 202-220, WB Saunders, 1994.

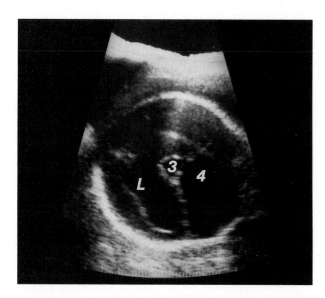

Dandy-Walker cyst. Axial view shows a large cystic structure below the tentorium (*4*). No cerebellar tissue remains. The lateral ventricles (*L*) and the third ventricle (*3*) are secondarily dilated.

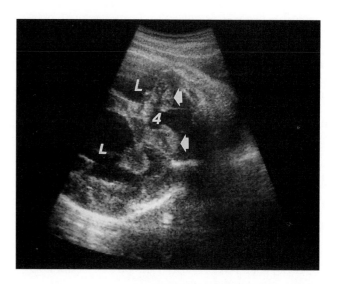

More mild example showing small dysplastic cerebellar configuration (*arrows*) adjacent to the cyst (*4*). Again there is secondary lateral ventricular dilatation (*L*).

2.7 ENCEPHALOCELE

EPIDEMIOLOGY/GENETICS

Definition Encephaloceles are neural tube defects that affect the cranium and result in a midline mass overlying a skull defect.

Epidemiology 1 out of 2000 live births (M1:F1). Varies with ethnic group and geographic region.

Embryology Encephaloceles are the result of failure of neural tube closure in the cranial region during the first month of fetal development. They are frequently associated with other brain malformations, hydrocephalus, iniencephaly, facial clefts, cardiac abnormalities, and genital malformations. Over 30 genetic, sporadic, and chromosomal syndromes have been described with encephaloceles including trisomy 13, amniotic band disruption syndrome, Meckel-Gruber syndrome (autosomal recessive disorder with encephalocele, polycystic kidneys, and polydactyly) and the Roberts' pseudothalidomide syndrome (autosomal recessive [AR]).

Inheritance Patterns Most often sporadic with multifactorial recurrence risks (2% to 5%). Otherwise related to specific syndrome diagnosis.

Teratogens Cocaine, rubella, and maternal hyperthermia.

Prognosis Dependent on the associated brain malformations and syndrome diagnosis. Size is not important prognostically as large encephaloceles may not contain neural elements or be associated with brain abnormalities.

SONOGRAPHY

Findings
1. **Fetus**
   a. A paracranial mass is present. In 75% of cases the mass is occipital, in 12% the mass is frontal, and in 13% it is parietal. The mass may be fluid filled, entirely brain filled, or both fluid and brain. If much or most of the brain is in the encephalocele, microcephaly occurs. A "cyst within a cyst" appearance indicates that the apparent cranial meningocele contains brain enclosing a prolapsed fourth ventricle.
   b. There is often hydrocephalus that becomes more likely if much brain is in the encephalocele.
   c. It is important to decide how much and what area of brain tissue lies in the encephalocele because both are factors that can affect the prognosis. Often the brain substance within the mass is the cerebellum, because most encephaloceles are occipital.
   d. In a relatively rare subgroup, mainly those encephaloceles in a parietal location, the encephalocele is due to the amniotic band syndrome. Amniotic bands may be visible attached to the encephalocele.
   e. The skull may assume the lemon shape normally thought to be characteristic of myelomeningocele.
2. **Amniotic Fluid:** Polyhydramnios may be present.
3. **Placenta:** Normal.
4. **Measurement Data:** The head size is usually small despite ventriculomegaly.
5. **When Detectable:** Usually detectable at 12-13 weeks using the vaginal probe.

Pitfalls
1. Occipital masses are especially likely to be overlooked and the condition thought to be hydrocephalus only.
2. Small amounts of brain in an apparently fluid-filled encephalocele may be overlooked.
3. The fetal ear has been mistaken for an encephalocele.

Differential Diagnosis
1. Nuchal edema—The skull will be intact.
2. Cystic hygroma—bilateral posterolateral cysts with intact skull.
3. Dandy-Walker cyst —The skull will be intact.
4. Cephalohematoma—The skull will be intact and the brain normal. Cephalohematoma only occur in labor.
5. Frontal encephaloceles may be mistaken for facial teratoma (epignathus).
6. Occipital hemangioma.

Where Else to Look
1. Look for Meckel-Gruber syndrome—large echogenic kidneys with visible cysts; polydactyly; encephalocele attached by a thin neck.
   Less common findings are: congenital heart disease; cleft lip and palate; microcephaly; and liver cysts.
2. Look for other findings of amniotic band syndrome, such as gastroschisis and absent limbs.
3. Agenesis of the corpus callosum is common with encephalocele and worsens the prognosis.
4. Dandy-Walker syndrome may occur with encephalocele.
5. Cervical rachischisis and cerebellar hypoplasia can be associated with encephalocele.

PREGNANCY MANAGEMENT

Investigations and Consultations Required In addition to the sonographic search for associated abnormalities, chromosome studies should be performed. Trisomy 13 is an etiology for a few encephaloceles (1% to 5%). Fetal echocardiography should be done to exclude cardiac malformations, which are a common feature of many of the syndromes with encephalocele. The family should also be referred to a pediatric neurosurgeon for discussion regarding prognosis and neonatal management.

Fetal Intervention   No in utero therapy is indicated. Decompression of the encephalocele under ultrasound control prior to delivery may be required.

Monitoring   To assess the development or progression of ventriculomegaly or hydrocephalus, serial ultrasound examinations should be done monthly. Management of IUGR should be based on the overall prognosis of the primary condition. In the absence of an apparent syndrome to explain growth retardation, standard obstetric protocols are appropriate.

Pregnancy Course   Many of the syndromes, of which encephalocele is a feature, may also have prenatal growth deficiency as a component. Management should be based on the prognosis for the underlying condition, not the presence of IUGR.

Pregnancy Termination Issues   Because of the large number of syndromes that may have encephalocele as a component, and the wide range of inheritance patterns seen in these conditions, termination should be done by a nondestructive technique in an institution with special expertise in fetal pathology.

Delivery   Delivery management depends on the size of the defect, the amount of herniated brain, and associated abnormalities. Nonaggressive management is recommended when severe microcephaly is present. In cases with normal head size cesarean section might improve prognosis by avoiding trauma to the herniated brain tissue.

NEONATOLOGY

Resuscitation   Most cases do not require assistance with the onset of respiration, unless the mass is very large and contains mostly brain tissue. Intubation may be difficult with large posterior masses impeding proper positioning for visualization of the cords. Bag-and-mask–assisted ventilation with the infant in a side-lying position is often sufficient.

With prenatal diagnostic evaluations confirming associated intracranial malformations, microcephaly with the bulk of the brain tissue in the mass, or other severe organ abnormalities, a predelivery discussion with the family concerning nonintervention, if spontaneous onset of respiration does not occur, is appropriate.

Special care to avoid trauma to the mass is important when the attachment is pedunculated or there is only a membranous tissue covering the surface.

Transport   Referral to a tertiary center with pediatric neurology and neurosurgery capabilities is indicated.

Testing and Confirmation   Diagnostic imaging, either cranial CT or MRI, to define the defect and to delineate any associated CNS abnormalities, is important. Chromosomal analysis, echocardiogram, and abdominal sonograms are indicated contingent upon physical findings and clinical course, if not obtained prenatally.

Nursery Management   Postoperatively, seizures and hydrocephalus are the more common neurologic complications requiring intervention.

SURGERY

Preoperative Assessment   The size and location of the lesion, its contents, and relationship to the midline and vascular structures are important for surgical planning. The volume of the remaining intracranial contents, hydrocephalus, and the head circumference are also important information.

Magnetic resonance imaging is useful to define the encephalocele contents and its relationship to vital structures. The relationship of the encephalocele to the structures of the posterior fossa and venous sinuses are important from the surgical standpoint and can be determined by MRI and magnetic resonance angiography (MRA).

Operative Indications   Small, entirely skin-covered lesions can be repaired electively. Large lesions or those that are leaking spinal fluid need to be repaired urgently.

Types of Procedures   Surgical treatment involves resection of the encephalocele contents, closure of the dural defect along with the scalp, skull, and dura. Larger defects, such as those in which the majority of the brain is in the encephalocele sac, or in which vital structures such as the brain stem are extracranial, cannot be treated surgically and are associated with a very poor outcome. If hydrocephalus is present, then a ventricular shunt is placed at the same procedure.

Surgical Results/Prognosis   Outcome is dependent on the size and contents of the encephalocele and, in addition, its location. Large lesions in which the majority of the brain is extracranial, or in which essential structures are included in the encephalocele sac, have a very poor functional outcome and are treated expectantly. Despite this, a good overall prognosis is possible with smaller lesions, those with relatively little neural contents, and those not involving major vascular structures.

BIBLIOGRAPHY

Bronshtein M, Bar-Hava I, Blumenfeld Z: Early second-trimester sonographic appearance of occipital haemangioma simulating encephalocele. *Prenat Diagn* 1992; 12:695-698.

Brown MS, Sheridan-Pereira M: Outlook for the child with a cephalocele. *Pediatrics* 1992; 90:914-919.

Curnes JT, Oakes WJ: Parietal cephaloceles: radiographic and magnetic resonance imaging evaluation. *Pediatr Neurosci* 1988; 14:71.

Fink IJ, Chinn DH, Callen PW: A potential pitfall in the ultrasonographic diagnosis of fetal encephalocele. *J Ultrasound Med* 1983; 2:313-314.

Goldstein RB, LaPidus AS, Filly RA: Fetal cephaloceles: diagnosis with US. *Radiology* 1991; 180:803-808.

Graham D, Johnson TRB Jr, Winn K et al: The role of sonography in the prenatal diagnosis and management of encephalocele. *J Ultrasound Med* 1982; 1:111-115.

Jeanty P, Shah D, Zaleski W et al: Prenatal diagnosis of fetal cephalocele: A sonographic spectrum. *Am J Perinatol* 1991; 8:144-149.

Nyberg DA, Hallesy D, Mahony BS et al: Meckel-Gruber syndrome: importance of prenatal diagnosis. *J Ultrasound Med* 1990; 9:691-696.

Saw PD, Rouse GA, DeLange M: Meckel syndrome: sonographic findings. *JDMS* 1991; 7:8-11.

Wiswell TE, Tuttle DJ, Northan RS et al: Major congenital neurologic malformations: a 17 year survey. *Am J Dis* 1990; 144:61.

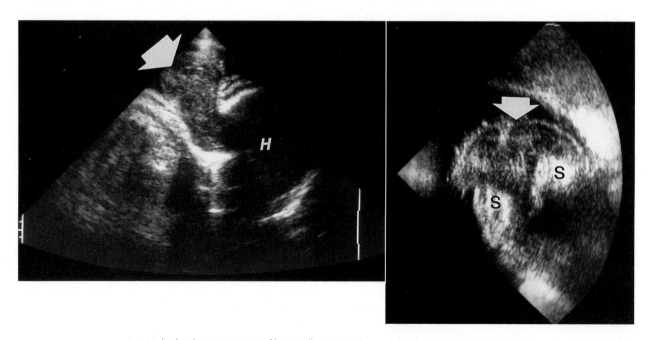

Longitudinal and transverse views of large midline occipital encephalocele (*arrow*). *H,* head; *S,* skull.

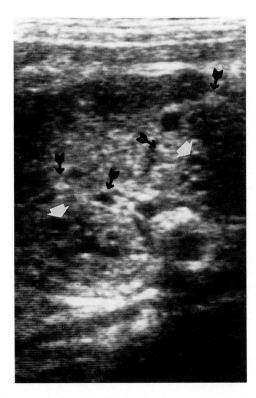

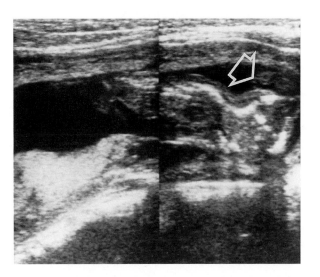

Parietal encephalocele due to amniotic bands. Note that the encephalocele (*arrow*) arises from the top of the head.

Meckel-Gruber kidneys—enlarged kidneys containing numerous visible cysts (*arrows*).

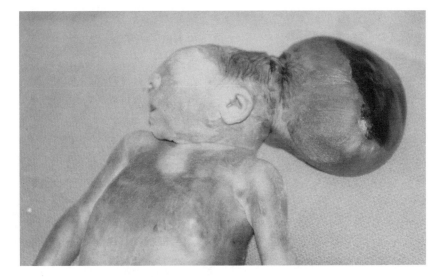

28-week stillborn with large isolated occipital encephalocele.

2.8 HOLOPROSENCEPHALY
ALOBAR, LOBAR, SEMILOBAR

EPIDEMIOLOGY/GENETICS

Definition   Holoprosencephaly is the term used for the spectrum of severe early abnormalities in forebrain cleavage. These cleavage abnormalities can occur both sagittally, resulting in fusion of the cerebral hemispheres, and horizontally, resulting in abnormalities of the optic and olfactory bulbs.

Epidemiology   1 to 2 out of 10,000 liveborns. 1 out of 250 embryos. (M1:F3 for alobar holoprosencephaly; M1:F1 for lobar form).

Embryology   Holoprosencephaly is an early arrest in prosencephalon cleavage. Most cases are sporadic, but chromosomal, genetic, and teratogenic causes have been described. One quarter of cases with multiple malformations are due to chromosomal abnormality, with trisomy 13, trisomy 18, 13q– and 18p– being the most common. An empiric recurrence risk for sporadic cases is approximately 6%.

Inheritance Patterns   Rare families showing autosomal dominant and autosomal recessive inheritance have been described. Multiple malformation syndromes, including the Meckel syndrome (AR), the Aicardi syndrome (X-linked dominant), the Fryn's syndrome (AR), and the hydrolethalus syndrome (AR), have been described with holoprosencephaly.

Teratogens   Alcohol, phenytoin, retinoic acid, maternal diabetes, and congenital infections have been reported with holoprosencephaly.

Prognosis   Most severely affected patients die at birth or in the first six months of life. Survival, with variable mental retardation, occurs in mild cases.

SONOGRAPHY

Findings
1. **Fetus**
    Brain changes. Three subtypes: a) alobar—virtually no cortical mantle; b) semilobar—single horseshoe-shaped ventricle with much mantle; c) lobar—the single ventricle is fused anteriorly only with incomplete falx and intrahemispheric fissure. The frontal horns are squared off. A third ventricle may be seen with a small echogenic area separating the third ventricle from the central ventricle.
    In the alobar and semilobar forms, the findings are: a) fused or partially fused thalamus with absence of the third ventricle; b) single ventricle with a horseshoe configuration; c) dorsal cyst—expansion of the posterior aspect of the common ventricle; d) hip-pocampal ridge—a bulge on the lateral aspect of the common ventricle at the midpoint; and e) absent cavum septum pellucidum, corpus callosum, and intrahemispheric fissure.
    Facial deformities are almost always seen: a) close-set eyes with either hypotelorism or a single orbit with one or two globes (cyclops deformity); b) median cleft lip and palate (see chapter 7); c) flattened nose with a single nostril; and d) there may be a proboscis superior to the level of the eyes with an absent nose and hypotelorism, yielding a markedly abnormal profile (ethmocephaly).
2. **Amniotic Fluid:** Polyhydramnios may occur.
3. **Placenta:** Normal.
4. **Measurement Data**
    1. The fetal head size is often enlarged, but may be normal or small despite ventricular enlargement.
    2. IUGR is often present
    3. The intraorbital distance is usually reduced.
5. **When Detectable:** With the vaginal probe at 13 weeks.

Pitfalls   See differential diagnosis.

Differential Diagnosis
1. Hydranencephaly can be confused with the alobar form. The thalamus will not be fused and a third ventricle should be visible in hydranencephaly.
2. The alobar form can be confused with aqueductal stenosis if the posterior fusion of the ventricles and the absent third ventricle are overlooked.
3. Schizencephaly—the cystic defect in schizencephaly may involve both hemispheres, but it will be asymmetrically shaped and the remaining ventricles will appear normal.
4. Dandy-Walker cyst—a massive Dandy-Walker cyst can give the impression of a dilated common ventricle, but the normal supratentorial system will be visible.
5. Agenesis of the corpus callosum can mimic the lobar form. The third ventricle will be separate from the lateral ventricles and will be at a high level.

Where Else to Look   Look for the stigma of trisomy 13—abnormal hands, feet, and omphalocele. Other associated problems are: congenital heart disease—particularly double outlet problems; omphalocele; and Dandy-Walker malformation.

PREGNANCY MANAGEMENT

Investigations and Consultations Required   The high incidence of cytogenetic abnormalities makes chromosome evaluation of the fetus mandatory, even late in pregnancy. Maternal evaluation for diabetes should be done. Fetal echocardiography is useful only to document additional malformations, but is not essential. Consultations with the neonatology staff should be arranged to discuss nonaggressive management at birth.

Fetal Intervention   In utero therapeutic procedures are contraindicated except to facilitate delivery (see Delivery below).

Monitoring   No pregnancy intervention such as early delivery or cesarean section is appropriate. All forms of holoprosencephaly have a very poor prognosis, therefore monitoring, except at the parent's request, is unwarranted. The head size needs to be assessed before delivery to make sure vaginal delivery is possible.

Pregnancy Course   Polyhydramnios may be associated with holoprosencephaly, resulting in preterm labor.

Pregnancy Termination Issues   The heterogeneous etiologies for holoprosencephaly require that a complete external and internal examination of the fetus be performed by individuals with training in fetal pathology and dysmorphology.

Delivery   Vaginal delivery should be accomplished in all cases. Cephalocentesis is appropriate in circumstances where a large head results in dystocia.

NEONATOLOGY

Resuscitation   With an established diagnosis of holoprosencephaly, the decision to initiate resuscitative measures should be discussed with the family prior to delivery. If the diagnosis is uncertain or associated anomalies not delineated, it is appropriate to support respiration to allow time for the diagnostic evaluation and parental adaptation to occur.

Transport   If the diagnostic evaluation has not been completed prior to delivery, transfer to a tertiary center with pediatric neurology capability is appropriate to confirm diagnosis and provide counselling and support to the family.

Testing and Confirmation   The clinical presentation of holoprosencephaly includes a spectrum of facial abnormalities including cyclopia, hypotelorism, and facial clefts. Newborns may have hydrocephalus and signs of neurologic dysfunction. Postnatal CT or MRI clearly defines these abnormalities.

Nursery Management   The priority is to obtain a definitive diagnosis as promptly as possible. If chromosomal analysis was not performed prenatally, blood should be collected prior to any major invasive procedure or blood transfusion. Respiratory support is indicated pending confirmation of diagnosis and giving the family time to make a decision about life-support and long-term care.

BIBLIOGRAPHY

Berry SM, Gosden C, Snijders RJ et al: Fetal holoprosencephaly: associated malformations and chromosomal defects. *Fetal Diagn Ther* 1990; 5:92-99.

Cohen MM: Perspectives on holoprosencephaly. Part I: epidemiology, genetics and syndromology. *Teratology* 1989; 40:211-235.

Cohen MM Jr: An update on the holoprosencephalic disorders. *J Pediatr* 1982; 101:865-869.

Filly RA, Chinn DH, Callen PW: Alobar holoprosencephaly: ultrasonographic prenatal diagnosis. *Radiology* 1984; 151:455-459.

Greene M, Benacerraf B, Frigoletto FD Jr: Reliable criteria for the sonographic diagnosis of alobar holoprosencephaly. *Am J Obstet Gynecol* 1987; 156:687-689.

Kobori JA, Herrick MK, Urich H: Arhinencephaly: the spectrum of associated malformations. *Brain* 1987; 110:237-260.

Munke M: Clinical, cytogenetic and molecular approaches to the genetic heterogeneity of holoprosencephaly. *Am J Med Genet* 1989; 34:237-245.

Nyberg DA, Mack LA, Bronstein A et al: Holoprosencephaly: prenatal sonographic diagnosis. *Am J Roentgenol* 1987; 149:1051-1058.

Pilu G, Ambrosetto P, Sandri F et al: Intraventricular fused fornices: a specific sign of fetal lobar holoprosencephaly. *Ultrasound Obstet Gynecol* 1994; 4:65-67.

Pilu G, Sandri F, Perolo A et al: Prenatal diagnosis of lobar holoprosencephaly. *Ultrasound Obstet Gynecol* 1992; 2:88-94.

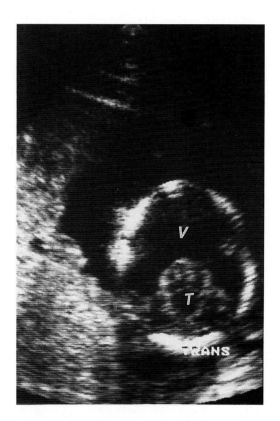

Alobar holoprosencephaly. The most severe form of holoprosencephaly with no cortical mantle and very large single ventricle (*V*). The thalamus (*T*) is fused on this coronal view.

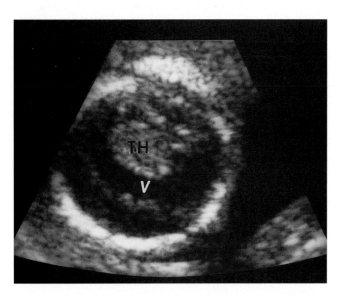

Semilobar holoprosencephaly. Single horseshoe-shaped ventricle (*V*) with considerable cortical mantle present. Again there is a fused thalamus (*TH*) with no septum pellucidum present.

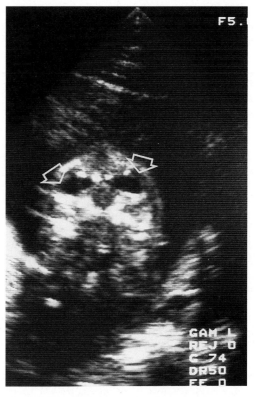

Hypotelorism with the eyes (*arrows*) unduly close together in a case of holoprosencephaly.

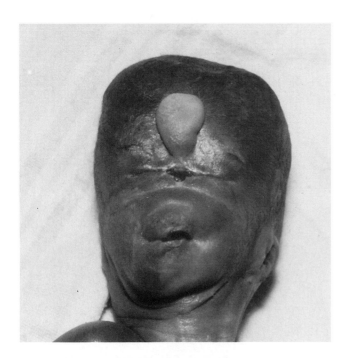

19-week fetus with isolated holoprosencephaly. Face shows proboscis, fused eyes, and absent nose.

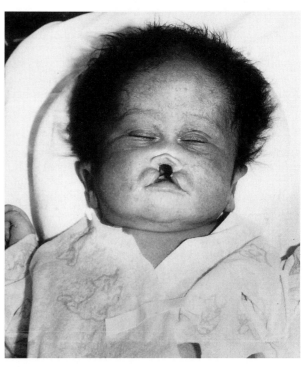

Newborn with median facial cleft, absent nose, and hypotelorism resulting from holoprosencephaly.

2.9 HYDRANENCEPHALY

EPIDEMIOLOGY/GENETICS

Definition   Hydranencephaly is a severe brain abnormality in which most or all of the cerebral hemispheres are absent and the cranium is filled with fluid.

Epidemiology   Rare occurrence (M1:F1).

Embryology   The etiology is heterogeneous, but most cases are thought to be due to generalized brain ischemia or overwhelming antenatal infection with resultant destruction of brain parenchyma. Ischemia may be due to hypotension, vascular agenesis/dysgenesis, arterial occlusion from twin to twin emboli, and occlusion of the vein of Galen. Most people differentiate hydranencephaly from extreme porencephaly by the former's symmetry and lack of cystic cavities, although they may represent a continuum. Extreme hydrocephalus differs from hydranencephaly in having a lining of cortex at the outside of its sac. Chromosomal abnormalities, especially trisomy 13, have been reported with hydranencephaly.

Inheritance Patterns   Rare familial recurrence has been reported. About 20 multiple malformation syndromes have been reported with hydranencephaly or porencephaly.

Teratogens: Congenital infections, including CMV and toxoplasmosis, and cocaine.

Prognosis   Hydranencephaly is usually lethal with neonatal survivors having profound mental retardation.

SONOGRAPHY

Findings
1. **Fetus**
   a. Almost all brain structures, above the brain stem and midbrain, are absent. The midbrain is variably present. In some instances, there is a central linear structure composed of the remnants of the brain, but usually even the falx and septum pellucidum are partially or completely absent.
   b. The brain stem, on coronal views, has a characteristic appearance as it protrudes into the completely fluid filled calvarium.
   c. The absence of cortex is due to a global cortical infarct. Infarction takes place sometime between 12 and 30 weeks. During the phase when infarction occurs, the brain becomes echogenic with loss of landmarks. The cortical brain, once infarcted, is fairly rapidly removed and eventually fluid replaces the brain.

2. **Amniotic Fluid:** Normal or increased.
3. **Placenta:** Normal.
4. **Measurement Data:** The head size is normal size or slightly enlarged.
5. **When Detectable:** Some time between 20 and 30 weeks as a rule, although an example at 12 weeks has been described.

Pitfalls   Because the dura and arachnoid are preserved, there may be confusion with very severe hydrocephalus. In the latter situation, the brain stem and midbrain are complete. Usually, with severe hydrocephalus, the ventricular enlargement is assymetrical and the third ventricle is dilated.

Differential Diagnosis
1. Lobar holoprosencephaly—the third ventricle will be absent, but the thalami are present.
2. Severe hydrocephalus—see Pitfalls above.
3. Porencephaly—only confusing if the normal brain (close to the transducer) is shadowed out by skull reverberations.

Where Else to Look   Usually not associated with problems elsewhere.

PREGNANCY MANAGEMENT

Investigations and Consultations Required   Although rare, disseminated fetal viral infections, especially herpes, can cause extensive cerebral destruction. Therefore, viral titers should be done. Chromosome studies should also be performed because of the potential for a misclassification of severe hydrocephalus as hydranencephaly.

Monitoring   Serial ultrasound examinations to monitor head size are quite appropriate. Because hydranencephaly should not be an "increased pressure" form of ventriculomegaly, an enlarging head relative to other fetal parameters should prompt a reassessment of the diagnosis.

Pregnancy Course   Hydranencephaly should not be associated with specific obstetric complications.

Pregnancy Termination Issues   Termination of pregnancy is an appropriate option, and it should be done by a nondestructive procedure at an institution with expertise in fetal neuropathology.

Delivery   Vaginal delivery is appropriate in all cases. In the presence of a relatively large head, cephalocentesis may be indicated to accomplish vaginal delivery of the infant.

NEONATOLOGY

Resuscitation   The decision to initiate resuscitative efforts should be discussed with the family prior to delivery. With a definitive diagnosis of hydranencephaly of known etiology, nonintervention is appropriate if spontaneous onset of respiration does not occur. If there is uncertainty of the diagnosis, support is indicated to allow time for confirmation.

Transport   Transfer to a tertiary center with pediatric neurology and neurosurgery capabilities is indicated for confirmation of diagnosis.

Testing and Confirmation   Affected infants may initially appear normal at birth or have signs of CNS dysfunction like seizures, poor feeding, and development delay. Postnatally the diagnosis is confirmed by MRI or CT scan. Serologic and microbiologic testing for congenital infections are indicated if not obtained prenatally.

Nursery Management   The major priorities are the confirmation of the diagnosis and etiology and facilitation of parental adaptation to the severe prognosis. Decisions regarding long-term custodial care may be required as some infants may survive the neonatal period.

BIBLIOGRAPHY

Belfar HB, Kuller JA, Hill LM et al: Evolving fetal hydranencephaly mimicking intracranial neoplasm. *J Ultrasound Med* 1991; 10:231-233.

Greene MF, Benacerraf B, Crawford JM: Hydranencephaly: US appearance during in utero evolution. *Radiology* 1985; 156:779-780.

Halsey JH Jr, Allen N, Chamberlin HR: The morphogenesis of hydranencephaly. *J Neurol Sci* 1971; 12:187-217.

Halsey JH Jr, Allen N, Chamberlin HR: Hydranencephaly. In: Vinken PJ, Bruyn GW (eds): Congenital malformations of the brain and skull. *Handbook Clin Neurol* 1977; 30:661.

Lin YS, Chang FM, Liu CH: Antenatal detection of hydranencephaly at 12 weeks, menstrual age. *J Clin Ultrasound* 1992; 20:62-64.

Pilu G, Rizzo N, Orsini LF et al: Antenatal recognition of cerebral anomalies. *Ultrasound Med Biol* 1986; 12:319-326.

Spirit BA et al: Fetal central nervous system abnormalities. *Fet Ultrasound* 1990; 28:59-73.

Hydranencephaly. No cortical mantle is present. No midline structures above the level of the cerebral peduncles (*P*) are present.

2.10 INIENCEPHALY

EPIDEMIOLOGY/GENETICS

Definition   Iniencephaly is an abnormality in cervical vertebrae associated with an excessive lordosis of the cervicothoracic spine and neural tube closure defects.

Epidemiology   Rare (M1:F10).

Embryology   The pathogenesis is unknown. It is possible that iniencephaly is a primary defect in fetal cervical development and the resulting lordosis causes a failure of neural tube closure. Alternatively, it may be a primary defect in neural tube closure. Anencephaly, encephalocele, hydrocephaly, and other anomalies have been associated with iniencephaly.

Inheritance Patterns   Sporadic, no known syndrome associations.

Teratogens   None known.

Screening   Alpha-fetoprotein (AFP) elevation may be present.

Prognosis   Iniencephaly, when diagnosed in utero, is almost always lethal.

SONOGRAPHY

Findings
1. **Fetus**
    a. There is a very short cervical spine with missing vertebrae—the fetal head is often extended.
    b. The cervical spine is open (cervical rachischisis), often with a large cervical meningocele.
    c. Anencephaly is often present.
    d. An additional lumbosacral meningomyelocele or caudal regression may be present.
2. **Amniotic Fluid:** Normal.
3. **Placenta:** Normal.
4. **Measurement Data:** Normal.
5. **When Detectable:** At 13 weeks using the endovaginal probe.

Pitfalls
A fetus with an extended neck for other reasons may be confused with iniencephaly because the cervical spine vertebrae are often difficult to see when the head is extended. Because the number of vertebrae is reduced in iniencephaly, locating and counting vertebral bodies is essential.

Differential Diagnosis
1. Masses arising from the front of the neck, such as goiter or teratoma, also cause neck extension.

2. It can be hard to distinguish a low posterior encephalocele from iniencephaly. The vertebrae may be difficult to examine due to position.

Where Else to Look
1. Look at the spine for other myelomeningocele.
2. Look at the intracranial structures; anencephaly is often seen.

PREGNANCY MANAGEMENT

Investigations and Consultations Required   The distinctive ultrasound features should preclude the need for any additional evaluation.

Monitoring   There are no special considerations for prenatal care, except supportive emotional care for the family. This is almost always a lethal anomaly, so ultrasonic monitoring is inappropriate except to ensure that massive hydrocephalus preventing vaginal delivery does not occur.

Pregnancy Course   The incidence of complicated labor and delivery is high with iniencephaly because of the high likelihood of fetal malpresentations.

Pregnancy Termination Issues   There are no indications for special pathologic examination. However, nondestructive methods of termination may be complicated by obstructed labor secondary to malpresentations of these fetuses.

Delivery   Cephalocentesis should be performed in the presence of severe hydrocephalus. In cases where obstructed labor occurs, embryotomy may be necessary to avoid cesarean section.

NEONATOLOGY

Resuscitation   Not indicated as the lesion is uncorrectable.

Transport   Not indicated as the lesion is uncorrectable.

Testing and Confirmation   The abnormality is obvious at birth.

Nursery Management   Provision of comfort care and support of family are the only appropriate care measures.

BIBLIOGRAPHY
Aleksic S, Budzilovich G, Greco MA et al: Iniencephaly: a neuropathologic study. *Clin Neuropathol* 1983; 2:55-61.
Foderaro AE, Abu-Yousef MM, Benda JA et al: Antenatal ultrasound diagnosis of iniencephaly. *J Clin Ultrasound* 1987; 15:550-554.

Katz VL, Aylsworth AS, Albright SG: Iniencephaly is not uniformly fatal. *Prenat Diagn* 1989; 9:595-599.

Meizner I, Bar-Ziv J: Prenatal ultrasonic diagnosis of a rare case of iniencephaly apertus. *J Clin Ultrasound* 1987; 15:200-203.

Meizner I, Press F, Jaffe A et al: Prenatal ultrasound diagnosis of complete absence of the lumbar spine and sacrum. *J Clin Ultrasound* 1992; 20:77-80.

Persutte WH, Lenke RR, Kurczynski TW et al: Prenatal ultrasonographic diagnosis of iniencephaly aperta. *JDMS* 1991; 7:208-212.

Sherer DM, Hearn-Stebbins B, Harvey W et al: Endovaginal sonographic diagnosis of iniencephaly apertus and craniorachischisis at 13 weeks, menstrual age. *J Clin Ultrasound* 1993; 21:124-127.

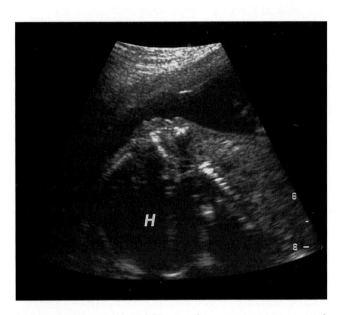

Iniencephaly. Retroverted head (*H*) because there were many missing cervical vertebrae. Cervical rachischisis was present.

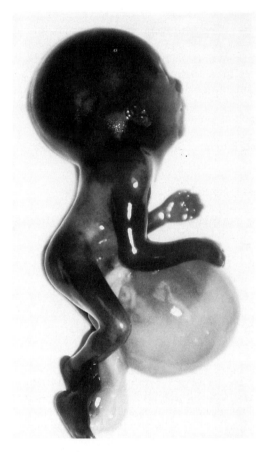

16-week fetus with severe neck extension due to iniencephaly. Note associated abdominal omphalocele.

2.11 INTRACRANIAL HEMORRHAGE

EPIDEMIOLOGY/GENETICS

Definition   Intracranial hemorrhage is the extravasation of blood from a blood vessel into the parenchyma or ventricles of the brain or spaces surrounding the brain.

Epidemiology   Unknown, but very rare.

Embryology   Maternal-fetal pregnancy complications, including hypotension and preeclampsia, are felt to be the most common etiologic factors. Twin to twin complications, antenatal infection, vascular malformations, alloimmune antibodies, and trauma are other possible causes of antenatal intracranial hemorrhage.

Inheritance Patterns   Sporadic.

Teratogens   Cocaine and congenital infections including CMV, herpes, and toxoplasmosis.

Prognosis   Dependent on the severity of damage to the CNS. Extensive hemorrhages are fatal. Permanent neurologic damage, moderate to severe mental retardation, hydrocephalus, and porencephalic cysts can be seen in survivors.

SONOGRAPHY

Findings
1. **Fetus**
    a. Intrabrain bleeds—Initially, an echogenic area within the brain is seen, which later becomes cystic. If it borders on a lateral ventricle, a bulge from the lateral ventricle known as a porencephalic cyst develops.
    b. Intraventricular bleeds—Blood within the ventricles has low level echoes for a brief period of time. Echogenic clots soon develop.
    c. Subdural bleeds—Echopenic and echogenic blood between the skull and the brain has been reported.
    d. Reactive hydrocephalus—If the blood clot does not obstruct the aqueduct of Sylvius, only lateral ventricular dilatation is seen. With aqueduct blockage, the third and lateral ventricles are all dilated.
2. **Amniotic Fluid:** Normal.
3. **Placenta:** Normal.
4. **Measurement Data:** Normal.
5. **When Detectable:** Bleeding generally occurs in the third trimester. It is easily detectable as soon as clot develops.

Pitfalls
1. If blood clot is not seen, the ventricular dilatation may be thought to be due to aqueduct stenosis.

2. A space between the brain and the skull is often seen as a normal variant in utero. Asymmetry and a local cranial bulge favor a subdural bleed. Doppler will show increased resistance in neighboring intracranial vessels.

Differential Diagnosis
1. Aqueductal stenosis—see Pitfalls above.
2. An echogenic intrabrain mass, due to clot, may be mistaken for tumor. No blood flow is seen with Doppler.
3. A brain infarct may resemble clot.

Where Else to Look
1. Other sites of bleeding—Liver and lungs in case the fetus has a bleeding diathesis.
2. Hydrops—The fetus may be very anemic.

PREGNANCY MANAGEMENT

Investigations and Consultations Required
1. Analysis of fetal platelet count and hematocrit by percutaneous umbilical blood sampling should be done.
2. Toxoplasmosis, other, rubella, cytomegalovirus, and herpes simplex virus (TORCH) titers and appropriate confirmation studies of abnormal results complete the work-up.
3. The family should be referred to a neonatologist for a thorough discussion of the neonatal management options and subsequent therapy.

Monitoring   In severe bleeds, the use of fetal assessment methods, such as nonstress testing, should not be used, as no benefit can be expected from early intervention. Frequent ultrasound studies are appropriate to see evolution of bleeds, to make sure no other bleeds occur, and to monitor the head for size increases related to hydrocephalus.

Pregnancy Course   Intracranial bleeds with resultant hydrocephalus may result in macrocephaly.

Pregnancy Termination Issues   Termination should occur by nondestructive procedures in a center with expertise in neuropathology.

Delivery   The pregnancy complicated by a fetal intracranial bleed requires delivery in a center with capabilities for neonatal resuscitation. In the case of alloimmune thrombocytopenia, consideration should be given to cesarean section to prevent further hemorrhage. Consideration of cephalocentesis versus cesarean section may arise if the degree of cerebral destruction is severe and severe hydrocephalus develops.

NEONATOLOGY

Resuscitation   The decision to initiate resuscitation in the presence of documented antenatal intracranial hemorrhage is contingent upon the extent of the hemorrhage, the degree of resultant brain destruction (porencephaly), the duration of the gestation at delivery, and the cumulative effect of the listed factors on the long-term prognosis. Prenatally, it is appropriate to discuss nonintervention with the family, should there be no spontaneous onset of respirations and the prognosis for severe disability is certain.

  If active resuscitation is to be instituted, there are no specific technical issues other than preparation for acute packed red cell transfusion if the hemorrhage is known to have been recent and severe.

Transport   Transfer to a tertiary perinatal center is appropriate to confirm diagnosis and prognosis.

Testing and Confirmation   Serologic testing for intrauterine coagulopathy secondary to congenital infections, coagulation defects, or isoimmune thrombocytopenia should be considered if the physical examination and clinical course are suggestive of any of the above disorders. The extent of the hemorrhage and resultant brain injury can be demonstrated by cranial CT or MRI. The latter may be preferable as vascular lesions are more easily identified.

Nursery Management   The initial priority is to establish cardiorespiratory adaptation. Support of perfusion and oxygen delivery by transfusion as noted above may be required. Post hemorrhagic hydrocephalus may complicate the course both prenatally and in the neonatal period.

BIBLIOGRAPHY

Ben-Chetrit A, Anteby E, Lavy G. et al: Increased middle cerebral artery blood flow impedance in fetal subdural hematoma. *Ultrasound Obstet Gynecol* 1991; 1:357-358.

Bowerman RA, Donn SM, Silver TM et al: Natural history of neonatal periventricular/intraventricular hemorrhage and its complications: sonographic observations. *Am J Roentgenol* 1984; 143:1041-1052.

Chinn DH, Filly RA: Extensive intracranial hemorrhage in utero. *J Ultrasound Med* 1983; 2:285-287.

Cochrane DD, Myles ST, Nimrod C et al: Intrauterine hydrocephalus and ventriculomegaly: associated anomalies and fetal outcome. *Can J Neurol Sci* 1985; 12:51-59.

Filly RA: The fetus with a central nervous system malformation: ultrasound evaluation. In: Harrison MR, et al (eds): *The unborn patient: prenatal diagnosis and treatment*. Philadelphia. WB Saunders, 1991. pp. 424-425.

Fogarty K: Sonography of fetal intracranial hemorrhage: unusual causes and a review of the literature. *J Clin Ultrasound* 1989; 17:366-370.

Minkoff H, Schaffer RM, Delke I et al: Diagnosis of intracranial hemorrhage in utero after a maternal seizure. *Obstet Gynecol* 1985; 65:22S-24S.

Mintz MC, Arger PH, Coleman BG: In utero sonographic diagnosis of intracerebral hemorrhage. *J Ultrasound Med* 1985; 4:375-376.

Naidu S, Messmore H, Caserta V et al: CNS lesions in neonatal isoimmune thrombocytopenia. *Arch Neurol* 1983; 40:552-554.

Zalneraitis EL, Young RS, Krishnamoorthy KS: Intracranial hemorrhage in utero as a complication of isoimmune thrombocytopenia. *J Pediatr* 1979; 95:611-614.

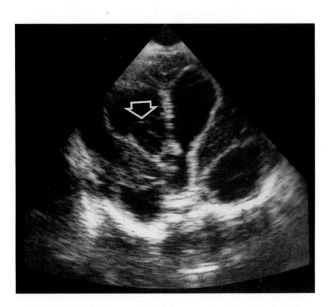

Intraventricular hemorrhage. The lateral and third ventricles are much enlarged. They have an echogenic border as is often seen with hemorrhage. Clot (*arrow*) can be seen within the right lateral ventricle and foramen of Monro.

2.12 INTRACRANIAL TERATOMA

EPIDEMIOLOGY/GENETICS

Definition   Teratomas are germ cell tumors that are derived from totipotent stem cells. These tumors contain cells representing all three embryonic germ cell layers: ectoderm, endoderm, and mesoderm.

Epidemiology   Very rare (M5:F1).

Embryology   Although the pathogenesis is unknown, teratomas may represent abnormalities in twinning. Commonly gastrointestinal, respiratory, and nervous system tissue elements are present. They occur most often in a paraaxial location from the brain to the sacral area. Primary sites in infants and children include sacrococcyx (60%), gonads (20%), chest and abdomen (15%), and intracranial (3%). Fifty percent of brain tumors detected in utero are teratomas.

Inheritance Patterns   Sporadic.

Teratogens   None.

Prognosis   Dependent upon the size and location of the tumor. So far, all prenatally diagnosed intracranial teratomas have been lethal.

SONOGRAPHY

Findings
1. **Fetus:** Structures within the fetal head are disorganized with areas of calcification and cystic areas. Few recognizable structures are visible. Almost all intracranial teratomas diagnosed in utero have been very advanced, filling much of the skull.
2. **Amniotic Fluid:** Amniotic fluid is often increased because the tumor may involve swallowing control.
3. **Placenta:** Normal.
4. **Measurement Data:** The fetal head size may be greatly increased.
5. **When Detectable:** Most often in the late second and third trimester.

Pitfalls
Intracranial bleeds can cause echogenic areas that may be mistaken for areas of intracranial calcification.

Differential Diagnosis
1. Other forms of intracranial tumor, for example, choroid plexus papilloma (characteristic intrachoroidal location), glioblastoma, craniopharyngioma, and neuroblastoma have been reported. Calcifications and cystic areas are indicative of intracranial teratoma.
2. Focal infarction or bleed—The appearance of the apparent mass will change relatively quickly.
3. Choroid plexus and corpus callosum lipoma are benign lesions with a typical echogenic appearance and location.

Where Else to Look   Teratomas may involve the mouth, so look closely at the face.

PREGNANCY MANAGEMENT

Investigations and Consultations Required   Because of the inability to make a precise diagnosis, other etiologies must be considered for the sonographic features. Disseminated viral infections and massive intracranial hemorrhage could present a similar picture. Maternal viral titers and percutaneous umbilical blood sampling for determination of fetal hematologic status may be helpful in excluding these conditions. A targeted computed axial tomography (CAT) scan with ultrasonic guidance can be helpful in establishing calcification and the presence of fat. Because of the grave prognosis, consultation with the neonatologist is essential for the planning of neonatal management. Likewise, a neurosurgical consult may provide the family additional information regarding the expected course in these infants.

Fetal Intervention   If the tumor is associated with hydrocephalus and an enlarged head, consideration should be given to cephalocentesis prior to delivery.

Monitoring   Because the head may grow to an unmanageable size, serial ultrasound studies to determine the time of delivery are desirable. Signs of fetal hydrops or polyhydramnios may be detected with ultrasound.

Pregnancy Course   Obstetric complications, including polyhydramnios, fetal hydrops, and cephalopelvic disproportion, are likely.

Pregnancy Termination Issues   As with other CNS malformations, the method of choice should allow a precise pathologic diagnosis of the sonographic findings.

Delivery   There are no benefits to cesarean section. Delivery should be vaginal if possible, even with an enlarged head (*see* Fetal Intervention and Monitoring above). Consideration should be given to management of labor without electronic heart rate monitoring, as evidence of "fetal distress" would not be unusual, given the significant CNS malformations. Decisions regarding mode of delivery should not be made on basis of fetal heart rate changes.

NEONATOLOGY

Resuscitation   A prenatal discussion with the family regarding nonintervention is appropriate should there be fetal distress or delay in spontaneous onset of respiration. If the decision is made to intervene, there are no specific resuscitation techniques required. The prenatal development of either hydrocephalus or hydrops can also complicate resuscitation.

Transport   Referral to a tertiary center with pediatric neurosurgery capabilities is indicated.

Testing and Confirmation   Intracranial teratomas can be associated with obstructive hydrocephalus, signs of increased intracranial pressure, and focal neurologic abnormalities. Half are found in the pineal region. Postnatal CT or MRI scan can confirm the diagnosis.

Nursery Management   As mortality from this lesion is almost 100%, the major issue is the accessibility of the tumor to operative resection.

SURGERY

Preoperative Assessment   These tumors are found primarily in the midline as are most congenital CNS tumors. The most common sites are the pineal region, suprasellar, and the fourth ventricle. There is a striking male predominance that has been reported to range between 1 in 5 and 1 in 10. MRI scanning of the head and spine are performed, plus a careful search for tumor outside the CNS.

Operative Indications   All intracranial mass lesions suspicious for neoplasm require surgical treatment for the purpose of diagnosis and therapy.

Types of Procedures   Some intracranial tumors depending upon the location and size may warrant biopsy alone. Open surgical biopsy and radical resection is indicated if a reasonable prognosis is anticipated.

Surgical Results/Prognosis   Teratomas can be divided pathologically into mature and immature forms. Mature teratomas have well differentiated components and a good prognosis if complete resection is possible. Immature teratomas show evidence of germinomatous or poorly differentiated components. These tumors have relatively poor prognosis with a significant recurrence rate and a tendency to spread along CSF pathways. Teratomas that present in the pineal or suprasellar region are more likely to be of the mature type whereas those in the fourth ventricle tend to be immature with a relatively poor prognosis. These tumors can attain tremendous size and the size does not necessarily reflect the pathology.

BIBLIOGRAPHY

Billmore DF, Grosfeld JL: Teratomas in childhood: analysis of 142 cases. *Pediatr Surg* 1986; 21:548-551.

Body G, Darnis E, Pourcelot D et al: Choroid plexus tumors: antenatal diagnosis and follow-up. *J Clin Ultrasound* 1990; 18:575-578.

Chervenak FA, Isaacson G, Touloukian R et al: Diagnosis and management of fetal teratomas. *Obstet Gynecol* 1985; 66:666-671.

Dolkart LA, Balcom RJ, Eisinger G: Intracranial teratoma: prolonged neonatal survival after prenatal diagnosis. *Am J Obstet Gynecol* 1990; 162:768-769.

Lipman SP, Pretorius DH, Rumack CM et al: Fetal intracranial teratoma: US diagnosis of three cases and a review of the literature. *Radiology* 1985; 157:491-494.

McConachie NS, Twining P, Lamb MP: Case report: antenatal diagnosis of congenital gliobastoma. *Clin Radiol* 1991; 44:121-122.

Mulligan G, Meier P: Lipoma and agenesis of the corpus callosum with associated choroid plexus lipomas. *J Ultrasound Med* 1989; 8:583-588.

Russel D, Rubinstein L: *Pathology of tumors of the nervous system*, 5th edition, Williams & Wilkins, 1989; p. 681.

Suresh S, Indrani S, Vijayalakshmi S et al: Prenatal diagnosis of cerebral neuroblastoma by fetal brain biopsy. *J Ultrasound Med* 1993; 12:303-306.

Ulreich S, Hanieh A, Furness ME: Positive outcome of fetal intracranial teratoma. *J Ultrasound Med* 1993; 3:163-165.

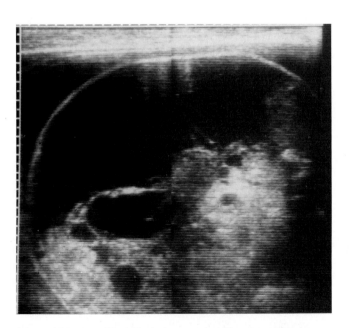

Intracranial teratoma. The entire brain was replaced by a tumor that was partially cystic and partially solid. The biparietal diameter was 18 cm (10 cm at term).

2.13 Microcephaly

EPIDEMIOLOGY/GENETICS

Definition Microcephaly is defined as a head circumference two standard deviations below the mean (i.e., less than 5%). Most cases are secondary to a small brain.

Epidemiology 1 out of 10,000 births (M1:F1) for isolated microcephaly. Much more common as an associated abnormality.

Embryology Microcephaly most often occurs secondary to a small brain. It can have antenatal or postnatal onset and is associated with various brain malformations, disruptions, and over 300 sporadic, genetic, and chromosomal syndromes.

Inheritance Patterns Both autosomal recessive and autosomal dominant families have been reported with isolated microcephaly.

Teratogens Most human teratogens, including intrauterine infection (cytomegalovirus, rubella, and toxoplasmosis), radiation, drugs, hypoxia, and alcohol, can cause microcephaly.

Prognosis Dependent on the etiology of the microcephaly and any associated brain malformations. Most microcephaly syndromes and isolated genetic microcephalies result in moderate to severe mental retardation.

SONOGRAPHY

Findings
1. **Fetus:** The head is small yet the facial structures remain normal sized. Diagnosis is easier if there is ventriculomegaly. Without ventriculomegaly the diagnosis should not be made in utero unless the head size is at least three standard deviations below normal. A slanting forehead supports the diagnosis.
2. **Amniotic Fluid:** Usually normal.
3. **Placenta:** If the microcephaly is due to CMV, there may be placentomegaly or oligohydramnios.
4. **Measurement Data:** The biparietal diameter and the head circumference are below three standard deviations for a given gestational age. Measurement of the frontal lobe size is said to be helpful in microcephaly detection. A measurement is made from the medial wall of the lateral ventricle to the front of the skull on a standard biparietal diameter view.
5. **When Detectable:** Usually not detectable until after 24 weeks. The diagnosis becomes progressively easier as the pregnancy proceeds.

Pitfalls After 30 weeks, it is common to see the head circumference and the biparietal diameter below the tenth percentile as a normal variant. Usually, there is a family history of small heads.

Differential Diagnosis
1. Normal variant small head. Ask for a family history of a small hat size.
2. Anencephaly, because the base of the brain persists.

Where Else to Look
1. Cytomegalovirus—Look at the lateral ventricular walls and if they are unduly echogenic calcification related to CMV may be present.
2. Look to see that the intracranial structures and head shape are symmetrical. If they are not, consider brain infarction. The lateral ventricle on the involved side may be enlarged.
3. Microcephaly is associated with Arnold-Chiari malformation and myelomeningocele. Look at the cerebellum and skull shape and the lower lumbar spine.
4. Microcephaly is associated with many syndromes, (e.g., Pena Shokeir 1), so look carefully at the rest of the fetus, especially the heart.
5. Neu Laxova syndrome is characterized by IUGR, sloping forehead, externalized eyes, short neck, and microcephaly.
6. Maternal phenylketonuria (PKU)—microcephaly, cardiac anomalies, micrognathia.

PREGNANCY MANAGEMENT

Investigations and Consultations Required
1. A careful history of drug or environmental exposures should be taken.
2. Biochemical evaluation of mother should be done to exclude maternal PKU.
3. Testing for maternal infections (CMV, toxoplasmosis, etc.). Viral titers should be performed with appropriate confirmational studies, if positive titers are found.
4. Congenital heart defects are commonly associated with conditions having microcephaly as a feature, therefore, fetal echocardiography should be a part of the initial evaluation.
5. Fetal karyotype is recommended, especially if the microcephaly is part of multiple malformations.

Monitoring There are no specific needs beyond usual obstetric care. Because the diagnosis is difficult to make, repeat ultrasound studies are helpful to confirm diminished cranial growth and may reveal additional anomalies.

Pregnancy Course   No specific obstetric complications would be expected secondary to this fetal malformation.

Pregnancy Termination Issues   If a diagnosis has not been established, a nondestructive procedure should be performed and a careful external examination of the fetus by a dysmorphologist should be a part of the autopsy protocol.

Delivery   Delivery at a tertiary center is appropriate if a precise diagnosis has not been made prenatally. Special care and evaluation may be necessary following birth.

NEONATOLOGY

Resuscitation   No specific measures are required with isolated microcephaly.

Transport   Neonatal referral to a perinatal tertiary center for isolated microcephaly is not indicated. Subsequent referral to a pediatric neurologist for consultation is appropriate.

Testing and Confirmation   In the genetic isolated microcephalies, brain growth may be normal throughout pregnancy or fall off shortly before term. Therefore, normal fetal ultrasounds are not necessarily reassuring. Measurement of head circumference and CT or MRI for brain morphology are indicated. Screening evaluations for isolated microcephaly include TORCH titers, blood and urinary testing for metabolic disorders, and cranial CT.

Nursery Management   As noted above, microcephaly is often associated with other malformations or diseases that will dictate the neonatal management.

BIBLIOGRAPHY

Broderick K, Oyer R, Chatwani A: Neu-Laxova syndrome: a case report. *Am J Obstet Gynecol* 1988; 158:574-575.

Chervenak FA, Rosenberg J, Brightman RC et al: A prospective study of the accuracy of ultrasound in predicting fetal microcephaly. *Obstet Gynecol* 1987; 69:908-910.

Goldstein I, Reece A, Pilu G et al: Sonographic assessment of the fetal frontal lobe: a potential tool for prenatal diagnosis of microcephaly. *Am J Obstet Gynecol* 1988; 158:1057-1062.

Kurtz AB, Wapner RJ, Rubin CS et al: Ultrasound criteria for in utero diagnosis of microcephaly. *J Clin Ultrasound* 1980; 8:11-16.

Martin HP: Microcephaly and mental retardation. *Am J Dis Child* 1970; 119:128-131.

Rossi LN, Candini G, Scarlatti G et al: Autosomal dominant microcephaly without mental retardation. *Am J Dis Child* 1987; 141:655-659.

Tolmie JL, McNay M, Stephenson JB et al: Microcephaly: Genetic counseling and antenatal diagnosis after the birth of an affected child. *Am J Med Genet* 1987; 27:583-594.

Volpe JJ: Neuronal proliferation, migration, organization, myelination. In: Neurology of the newborn. Philadelphia. WB Saunders, 1987. p. 35.

Warkany J, Lemire RJ, Cohen MM: Mental retardation and congenital malformations of the central nervous system. In: Microcephaly. Chicago. Mosby–Year Book, 1981.

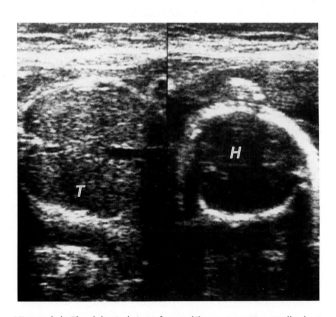

Microcephaly. The abdominal circumference (*T*) measurement, normally about the same size as the head circumference at term, is much larger. The head (*H*) circumference needs to be at least below the fifth percentile before microcephaly is considered, unless there is also ventriculomegaly (see example under cytomegalovirus).

2.14 SPINAL DYSRAPHISM
MYELOMENINGOCELE, MYELOSCHISIS, MENINGOCELE

EPIDEMIOLOGY/GENETICS

Definition Myelomeningocele, the most common type of neural tube defect, is defined by: 1. protrusion of neural elements and meninges through open vertebral arches; and 2. associated neurologic deficits.

Epidemiology The incidence is very geographic and population dependent and ranges from about 1 out of 500 to 1 out of 2000 births in the United States (M1:F>1).

Embryology Meningomyeloceles result from the failure of the vertebral arches to close prior to the sixth week of pregnancy secondary to a failure of normal neural ectodermal development. They most often occur in the lumbosacral area and are associated with hydrocephalus due to an Arnold-Chiari malformation in 90% of patients. Genitourinary tract and cardiac abnormalities are the most frequent associated malformations. Although most myelomeningoceles are isolated abnormalities, over 25 genetic, sporadic, and chromosomal multiple malformation syndromes have been described, including trisomy 18.

Inheritance Patterns Multifactorial inheritance with a combination of genetic and environmental influences. The risk of recurrence, after one affected pregnancy, is about 2% to 3%.

Teratogens Two percent of fetuses exposed to valproic acid will have neural tube defects. Folic acid antagonists (methotrexate and aminopterin), vitamin A, thalidomide, maternal diabetes, hyperthermia, and folic acid deficiency are also associated with an increased risk for neural tube defects.

Screening Maternal serum alpha-fetoprotein screening will detect approximately 80% of meningomyeloceles.

Prognosis Dependent on the size and location of the defect and the presence of associated abnormalities. In simple isolated defects, there is a 10% risk for mental retardation. Modern surgical and medical treatment has resulted in better long-term function, but urinary tract and orthopedic disability is a common long-term problem.

SONOGRAPHY

Findings
1. **Fetus**
   a. The cord is tethered and often split into two components. At the site of the cord abnormality, the bony canal is widened and forms a U shape.
   In the most common form of myelomeningocele, there is a cystic pouch posterior to the spine that contains some linear structures representing nerve fibers. In another form, the cystic pouch contains no nerves (meningocele). In a third form (myeloschisis), there is no pouch, but the nerves are tethered and exposed to the amniotic fluid because they are not covered with skin.
   b. Most spinal dysraphism occurs in the lower lumbar and upper sacral areas, but a few spinal defects are at a higher level. It is important to assess the level accurately as it affects prognosis. The iliac superior crest aspect is at L5 level. The superior vertebral level at which the abnormality first occurs can be established by counting up from this level.
   c. Findings that worsen the prognosis are a marked angulation of the spine at the level of the deformity (a gibbous deformity), a very large or long defect, or a defect at a higher vertebral level than L2.
   d. Technical aspects—Three bony structures compose the surroundings of the spinal canal. The posterior ossification center of the vertebral body and bilateral ossification centers related to the junction of the lamina and pedicle known as the posterior elements. A transverse spinal view will show these latter structures as echogenic areas that are splayed. A sagittal, posterior view will show a cystic pouch posterior to the spine. If no pouch is present, a depression at the abnormal level will be seen. A coronal view of the spine will show the posterior elements more widely separated at the level of the defect.
   e. Cranial changes
      i. Typically, the head is bilaterally flattened in the frontal region to give a "lemon" or "bullet" shape.
      ii. The cerebellum is rounded to form a "banana" shape. Its width is decreased.
      iii. The cisterna magna is effaced—this is the strongest sign. These are the components of the Arnold-Chiari type 2 complex.
      iv. Bilateral, lateral, and third ventricular dilatation may occur.
   f. Leg changes—With severe myelomeningocele, there is absent leg movement and clubfoot, prognostic of poor long-term result. Good leg movement in utero may be followed by lower limb paralysis at birth and has no prognostic significance.
2. **Amniotic Fluid:** Usually normal.
3. **Placenta:** Usually normal.
4. **Measurement Data:** Even though the lateral ventricles may be dilated, the head size is small. Intrauterine growth retardation may occur.

5. When Detectable: Can be detected at 11 weeks by vaginal sonography, but usually detected at 16 to 18 weeks. Approximately 98% are detected by the recognition of the sonographic signs in the head and spine.

Pitfalls
1. Defects involving a single vertebral body or those located in the sacral vertebrae can be difficult to detect.
2. Sacral defects may not be detectable until later because the sacral bones are not ossified until 20 weeks.
3. Occasional spina bifida do not show a lemon deformity and even more rarely do not show a banana cerebellar change. Conversely, a lemon sign may be seen in a normal fetus.
4. Oblique views through the lumbar spine region can make the gluteus muscles look like a myelomeningocele.
5. Oligohydramnios or obesity may prevent the meningocele sac from being seen.
6. A slanting transducer angulation can create an impression of a widened interpedicular distance.

Differential Diagnosis   Sacrococcygeal teratoma—the primary region of abnormality in myelomeningocele is superior to the coccyx, partially fluid filled and more or less symmetrical.

Where Else to Look
1. The lower limbs (see Fetus above).
2. The head (see Fetus above).
3. The kidneys for hydronephrosis, however, the genitourinary system is almost always normal.
4. Other findings of trisomy 18, which is associated with myelomeningocele.

PREGNANCY MANAGEMENT

Investigations and Consultations Required   Amniocentesis should be performed for chromosome studies (approximately a 10% risk of aneuploidy) and for confirmation of the diagnosis by amniotic fluid AFP and acetylcholinesterase. A history of medication exposure should be taken, with special emphasis on anticonvulsants. Congenital heart malformations are associated with neural tube defects, therefore, fetal echocardiography should be done. Consultation with a neurosurgeon and a developmental pediatrician will prepare the family for the multidisciplinary approach necessary for the most favorable outcome in their child.

Fetal Intervention   In utero therapy is not indicated. However, as noted below, active pregnancy management may be beneficial.

Monitoring   Serial ultrasound examinations every 3 to 4 weeks to assess the degree or progression of ventriculomegaly are necessary.

Pregnancy Course   For lesions above the lumbar area, the likelihood of progressive ventriculomegaly and macrocephaly is high.

Pregnancy Termination Issues   If chromosome studies can be completed on abortus material and no associated anomalies are seen by ultrasound, suction dilatation and evacuation procedures are appropriate.

Delivery   The presence of progressive and severe ventriculomegaly may be justification for early delivery after 32 weeks gestation. The potential benefit of early shunting, however, must be weighed against the risk of prematurity. In the absence of progressive ventriculomegaly, delivery should be at term. The mode of delivery for the fetus with myelomeningocele is controversial. Recent information seems to favor cesarean section because of evidence suggesting a better prognosis for motor function in these infants. Unfortunately, no well-controlled prospective studies have been done.

NEONATOLOGY

Resuscitation   In the third trimester and prior to the onset of labor, a discussion with the parents of the options for intervention is mandatory. By this point, the presence of other CNS and unrelated organ system anomalies affecting prognosis should be delineated, allowing for a more accurate assessment of potential outcome. Fetal distress in labor and respiratory depression at birth occur frequently and an antepartum decision regarding resuscitation is helpful.

Protection of the lesion from trauma and surface contamination is imperative. Use of sterile sheets on the resuscitation table and having one member of the team prepared to cover and pad the lesion using strict aseptic technique are important measures.

Transport   Referral to a tertiary center with a multidisciplinary team for management is always indicated. Protection of the lesion as described above during transport is essential.

Testing and Confirmation   The first priority is the complete assessment of the infant to identify all abnormalities and determine severity of dysfunction. This should include thorough neurologic examination, cranial CT to delineate associated CNS malformations, and evaluation for other organ system anomalies if there are other dysmorphic physical findings.

Nursery Management   The decision regarding direct intervention beginning with surgical closure should again be reviewed with the family as the projected outcome after full evaluation of the infant may not coincide with that from prenatal assessment.

Closure of the defect within 48 hours or broad spectrum antibiotic treatment have been shown to preserve existing peripheral neurologic function.

Following closure of the defect, the three primary management issues, depending on the location and extent of the spinal defect, are concomitant hydrocephalus in 65% to 95% of infants; urinary tract structural and functional abnormalities; and orthopedic deformities and dysfunction. All require management by the appropriate subspecialties.

SURGERY

Preoperative Assessment The location and size of the myelomeningocele defect as well as the presence of a kyphotic deformity are important from the neurosurgical standpoint. The presence of associated cranial and extracranial anomalies, particularly hydrocephalus, are also important prenatal information.

General physical assessment with special attention to the cardiac, pulmonary, and renal systems are important in the decision to proceed with closure of the myelomeningocele and in determining the timing of surgery. A head sonogram is necessary to establish the ventricular size. In addition, careful inspection of the myelomeningocele lesion is essential. If the defect is open and leaking spinal fluid, then despite small ventricular size by sonogram, hydrocephalus may still be present and a ventricular shunt necessary.

Operative Indications All open (i.e., not completely skin-covered) defects require early closure to minimize the risk of infection.

Types of Procedures Repair involves release of the exposed spinal cord from the surrounding skin with closure of the dural tube, muscle, and subcutaneous tissue over the cord. Ventricular shunting, if indicated, is performed at the same procedure.

Surgical Results/Prognosis The functional outcome of a child born with a myelomeningocele is, in general terms, related to the size and level of the defect. The larger and higher (thoracic or thoracolumbar) lesions are associated with paraparesis or paraplegia, sphincter dysfunction, and a greater risk of spinal deformity. Careful monitoring for signs of lower cranial nerve or brainstem dysfunction can identify those children who develop symptomatic Chiari II malformation that may require surgical decompression. Children with myelomeningocele will require careful long-term follow-up from the neurosurgical, orthopedic, urologic, and pediatric standpoint.

BIBLIOGRAPHY

Ball RH, Filly RA, Goldstein RB et al: The lemon sign: not a specific indicator of meningomyelocele. *J Ultrasound Med* 1993; 3:131-134.

Benacerraf BR, Stryker J, Frigoletto FD Jr: Abnormal US appearance of the cerebellum (banana sign): indirect sign of spina bifida. *Radiology* 1989; 171:151-153.

Dennis MA, Drose JA, Pretorius DH et al: Normal fetal sacrum simulating spina bifida: "Pseudodysraphism". *Radiology* 1985; 155:751-754.

Goldstein RB, Podrasky AE, Filly RA et al: Effacement of the fetal cisterna magna in association with myelomeningocele. *Radiology* 1989; 172:409-413.

Hall JG, Friedman JM, Kenna BA et al: Clinical, genetic, and epidemiological factors in neural tube defects. *Am J Hum Genet* 1988; 43:827-837.

Kollias SS, Goldstein RB, Cogen PH et al: Prenatally detected myelomeningoceles: sonographic accuracy in estimation of the spinal level. *Radiology* 1992; 185:109-112.

Lirette M, Filly RA: Relationship of fetal hydronephrosis to spinal dysraphism. *J Ultrasound Med* 1983; 2:495-497.

Morrow RJ, McNay MB, Whittle MJ: Ultrasound detection of neural tube defects in patients with elevated maternal serum alpha-fetoprotein. *Obstet Gynecol* 1991; 78:1055-1057.

Neutzel MJ: Myelomeningocele: current concepts of management. *Clin Perinatol* 1989; 16: 311.

Nyberg DA, Mack LA, Hirsch J et al: Abnormalities of fetal cranial contour in sonographic detection of spina bifida: evaluation of the lemon sign. *Radiology* 1988; 167:387-392.

Pilu G, Romero R, Reece EA et al: Subnormal cerebellum in fetuses with spina bifida. *Am J Obstet Gynecol* 1988; 158:1052-1056.

Riegel D, Rotenstein D: In: Pediatric Neurosurgery, 3rd edition, WB Saunders, 1994. p.51.

Van Allen MI, Kalousek DK, Chernoff GF et al: Evidence for multisite closure of the neural tube in humans. *Am J Med Genet* 1993; 47:723-743.

Van den Hof MC, Nicolaides KH, Campbell J et al: Evaluation of the lemon and banana signs in one hundred thirty fetuses with open spina bifida. *Am J Obstet Gynecol* 1990; 162:322-327.

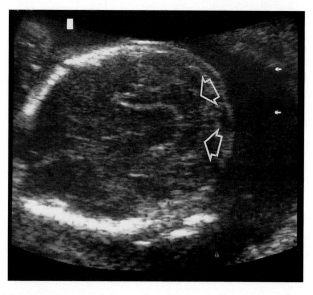

Spinal dysraphism. Cranial changes of Arnold-Chiari malformation; the cerebellum (*arrows*) forms a "banana" shape and there is no visible cisterna magna. The anterior aspect of the skull is flattened so that the skull assumes a lemon shape.

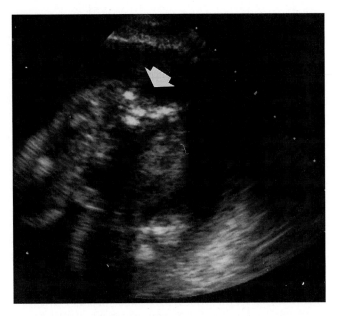

Transverse view of myeloschisis. The lumbar spine lateral ossification centers are separated and there is a dip between them (*arrow*).

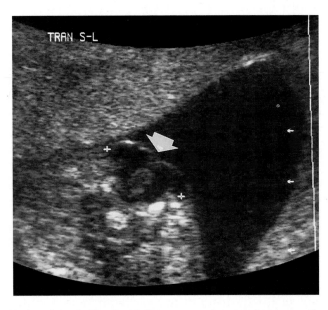

Myelomeningocele. There is a similar appearance, but a membrane covers the defect (*arrow—between +'s*). Some nerves can be seen within the meningocele.

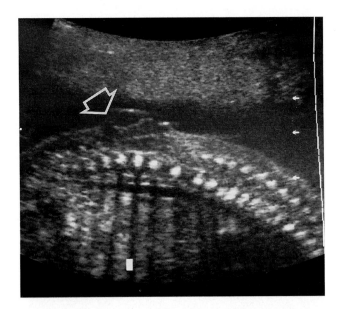

Sagittal view. The septated cystic mass (*arrow*) can be seen in the L4/L5 area.

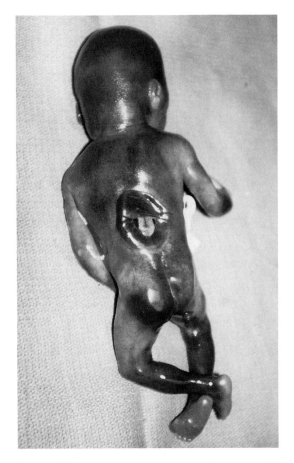

20-week fetus with lower thoracic–upper lumbar meningomyelocele. Neural elements are visible below the ruptured sac.

2.15 Vein of Galen Malformation

EPIDEMIOLOGY/GENETICS

Definition   Aneurysms of the vein of Galen are dilatations of the vein ranging from large single aneurysms to multiple smaller communications.

Epidemiology   Rare (M2:F1).

Embryology   The cerebral vessels derive from a primitive plexus that differentiates into arteries and veins. It is not clear how, when, or why cerebral or other arteriovenous malformations arise. Pathologically the vein of Galen appears dilated and communicates with normal-appearing arteries. Most cases occur as isolated abnormalities. Congenital heart defects, cystic hygromas, and hydrops are associated with vein of Galen malformations.

Inheritance Patterns   Sporadic.

Teratogens   None suspected.

Prognosis   Infants presenting at birth with heart failure or hydrops have so far always died. Later childhood presentation is associated with a 20% surgical mortality rate. Successful survivors are normal.

SONOGRAPHY

Findings
1. **Fetus**
   a. CNS
      i. There is a large irregularly shaped, basically circular, cystic space in the posterior aspect of the brain in the midline. The aneurysm lies posterosuperior to the third ventricle. Multiple small feeder arteries can be seen with real-time and color flow Doppler imaging. A large tubular vein flows toward the occipital region. Careful color flow Doppler analysis of feeder arteries to the aneurysm helps surgical planning.
      ii. Secondary third and lateral ventriculomegaly may be present.
   b. Thorax—the cardiac size may be increased with large neck arteries and superior inferior vena cava.
   c. Abdomen
      i. Hepatosplenomegaly may be seen.
      ii. Secondary hydrops, due to arteriovenous shunting, may be the presenting feature. There may be ascites, pleural effusion, pericardial effusion, and skin thickening.
2. **Amniotic Fluid:** Normal.
3. **Placenta:** Normal.
4. **Measurement Data:** Normal.
5. **When Detectable:** About 14 weeks.

Pitfalls
1. Confusion with a quadrageminal cistern, a normal cystic structure posterior to the third ventricle, may occur until Doppler is used.
2. The cavum vergi and septum pellucidum usually extend anteriorly, but may persist only posteriorly.

Differential Diagnosis
1. Quadrageminal cistern.
2. Centrally placed arachnoid cyst.

Where Else to Look   Any central intracranial cystic structure of uncertain origin should be examined with Doppler and the heart and abdomen should be examined for cardiomegaly and hydrops. Hydrops and cardiomegaly should precipitate a look for a vein of Galen aneurysm.

PREGNANCY MANAGEMENT

Investigations or Consultations Required   No further diagnostic evaluation is necessary, if Doppler confirms the vascular nature of the lesion. Fetal echocardiography may be helpful in detecting early signs of congestive heart failure. A pediatric neurosurgeon should be consulted to assist with prenatal management, and to discuss the postnatal treatment options with the family.

Fetal Intervention   In utero therapy is not indicated.

Monitoring   Because of the high risk of fetal hydrops, and subsequent development of preeclampsia in some of these cases, careful follow-up by a perinatologist is appropriate. Frequent ultrasound studies should be performed (e.g., every 2 weeks) because more severe hydrops may precipitate early delivery.

Pregnancy Course   The high risk of fetal hydrops and subsequent preeclampsia or the development of obstructive hydrocephalus makes this fetal malformation one with significant risk for obstetric complications.

Pregnancy Termination Issues   As with all brain malformations, termination of pregnancy and subsequent fetal autopsy must be performed in institutions with special expertise in neuropathology.

Delivery   In severe cases nonaggressive management may be the best approach. In those cases without complications, elective delivery, when fetal lung maturity is attained, might improve prognosis. However, there is little information available on which to base recommendation regarding timing or mode of delivery.

NEONATOLOGY

Resuscitation   The approach to resuscitation is based on the extent of congestive heart failure and hydrops present prior to delivery, in addition to the anatomic characteristics and, therefore, surgical correctability of the lesion. Planned delivery after fetal lung maturity is achieved and avoidance of fetal distress followed by immediate and atraumatic resuscitation offers the best opportunity for a favorable outcome. Consideration should be given to early institution of ionotropic agents to improve myocardial function and paralysis to reduce oxygen consumption and fluctuations in cerebral vascular pressures. Drainage of serous fluid collusions, if present (pleural, pericardial, and peritoneal), may be needed to facilitate cardiorespiratory adaptation.

As with any abnormality in which there is a strong chance of neonatal death and of a poor long-term prognosis, a discussion with the parents prenatally regarding nonintervention is appropriate.

Transport   Referral to a tertiary center with pediatric cardiology and pediatric neurosurgery capabilities is imperative. Support of oxygenation and perfusion during transport is critical.

Testing and Confirmation   Vein of Galen aneurysms present in the newborn period with heart failure or hydrops. Later childhood presentations include headache or other CNS symptoms and are associated with a better prognosis. Occasionally, vein of Galen malformations are associated with hydrocephalus or porencephaly. Postnatal CT or MRI scans and arteriograms can define this abnormality.

Nursery Management   The priority issues are maintenance of adequate gas exchange and tissue perfusion and avoidance of wide fluctuations in cerebral intravascular pressure. Myocardial ischemia and intracranial hemorrhage are the reported causes of death. Measures to control congestive heart failure include ionotropic agents, diuretics and fluid restriction, and correction of metabolic abnormalities such as acidosis, hypoglycemia, and electrolyte imbalances.

Timing and techniques for closure of the feeding vessels to the aneurysm are determined both by the infant's clinical status and the vascular anatomy of the lesion. Magnetic resonance imaging is the preferable study to determine the latter.

SURGERY

Preoperative Assessment   Vein of Galen malformations can be divided into two distinct types.

1. True aneurysmal dilatations of the vein of Galen as a consequence of a true arteriovenous fistula with shunting of arterial blood into an embryologic venous precursor, the median vein of the prosencephalon.
2. Secondary enlargement of the vein of Galen as a consequence of an adjacent parenchymal arteriovenous malformation.

Assessment of cardiac status as well as associated intracranial vascular or structural anomalies, hydrocephalus, or hemorrhages is required.

Postnatal assessment involves MRI evaluation and cerebral angiography. Management in children who are asymptomatic, that is, without cardiac failure or hydrocephalus, is observation alone with follow-up ultrasound or MRI at 3 months and 6 months of age.

Operative Indications   If the malformation persists, then angiography and treatment is performed at 6 to 8 months of age. In children who present with cardiac failure or progressive hydrocephalus, immediate diagnostic angiography is indicated.

Types of Procedures   Treatment of vein of Galen malformations is either transarterial or transvenous endovascular embolization with obliteration of the arteriovenous fistula. In some situations, direct surgical obliteration may be necessary but this is associated with significant morbidity and mortality. Vein of Galen dilatations are treated by addressing the primary arteriovenous malformation.

Surgical Results/Prognosis   In general, excellent outcomes are obtained with modern endovascular treatment with two-thirds of children having an excellent outcome with minimal mortality and morbidity. Neonates who present with cardiac failure that cannot be managed medically fair poorly. This group includes almost all vein of Galen aneurysms diagnosed in utero.

BIBLIOGRAPHY

Dan U, Shalev E, Greif M et al: Prenatal diagnosis of fetal brain arteriovenous malformation: the use of color doppler imaging. *J Clin Ultrasound* 1992; 20:149-151.

Hoffman HJ, Chuang S, Hendrick EB et al: Aneurysms of the vein of Galen: experience at the Hospital for Sick Children, Toronto. *J Neurosurg* 1982; 57:316-322.

Jeanty P, Kepple D, Roussis P et al: In utero detection of cardiac failure from an aneurysm of the vein of Galen. *Am J Obstet Gynecol* 1990; 163:50-51.

Garcia-Monaco R, Lasjaunias P, Berenstein A: Therapeutic management of vein of Galen aneurysmal malformations. In: Vinuela F et al (ed): *Interventional neuroradiology: endovascular therapy of the central nervous system.* New York. Raven Press, 1992; p. 113.

Vintzileos AM, Eisenfeld LI, Campbell WA et al: Prenatal ultrasonic diagnosis of arteriovenous malformation of the vein of Galen. *Am J Perinatol* 1986; 3:209-211.

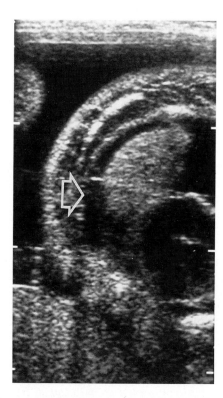

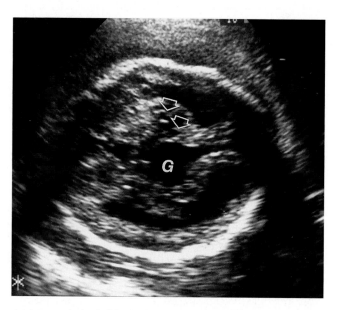

Axial view at the level of the third ventricle. The large black area (*G*) is the vein of Galen aneurysm. The small cystic areas (*arrows*) adjacent to the big cystic area represent feeder arteries.

Vein of Galen aneurysm. Transverse view through the chest. There is a pleural effusion (*arrow*) and skin thickening.

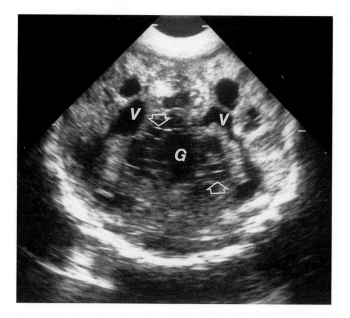

Coronal view shows the aneurysm (*G*) with feeder vessels (*arrows*). There is mild lateral ventriculomegaly (*V*).

3 Cardiac

3.1 BRADYCARDIAS

EPIDEMIOLOGY/GENETICS

Definition   Bradycardia is defined as a heart rate of less than 100 beats per minute.

Epidemiology   Occurs in 1 out of 20,000 neonates. Complete heart block is related to structural heart disease 50% of the time, most commonly complex lesions and heterotaxias. Fifty percent of heart blocks have an immunologic origin. Second degree heart block can progress to complete heart block especially if rheumatologic factors are positive.

Embryology   Bradycardia may be secondary to immunologic damage to the conduction system on the basis of maternal connective tissue disorders, such as lupus erythematosus or Sjögren's syndrome. In patients without connective tissue disorders, there is a high incidence of complex cardiac disease, usually involving defects of the atrioventricular septum.

Inheritance Patterns   If associated wth congenital heart defects, multifactorial inheritance is likely, and the risk is based on the specific defect. In the presence of antibody in the maternal serum, the risk of a subsequently affected child is 8%.

Teratogens   None.

Prognosis   Dependent upon etiology.
1. Atrial bigeminy has a good prognosis. Ectopic atrial beats frequently resolve spontaneously—1% will develop supraventricular tachycardia, requiring treatment with antiarrhythmics.
2. Sinus bradycardia—The prognosis depends on the underlying etiology. If this is an isolated finding, the prognosis is excellent because heart rates are usually 80 to 100 bpm.
3. Complete heart block—The prognosis is poor if the heart block is associated with structural heart disease or the development of hydrops. It is also poor if the ventricular rate is less than 55 bpm.
4. Second-degree heart block is well tolerated hemodynamically if complete heart block does not develop.

SONOGRAPHY

Findings
1. **Fetus:** M-mode echocardiography makes a definitive diagnosis. A sector pass that goes through the atrial wall and the aortic valve or ventricular wall simultaneously is diagnostic.
   a. Complete heart block—The atrium and ventricle are beating regularly, but are completely disassociated.
   b. Sinus bradycardia—There is a one-to-one relationship between the atrium and the ventricle.
   c. Blocked atrial bigeminy—Normally conducted beat alternates with an early atrial beat with no ventricular response.
   d. Second degree heart block—There are intermittently conducted atrial beats in 3 to 1, 2 to 1 or Wenckebach pattern.
2. **Amniotic Fluid:** Normal, except in the presence of hydrops.
3. **Placenta:** Normal, except in the presence of hydrops.
4. **Measurement Data:** Normal.
5. **When Detectable:** Second trimester.

Differential Diagnosis   Those cases that are associated with complex congenital heart defects must be excluded before embarking on an aggressive obstetrical management plan. Congenital heart block may be confused with severe fetal distress in rare instances.

Where Else to Look
1. Look for signs of hydrops (e.g., scalp edema, ascites, pleural effusion, pericardial effusion, etc.)
2. Look for structural cardiac abnormalities: atrioventricular (AV) canal, large ventricular septal defect (VSD), left or right atrial isomerism, abnormal systemic venous return.
3. If there is sinus bradycardia, look for central nervous system (CNS) abnormalities and intrauterine growth retardation (IUGR).

PREGNANCY MANAGEMENT

Investigations and Consultations Required Maternal serum studies to detect anti-SS-A/Ro and or anti-SS-B/La antibodies should be performed. In cases with congenital structural cardiac malformations, chromosome studies are essential. A pediatric cardiologist should be consulted to assist in pregnancy management. Complete heart block is associated with maternal collagen vascular disease. Anti-Ro and anti-La antibodies should be sent.

Fetal Intervention In the fetus greater than 32 weeks gestational age, early delivery and postnatal pacing is appropriate, if hydrops develops. In utero therapy for the previable fetus has included direct ventricular pacing, administration of steroids and plasmapheresis to decrease maternal antibody levels, and adrenergic drugs to increase cardiac output. The benefit of these treatment modalities is unknown. In the case of complete heart block, consider Decadron therapy in cases with immunologic cause if onset is recent, hydrops is present, and there are no maternal contraindications. Steroids must be continued after birth because there will be adrenal suppression.

Monitoring Pregnancy/Course Serial ultrasound examinations may be useful to detect early signs of fetal hydrops. Nonstress testing cannot be used. The biophysical profile can be used to assess fetal well-being. Prenatal care should be coordinated by a perinatologist and is dependent on underlying rhythm:

1. Blocked atrial bigeminy—Check the fetal heart rate 1 to 2 times a week depending on gestational age to be certain that supraventricular tachycardia (SVT) has not developed. Ectopic beats frequently will spontaneously resolve. Depending on ventricular rate, consider evaluating for hydrops every 1 to 3 weeks.
2. Sinus bradycardia—Evaluate for other signs of fetal well-being. Monitor for signs of hydrops.
3. Complete heart block—Repeat evaluation every 1-3 weeks, depending on gestational age, to evaluate for signs of hydrops. The prognosis is worse when the heart block is associated with structural heart disease or a fetal heart rate of less than 70.
4. Second-degree heart block—weekly follow-up to evaluate for hydrops and progression to complete heart block.

Pregnancy Termination Issues Termination of pregnancy is not indicated in the absence of associated structural heart disease in view of the potential for good prognosis with postnatal treatment. Consider termination in patients with complete heart block and cardiac structural abnormalities, given the overall poor prognosis.

Delivery Pregnancy management and delivery must occur in a tertiary center. The mode of delivery is controversial. Conventional fetal heart rate recording can-not diagnose fetal distress, and fetal scalp sampling gives limited information. Elective cesarean section should be performed in cases with fetal hydrops and may be the best option in all cases of congenital heart block. Delivery should be at a center where pediatric cardiology is available for a patient with a complete heart block.

From 35 weeks forward, atrial rates should be monitored as well as ventricular rates. Decreased atrial rate may be a sign of fetal distress. The same is true during labor and delivery. There is no contraindication to vaginal delivery, but it may be difficult to recognize fetal distress.

NEONATOLOGY

Resuscitation A skilled resuscitation team should be present for the delivery. Fetuses with bradyarrhythmias frequently have concurrent asphyxia with delay in onset of spontaneous breathing. Immediate electrocardiogram (ECG) monitoring may be necessary to differentiate bradycardia owing to distress from that secondary to a bradyarrhythmia. In addition, Doppler blood pressure and oxygen saturation by pulse oximetry should be monitored from the beginning. With evidence of inadequate perfusion or oxygenation use of chronotrope infusion such as isoprotenol may be helpful. Hydrops fetalis also may develop from fetal bradycardia. See Chapter 12.2 for management recommendations.

Transport Immediate referral to a tertiary center with full pediatric cardiac diagnostic capabilities is imperative. When inadequate perfusion is evident (i.e., hypotension and/or metabolic acidosis) assisted ventilation and chronotrope infusion should be initiated prior to and continued during the transport.

Testing and Confirmation The diagnosis and etiology are confirmed by electrocardiography and echocardiography to establish intracardiac anatomy.

Nursery Management Once the diagnosis and etiology are confirmed, management is determined by the conduction defect identified, the presence of hydrops fetalis, the presence of a structural cardiac lesion, and the degree of immaturity of the infant. Specific therapies for the various bradyarrhythmia are as follows.

1. Atrial bigeminy with block—No therapy is usually required.
2. Sinus bradycardia—No therapy is required.
3. Second degree heart—Monitor for progression to complete heart block during the neonatal period if the etiology is immunologic.
4. Complete heart block—Consider pacemaker therapy if the fetus is hydropic and the heart rate is less than 55 bpm or there are wide ventricular escape beats.

SURGERY

Preoperative Assessment   The dysrhythmia is confirmed by ECG. Postnatal echocardiography is performed to rule out concomitant structural heart disease. Lingering drug effects, metabolic disorders (hypothyroidism), and hypothermia should be considered.

Operative Indications   Symptomatic bradycardia is treated by pacemaker insertion. The presence of structural heart disease will lower the threshold for pacer insertion. Bradycardias should be reevaluated by Holter examinations and considered as a cause for poor growth.

Types of Procedures   Permanent pacemaker insertion is recommended. In neonates and small infants, epicardial lead systems are usually placed and the generators inserted in the abdominal wall.

Surgical Results/Prognosis   The prognosis is generally good, in the absence of structural heart disease. Pacemaker insertion is a low-risk procedure, but lead malfunction is common in small patients and generators must be replaced after several years due to battery exhaustion.

BIBLIOGRAPHY

Bierman FZ, Baxi L, Jaffe I et al: Fetal hydrops and congenital complete heart block: response to maternal steroid therapy. *J Pediatr* 1988; 112:646.

Crawford D, Chapman M, Allan L: The assessment of persistent bradycardia in prenatal life. *Br J Obstet Gynecol* 1985; 92:941-944.

Julkunen H, Kaaja R, Wallgren E et al: Isolated congenital heart block: fetal and infant outcome and familial incidence of heart block. *Obstet Gynecol* 1993; 82:11-16.

Kleinman CS: Prenatal diagnosis and management of intrauterine arrhythmias. *Fetal Ther* 1986; 1:92.

Kleinman CS, Copel JA, Hobbins JC: Combined echocardiographic and Doppler assessment of fetal congenital atrioventricular block. *Br J Obstet Gynecol* 1987; 94:967.

Michaelson M, Engle MA: Congenital complete heart block: an international study of the natural history. *Cardiovasc Clin* 1972; 4:86-101.

Shenker L, Reed KL, Anderson C et al: Congenital heart block and cardiac anomalies in the absence of maternal connective tissue disease. *Am J Obstet Gynecol* 1987; 157:248-253.

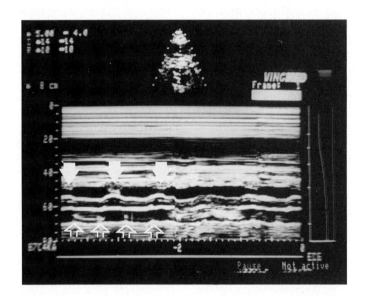

This is an M-mode through the ventricle, aortic valve, and atrium. The solid arrows point to ventricle wall motion and the open arrows point to atrial wall motion. There is no association and the ventricular rate is significantly slower (70 bpm versus 140 bpm).

3.2 CARDIAC RHABDOMYOMA

EPIDEMIOLOGY/GENETICS

Definition A cardiac rhabdomyoma is a benign, non-encapsulated tumor derived from striated cardiac muscle.

Epidemiology Approximately 1 out of 20,000 (M1:1F1). Although it is extremely rare, it is the most frequent cardiac tumor in children.

Embryology Cardiac rhabdomyoma is a benign cardiac tumor that is related to tuberous sclerosis in 50% to 86% of postnatally diagnosed cases. This may be even higher in prenatally diagnosed cases. It is estimated that over 50% of fetuses with tuberous sclerosis will have cardiac rhabdomyomas.

Inheritance Patterns Sporadic, unless associated with tuberous sclerosis that is autosomal dominant with 50% recurrence.

Teratogens None.

Prognosis The majority of cardiac rhabdomyomata regress with age and unless large and hemodynamically significant, do not require specific treatment. Tuberous sclerosis is associated with seizures, mental retardation, and a variety of tumors. The prognosis of cardiac rhabdomyomas depends on the number, size, and location of the tumors and presence or absence of arrythmia. The overall mortality rate approaches 30%.

SONOGRAPHY

Findings
1. **Fetus**
   a. Two-dimensional echocardiogram shows an intracardiac mass with an echogenic tissue density. The most common location is the interventricular septum.
   b. There may be a tachyarrhythmia.
   c. Doppler flow will help evaluate any outflow/inflow obstruction.
2. **Amniotic Fluid:** Normal, except with concurrent hydrops.
3. **Placenta:** Normal, except with concurrent hydrops.
4. **Measurement Data:** Normal
5. **When Detectable:** In the second trimester.

Pitfalls A mass attached to the heart may appear to lie in the lung. If the mass is of cardiac origin it will almost pulsate.

Differential Diagnosis Because of the strong association with tuberous sclerosis, and the propensity for associated supraventricular tachycardia, these tumors must be differentiated, if possible, from other cardiac tumors.

1. Fibroma—usually in the septal or parietal wall of the left ventricle and, rarely, in right ventricle. There may be intramass calcifications.
2. Teratoma—usually extracardiac. The occasional intracardiac mass may be associated with congenital heart disease.

Where Else to Look Central nervous system and kidneys for evidence of tuberous sclerosis. Examine the mother for tuberous sclerosis and facial-skin lesions.

PREGNANCY MANAGEMENT

Investigations and Consultations Required The family should be evaluated by a geneticist for signs of tuberous sclerosis. A detailed ultrasound examination should focus on the CNS and kidneys for other stigmata of tuberous sclerosis. Prenatal management should be planned in consultation with a pediatric cardiologist.

Fetal Intervention None is indicated unless fetal tachycardia develops. Management then would be similar to that outlined in the section on fetal tachycardias.

Monitoring Serial ultrasound examinations should be performed to detect signs of congestive heart failure, rhythm abnormalities, and outflow-tract obstruction. If any of these complications arise, the option of early delivery may be considered, but only after full discussion with the family regarding the high mortality rate and the complications of tuberous sclerosis.

Pregnancy Course No specific obstetric complications are to be expected in the absence of fetal hydrops.

Pregnancy Termination Issues Unless a diagnosis of tuberous sclerosis has been made in one of the parents, a full pathologic and morphologic examination of an intact fetus is essential.

Delivery No alteration in standard care is necessary, but delivery should occur in a tertiary center with a pediatric cardiologist immediately available.

NEONATOLOGY

Resuscitation Rhabdomyomas are unlikely to be symptomatic in the delivery room. In the absence of hydrops fetalis or fetal arrhythmia, infants with rhabdomyoma usually do not require assistance with the onset of breathing.

Transport Immediate referral to a tertiary perinatal center with full pediatric cardiac diagnostic capabilities is necessary only for either hydrops or arrhythmia during the fetal course.

Testing and Confirmation   Echocardiography will confirm both the anatomy and functional abberations. A 12-lead ECG is necessary to evaluate the potential for conduction defects.

Nursery Management   In the absence of hydrops, significant outflow-tract obstruction, or rhythm disturbance, no specific intervention is needed.

SURGERY

Preoperative Assessment   These tumors may affect the circulation by mass effect, compromising flow or ventricular chamber volume. Arrhythmias and coronary compression are other potential complications. These features should be assessed by postnatal echocardiogram.

Operative Indications   Surgery is indicated in the presence of outflow/inflow tract obstruction. These tumors are histologically benign, but may have dire effects. Surgery is indicated when there is obstruction to the circulation, thrombus formation, or serious arrhythmia. Some large tumors cannot be resected without removal of excessive ventricular muscle. In

some of these cases, cardiac transplantation has been performed. Most tumors spontaneously regress and if clinically stable, may be followed with echocardiography.

Types of Procedures   Simple excision is sometimes possible for small lesions; transplantation has been reserved for large lesions.

Surgical Results/Prognosis   Surgical experience is limited. The technical aspects of the procedure are straightforward unless the mass is large and impinges upon vital structures such as coronary arteries or valves.

BIBLIOGRAPHY

Dennis MA, Appareti K, Manco-Johnson ML et al: The echocardiographic diagnosis of multiple fetal cardiac tumors. *J Ultrasound Med* 1985; 4:327.

Gressen CD, Shime J, Rakowski H et al: Fetal cardiac tumor: a prenatal echocardiographic marker for tuberous sclerosis. *Am J Obstet Gynecol* 1987; 156:689-690.

Harvey WP: Clinical aspects of cardiac tumors. *Am J Cardiol* 1968; 21:328.

Ludomirsky A: Cardiac tumors. In: Garson A Jr, Bricker JT, McNamara DG (eds): The science and practice of pediatric cardiology. 1st edition. Philadelphia. Lea and Febiger, 1990.

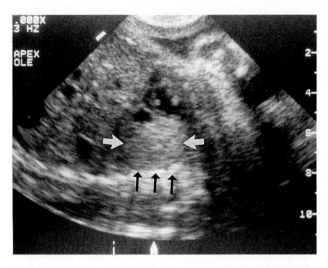

This is a sagittal view of the fetal heart. The white arrows point to the superior inferior margin of a large rhabdomyoma and the small, black arrows point to the posterior portion in the entire posterior wall of the left ventricle. There is a diminutive left ventricular cavity anterior to the mass.

3.3 Coarctation of the Aorta

EPIDEMIOLOGY/GENETICS

Definition   Narrowing of either a short or long segment of the aorta near the area of the ductus arteriosus.

Epidemiology   1 out of 1600 live births (M2:F1). Accounts for 8% of congenital heart disease. Forty percent of cases have associated cardiac anomalies and the recurrence risk is 2% if one sibling is affected and 6% if two siblings are affected.

Embryology   Heterogeneous. Some may result from decreased antegrade flow into the ascending aorta in utero. Coarctation and aortic valve abnormalities occur in 30% of girls with the Turner's syndrome. Aortic arch abnormalities have been seen in over 25 genetic syndromes including DiGeorge velocardiofacial, and the short-rib polydactylies.

Inheritance Patterns   Sporadic. Those due to the Turner's syndrome result from a variety of abnormalities of the X chromosome.

Teratogens   Maternal diabetes and vitamin A.

Prognosis   Isolated coarctation of the aorta requires surgery but the long-term outlook is excellent.

SONOGRAPHY

Findings
1. **Fetus**
   a. There is a discrete shelf or membrane that can be seen in the posterior lateral aspect of the descending aorta near the insertion of the ductus arteriosus.
   b. Frequently there is associated hypoplasia of the aortic arch, or the isthmus of the aorta, or an associated bicuspid aortic valve.
   c. Doppler examination shows a flow disturbance at the area of the coarctation and increased velocity of blood flow. There is often right atrial and right ventricular enlargement.
   d. The mitral valve and left ventricular size should be evaluated given the association with parachute mitral valves and left ventricular hypoplasia.
2. **Amniotic Fluid:** Normal.
3. **Placenta:** Normal.
4. **Measurement Data:** Normal.
5. **When Detectable:** This entity is difficult to detect and may not be detected until late in pregnancy.

Pitfalls
1. Frequently the presence of a wide open ductus arteriosus allows laminar blood flow around the posterior shelf, making it difficult to diagnose coarctation with certainty.
2. A tortuous aorta may give the false appearance of a coarctation.

Differential Diagnosis   Pulmonary stenosis may also result in right ventricular dilatation.

Where Else to Look
1. Coarctation can be associated with other congenital heart defects, most commonly a VSD or transposition of the great arteries.
2. Look for stigmata of Turner's syndrome such as abnormal renal position, cystic hygroma, isolated pleural effusion, or ascites.

PREGNANCY MANAGEMENT

Investigations and Consultations Required   Chromosome studies should be done because of the high incidence of Turner's syndrome and DiGeorge syndrome fluorescent in situ hybridization (FISH) studies in cases of interrupted aortic arch. The family should be referred to a pediatric cardiologist for discussion of prognosis and neonatal management.

Monitoring   Signs of progressive obstruction will be manifested by increasing right-heart size. As the patient approaches term, the ductus arteriosus begins to constrict and more frequent fetal monitoring is recommended.

Pregnancy Course   Coarctation is well tolerated in utero because the ductus arteriosus carries blood supply to the arch.

Pregnancy Termination Issues   The necessity of pathologic confirmation and detection of abnormalities not seen prenatally require that an intact fetus be delivered, unless a chromosomal etiology has been established.

Termination is not usually a consideration when coarctation is not associated with chromosomal abnormalities, given the high success rate of surgical repair.

Delivery   Delivery should be at an institution where pediatric cardiac surgery is available. The presence of a coarctation should not influence the method of delivery because the ductus arteriosus does not undergo complete constriction until after delivery is completed.

NEONATOLOGY

Resuscitation   The goal of neonatal resuscitation is major organ recovery prior to surgery.

Assistance with the onset of respiration is usually not required. However, if there is delay in the spontaneous onset of breathing, oxygen supplementation should be limited to 40% to 60% maximum and only for that time needed to establish adequate color to avoid closing the ductus. Infants should be immediately transported to the neonatal intensive care unit and prostaglandin E1 (PGE1) infusion begun.

Transport   Immediate transport to a tertiary center with full pediatric cardiac diagnostic and surgical capabilities is essential. During transport the infant should receive a continuous infusion of PGE1 to maintain patency of the ductus arteriosus. As apnea is a frequent side effect of prostaglandin infusion, intubation, and assisted ventilation may be necessary. Supplemental oxygen should not be given.

Testing and Confirmation   Confirmation is by postnatal echocardiography and four extremity blood pressure measurements. In simple cases of coarctation, cardiac catherization is rarely needed.

Nursery Management   The goal of initial neonatal management is to achieve and sustain a balance between pulmonary and systemic blood flow by maintaining patency of the ductus and a pulmonary to systemic shunt across the ductus to provide adequate perfusion to the lower body, particularly the liver and kidneys. Hyperventilation and supplemental oxygen decrease pulmonary resistance and thereby alter the direction and magnitude of ductal or intracardiac shunting through associated lesions. Both should be avoided. Acidosis should be treated aggressively with buffer. Dopamine infusion may be needed to improve cardiac output and renal perfusion. Recovery from surgical repair is enhanced by limiting organ damage from inadequate perfusion prior to surgery.

SURGERY

Preoperative Assessment   Echocardiography reliably identifies the site and morphology of the coarctation (long segment with isthmus hypoplasia versus "napkin-ring" short focal stenosis). Bicuspid aortic valve, VSD, subaortic obstruction, and adequate left ventricle (LV) size are features that may dictate simultaneous repair by means of a median sternotomy using a cardiopul-

monary bypass rather than a simple coarctation repair by means of a lateral thoracotomy.

Operative Indications   All true coarctations should be repaired. Coarctation producing symptoms (congestive heart failure [CHF] or poor peripheral perfusion) should be repaired at presentation, whereas mild to moderate coarctation without hypertension may be repaired later (age 3 to 5 years) when risk of recurrent coarctation is less. Mild coarctations may be followed for increasing gradients; stenoses may worsen as ductal tissue in the aortic wall involutes. Femoral pulse examination and Doppler interrogation of the coarctation provide reliable information with which to guide management.

Types of Procedures   Three types of repair are performed for isolated coarctation: simple excision with end-to-end anastomosis, extended resection with anastomosis of the descending aorta to the undersurface of the aortic arch, and patch enlargement of the narrowed site with ipsilateral subclavian artery ("subclavian flap"). The latter approach is more commonly used in neonates and small infants.

Surgical Results/Prognosis   Operative mortality is low in isolated coarctation repair (less than 5%), but increases significantly in the presence of other cardiac defects. Recurrent coarctation months to years later is a possibility following neonatal repair, regardless of technique, and complicates 10% to 20% of repairs. Long-term survival and quality of life are more likely to be determined by concurrent lesions such as VSD and aortic valve and mitral valve disease.

BIBLIOGRAPHY

Allan CD, Chita SK, Anderson RH et al: Coarctation of the aorta in prenatal life: an echocardiographic anatomical and functional study. *Br Heart J* 1988; 59:356-360.

Freed MD, Heymann MA, Lewis AB et al: Prostaglandin E1 in infants with ductus arteriosus-dependent congenital heart disease. *Circulation* 1981; 64:899-905.

Hornberger LK, Sahn DJ, Kleinman CS et al: Antenatal diagnosis of coarctation of the aorta: a multicenter experience. *J Am Coll Cardiol* 1994; 23:417-423.

Leoni F, Huhta JC, Douglas J et al: Effect of prostaglandin on early surgical mortality in obstructive lesions of the systemic circulation. *Br Heart J* 1984; 52:654-659.

Liberthson RR et al: Coarctation of the aorta: review of 234 cases and clarification of management problems. *Am J Cardiol* 1979; 43:835-840.

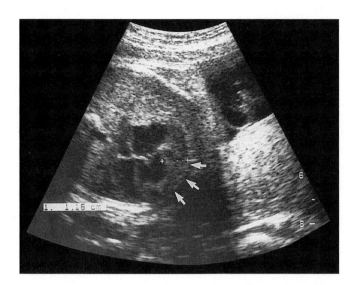

This is a fetal heart viewed in the four chamber view. The white arrows surround the right ventricle, which is thickened and hypertrophied and significantly larger than the left ventricle. The right atrium is also dilated. This is a patient with a coarctation and subsequent enlargement of the right heart. The views of the aorta show diminished aortic size.

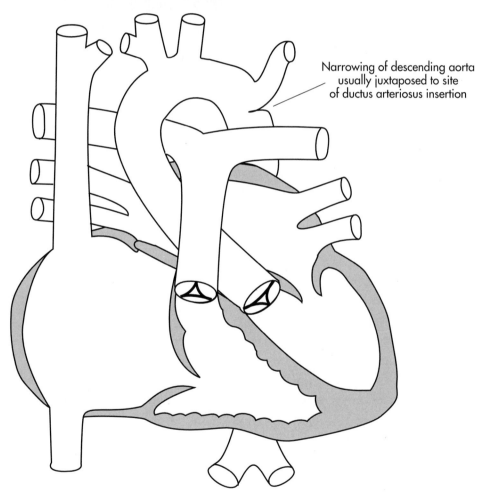

Narrowing of descending aorta usually juxtaposed to site of ductus arteriosus insertion

Diagram showing typical area of narrowing in the aorta. *Used with permission from Mullins CE, Mayer DC: Congenital heart disese: a diagnostic atlas. New York. Wiley-Liss, 1988.*

3.4 DOUBLE-OUTLET RIGHT VENTRICLE

EPIDEMIOLOGY/GENETICS

Definition   Heterogeneous group of congenital heart defects with the common feature that both great arteries arise primarily from the morphologic right ventricle. A VSD provides the only outlet from the left ventricle.

Epidemiology   Rare (M1:F1). 1.5% to 2% of congenital heart disease.

Embryology   Failure of leftward shift of the primitive conus results in both great vessels arising from the right ventricle. Double-outlet right ventricle (DORV) is associated with tracheoesophageal (TE) fistula and with chromosomal anomalies such as trisomy 18.

Inheritance Patterns   Generally sporadic. The risk of recurrence in siblings is 3% to 4% percent. Ten percent to 15% of cases are the result of chromosome abnormalities.

Teratogens   None known.

Prognosis   The prognosis varies greatly depending on the anatomical details, in particular:
1. The relationship of the great vessels to one another.
2. The morphology of the ventricles and their outflow tracts.
3. The presence of associated congenital cardiac defects.
    An accurate and complete diagnosis is of the utmost importance.

SONOGRAPHY

Findings
1. **Fetus:** There are three major forms of DORV.
    a. DORV with normally related great vessels. The VSD is usually subaortic.
    b. DORV with parallel great arteries and the aorta to the right. The VSD is usually subpulmonic.
    c. DORV with aorta anterior and leftward. The VSD is usually subaortic.
    The echocardiogram needs to define:
    a. The commitment of both great arteries, primarily to the right ventricle.
    b. The relationship of great vessels to one another—the aorta will have head and neck vessels arising from it (usually three). The pulmonary artery may be seen branching.
    c. The location of the VSD.
    d. The size of ventricles particularly to rule out left ventricular hypoplasia.
    e. Associated cardiac anomalies, especially pulmonary stenosis, coarctation, interrupted aortic arch, and AV valve abnormalities.

Doppler is needed to assess:
    a. Atrial ventricular valve incompetence.
    b. Atrioventricular valve stenosis, most commonly on the left.
    c. Outflow-tract obstruction.
2. **Amniotic Fluid:** Normal, unless hydrops develops.
3. **Placenta:** Normal, unless hydrops develops.
4. **Measurement Data:** Normal.
5. **When Detectable:** 17 to 20 weeks depending on maternal size and cardiac position during the ultrasound exam. 13 weeks transvaginally.

Pitfalls   It is important to distinguish between the ventricles by their morphology. The right ventricular wall will be trabeculated with a moderator band. The left ventricular wall is smooth.

Differential Diagnosis   It may be difficult to distinguish DORV with subaortic VSD from tetralogy of Fallot. Some believe that if there is more than 50% commitment of aorta to the right ventricle, the diagnosis is DORV. The great vessels are normally related in tetralogy of Fallot. Obstetrical management is similar for both malformations.

Where Else to Look   There is a strong association with chromosomal anomalies (10% to 15%), so a detailed examination of the remainder of the fetus should be performed. Polyhydramnios and a nonvisualized stomach make a TE fistula likely.

PREGNANCY MANAGEMENT

Investigations and Consultations Required   Cytogenetic studies should be performed to detect trisomies. Molecular studies with the DiGeorge FISH probe are appropriate in cases with "apparently normal" chromosome studies. A pediatric cardiologist should be consulted to plan perinatal management.

Fetal Intervention   None is indicated.

Monitoring   DORV is well tolerated in utero. Patients with associated AV canals and massive AV valve incompetence or patients with complete heart block may develop hydrops.

Pregnancy Course   Serial ultrasound examinations should be performed to search for evidence of congestive heart failure. However, the poor prognosis for the infant with structural cardiac malformations and hydrops should be discussed with the family before decisions regarding early delivery are made.

Pregnancy Termination Issues   Unless a precise cytogenetic or molecular diagnosis has been made prenatally, the method of termination should provide an intact fetus for a complete pathologic and morphologic evaluation.

Delivery   In the absence of fetal congestive heart failure, no change in standard obstetric management is warranted. There is no cardiac contraindication to vaginal delivery. Delivery should occur in a tertiary center with immediate access to a pediatric cardiologist.

NEONATOLOGY

Resuscitation   Infants are rarely symptomatic in the delivery room.

Transport   Following diagnosis, immediate referral to a tertiary center with full pediatric cardiac diagnostic and surgical capabilities is indicated. Consultation with a pediatric cardiologist prior to transport to determine the need for PGE1 infusion is appropriate.

Testing and Confirmation   When cyanotic congenital heart disease is suspected after birth the initial screening procedures beyond a careful physical examination of the cardiac and respiratory systems include: chest radiograph, twelve lead electrocardiogram, and a hyperoxia test. Cyanosis secondary to an anatomic shunt will not resolve by increasing the inspired oxygen concentration. Definitive confirmation of the anatomy is by postnatal echocardiography.

Nursery Management   Neonatal management is determined by anatomical details.
1. DORV with subaortic VSD will initially be stable and develop signs and symptoms of CHF as their pulmonary vasculature falls at 4 to 6 weeks.
2. DORV with subpulmonic VSD will present with varying degrees of cyanosis. Coarctation or aortic abnormalities are common in this group and will worsen the cyanosis. If coarctation is found, PGE1 should be started and the patient referred for urgent surgical repair. Stable patients should be referred for surgical repair at about 3 months.
3. DORV with pulmonary stenosis will be similar to patients with tetralogy of Fallot. If cyanosis is profound, PGE1 should be started to maintain ductal patency. This will also decrease pulmonary vascular resistance and increase pulmonary blood flow. These patients will need to be referred for urgent surgical intervention, either total repair or palliative shunting. Patients with stable saturations can be electively repaired at a later date.

SURGERY

Preoperative Assessment   Prior to surgery, a fetal echocardiogram should determine how close the great arteries are to each ventricle, whether the ventricles are "balanced," the presence of other anomalies such as aortic arch obstruction, and the anatomic relation of the VSD to the aorta.

Operative Indications   The timing and the nature of operation are dictated by whether pulmonary blood flow is excessive or inadequate, whether coarctation is present, and whether an extracardiac conduit or a complex intracardiac tunnel will be required. Complex cases may require a preliminary pulmonary artery shunt or band with later correction, whereas simpler forms (DORV with subaortic VSD) may be treated like an isolated VSD and undergo total correction in early infancy. All patients will require surgery, but in the absence of heart failure or cyanosis, repair can be deferred until 2 to 4 years of age.

Types of Procedures   About 50% of patients will be treated by simple VSD closure. The other half are more complex and may require arterial switch with VSD closure, complex intracardiac baffles or extracardiac conduits, or Fontan-type correction if the heart cannot be septated.

Surgical Results/Prognosis   The broad spectrum of the disorder makes a simple summary of results unsatisfactory, but patients with the simplest form do very well. Operative risk is low (1% mortality), quality of life is excellent, and freedom from further cardiovascular problems is possible.

BIBLIOGRAPHY
Berg KA, Clark EB, Astemborski JA et al: Prenatal detection of cardiovascular malformation by echocardiography: an indication for cytogenetic evaluation. *Am J Obstet Gynecol* 1988; 159:477-481.

DiSessa TG et al: Two-dimensional echocardiographic characteristics of double outlet right ventricle. *Am J Cardiol* 1979; 44:1146.

Sondheimer HH, Freedom RN, Olley PN: Double-outlet right ventricle. In: Keith JD, Rowe RD, Vlad P (eds): *Heart disease in infancy and childhood.* New York. MacMillan, 1978.

Sridaromount S, Feldt RH, Ritter DG et al: Double-outlet right ventricle: anatomic and angiographic correlations. *Mayo Clin Proceed* 1978; 53:555.

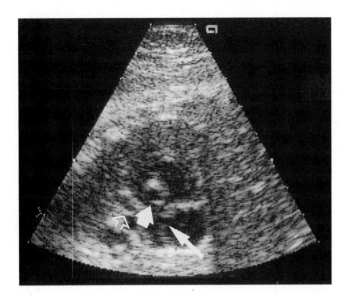

This is a patient with a double-outlet right ventricle. Notice the aorta is displaced far over to the right (*open arrow*) and both great vessels (*short arrow* = *pulmonary artery*) exit the right ventricle side by side. There is a subpulmonic ventricular septal defect partially covered with aneurysmal tissue (*long arrow*). This is a double-outlet right ventricle with a subpulmonic ventricular septal defect.

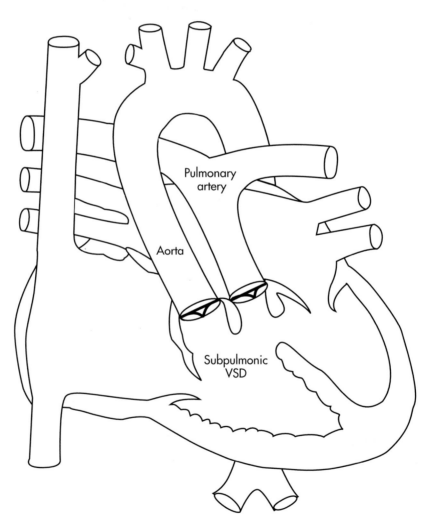

Diagram showing cardiac arrangement with double-outlet right ventricle. *Used with permission from Mullins CE, Mayer DC:* Congenital heart disease: a diagnostic atlas. *New York. Wiley-Liss, 1988.*

3.5 EBSTEIN'S ANOMALY

EPIDEMIOLOGY/GENETICS

Definition   Displacement of the septal and posterior leaflets of the tricuspid valve toward the apex of the right ventricle.

Epidemiology   1 out of 20,000 live births (M1:F1). Less than 1% of all congenital heart disease.

Embryology   The tricuspid valve leaflets and chordae are formed from the interior of the right ventricular myocardium by a process called delamination. This process, which is an undermining of the inlet zone of the ventricular wall, is thought to be arrested in Ebstein's anomaly.

Inheritance Patterns   The majority of cases are sporadic. The recurrence risk is 1% if one sibling is affected and 3% for two siblings. There are no known associated genetic syndromes.

Teratogens   Lithium.

Prognosis   The severity of the prognosis depends on the degree of tricuspid valve displacement and right ventricular outflow-tract obstruction. Patients with mild displacement usually have no outflow obstruction. These patients are usually asymptomatic and their prognosis is excellent. Frequently no intervention is needed. Patients with a great deal of displacement are born with a severely enlarged right heart and a right to left shunt through their patent foramen ovale/atrial septal defect causing profound cyanosis. Frequently there is associated pulmonary stenosis or atresia and the prognosis is extremely poor.

SONOGRAPHY

Findings
1. **Fetus:** Two-dimensional
   a. There is apical displacement of the tricuspid valve;
   b. A large tricuspid valve annulus, frequently with chordal attachments, is present;
   c. Secondary enlargement of the right atrium develops;
   d. Atrialization of part of the right ventricle occurs;
   e. Pulmonary stenosis or atresia may be seen.
   Doppler shows
   a. Tricuspid insufficiency;
   b. Pulmonary outflow obstruction.
2. **Amniotic Fluid:** Normal, unless there is hydrops.
3. **Placenta:** Normal, unless there is hydrops.
4. **Measurement Data:** Normal, unless there are associated anomalies.

5. **When Detectable:** 17 to 20 weeks. 13 weeks transvaginally.

Pitfalls
1. The tricuspid valve may be abnormal and incompetent but not displaced.
2. In a normal heart the tricuspid valve inserts more apically than the mitral valve. If the insertion is greater than 15mm from the tricuspid valve annulus to the distal point of septal leaflet attachment in systole the diagnosis is likely. This is further supported if there is tricuspid insuffiency.

Where Else to Look
Look in the heart for:
1. Ventricular septal defect
2. Ventricular inversion
3. Tetralogy of Fallot
4. Mitral valve abnormalities
5. Coarctation of the aorta
6. Atrial septal defect
7. Total anomalous pulmonary venous return
Outside the heart look for these associated problems:
1. Low-set ears
2. Micrognathia
3. Cleft lip and palate
4. Absent left kidney
5. Megacolon
6. Undescended testes

PREGNANCY MANAGEMENT

Investigations and Consultations Required   Although chromosome abnormalities are rare in Ebstein's anomaly, chromosome analysis of the fetus should be done. A pediatric cardiologist should be consulted to help plan perinatal management.

Monitoring   Patients with Ebstein's anomaly are at risk for Wolf-Parkinson-White and supraventricular tachycardia, two unusual forms of cardiac dysrhythmia. Patients with severe displacement and regurgitation of the tricuspid valve should be followed closely for signs of CHF, that is, ascites, hepatomegaly, pleural effusion.

Pregnancy Course   In the absence of hydrops the in utero course is normal.

Pregnancy Termination Issues   Because a precise diagnosis is essential for counseling, an intact fetus must be available for a complete pathologic examination.

Delivery   The optimal management for these patients has not been defined. However, the poor prognosis for the infant with a structural malformation and hydrops makes the option of early delivery a controversial one. There is no cardiac contraindication to vaginal delivery. Delivery in a tertiary center where a pediatric cardiologist is immediately available is mandatory.

NEONATOLOGY

Resuscitation   In the absence of fetal hydrops or cardiac dysrhythmia, assistance with the onset of breathing is usually not required. Neonates who are symptomatic from Ebstein's anomaly may exhibit intense cyanosis early after birth.

Transport   If the newborn is asymptomatic at birth except for cardiomegaly, referral for evaluation can be done at nursery discharge. If there is cyanosis, congestive failure, or rhythm disturbance, immediate referral to a tertiary perinatal center with full pediatric cardiac diagnostic capabilities is necessary. Consultation with a pediatric cardiologist prior to transport to determine management requirements during transport is recommended.

Testing and Confirmation   Echocardiography will confirm anatomic and functional abnormalities. A 12-lead ECG is necessary to exclude or diagnose dysrhythmia or potential for a conduction defect. Assessment of oxygenation by arterial Po_2 or pulse oximetry is indicated.

Nursery Management   Specific care requirements are determined by the clinical presentation. Usually cyanosis becomes less severe as pulmonary vascular resistance drops toward the end of the first week. If hypoxemia is severe, continuous infusion of PGE1 may be used on a temporary basis to improve pulmonary flow. Congestive failure can usually be controlled with diuretics and digitalis.

SURGERY

Preoperative Assessment   Postnatal assessment by echocardiography ascertains the degree of obstruction to blood flow through the right ventricle into the pulmonary circulation. Conduction abnormalities are common and may complicate management. A hugely dilated right atrium may compromise right lung function and necessitate surgical reduction.

Operative Indications   Life-threatening cyanosis, intractable arrhythmia, and right-lung compression mandate surgery. Many children have adequate pulmonary blood flow and grow to childhood or even adulthood. Later, chronic cyanosis, risk of stroke (from paradoxical embolism), and poor exercise tolerance may warrant consideration for surgical repair.

Types of Procedures   The tricuspid valve can sometimes be repaired to alleviate stenosis or regurgitation; alternatively the valve may be replaced with a tissue or mechanical prosthesis. Atrial septal defect closure eliminates the right-to-left shunt and treats cyanosis. Frequently the right ventricle remains dysfunctional. More radical approaches include a "Norwood" type conversion to a single ventricle heart or cardiac transplantation. Tachyarrhythmias due to aberrant conduction pathways may require catheter or operative ablation.

Surgical Results/Prognosis   The long-term results depend on the severity of the anatomic disturbance. Milder forms may survive into adulthood with moderate cyanosis and reduced exercise capacity but may not need surgery. Severe infantile forms carry high mortality and morbidity despite intervention.

BIBLIOGRAPHY

Brown J, Gunn TR, Mora JD et al: The prenatal ultrasonographic diagnosis of cardiomegaly due to tricuspid incompetence. *Pediatr Radiol* 1986; 16:440.

Park JM et al: Ebstein's anomaly of the tricuspid valve associated with prenatal exposure to lithium carbonate. *Am J Dis Child* 1980; 134:704-708.

Van Mierop LHS et al: Anomalies of the tricuspid valve resulting in stenosis or incompetence. In: Adams FH et al. (eds): *Heart disease in infants, children and adolescents*. 3rd edition. Baltimore. Williams & Wilkins, 1983.

Yeager SB, Parness IA, Sanders SP: Severe tricuspid regurgitation simulating pulmonary atresia in the fetus. *Am Heart J* 1988; 115:906-908.

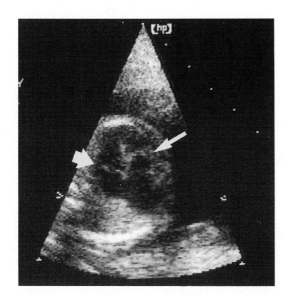

18-week fetus referred because of prenatal Lithium exposure. The long white arrow points to the displaced tricuspid valve and the short white arrow points to the mitral valve annulus.

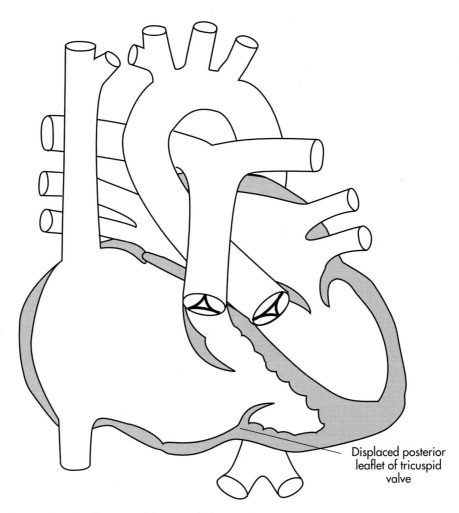

Displaced posterior leaflet of tricuspid valve

Diagram showing Ebstein's malformation of the tricuspid valve. *Used with permission from Mullins CE, Mayer DC:* Congenital heart disease: a diagnostic atlas. *New York. Wiley-Liss, 1988.*

3.6 ECTOPIA CORDIS
PENTALOGY OF CANTRELL

EPIDEMIOLOGY/GENETICS

Definition   The heart is partially or totally outside the thorax. Ectopia cordis can occur as part of other conditions such as limb-body wall complex and pentalogy of Cantrell. Pentalogy of Cantrell is composed of thoracoabdominal ectopia cordis, omphalocele-like supraumbilical wall defect, cleft sternum, pericardial defect, and other congenital heart defects.

Epidemiology   Very rare, less than 1 out of 100,000 (M2:F1).

Embryology   The embryology and etiology of ectopia cordis is heterogeneous. Some cases are the result of early amnion rupture with other limb-body wall abnormalities. The pentalogy of Cantrell is thought to be due to a failure of ventral wall closure due to defects in the mesodermal tissue elements. Failure of fusion of the sternal primordial bands occurs with a severity that varies from simple sternal cleft to true ectopia cordis.

Inheritance Patterns   Generally sporadic. Rare cases with trisomy 21 have been reported.

Teratogens   None known.

Prognosis   The prognosis is dependent upon the severity of intracardiac abnormalities as well as associated defects. Generally, the pentalogy of Cantrell and most limb body wall disruptions are lethal. Minor degrees of ectopia cordis resulting from failure of sternal closure may be surgically correctable.

SONOGRAPHY

Findings
1.   **Fetus:** There are two forms: The thoracic and the thoracoabdominal:
   a. In the thoracic form (classic form) there is:
      i. a sternal defect;
      ii. absence of the parietal pericardium;
      iii. cephalic orientation of cardiac apex (which often beats against the baby's chin);
      iv. a small thoracic cavity.
      In the thoracoabdominal form there is partial absence or a cleft of the lower sternum and there is usually a defect of the diaphragmatic parietal pericardium. An omphalocele is frequently seen.
   b. In the absence of structural heart disease Doppler flow patterns should be normal.
2.   **Amniotic Fluid:** Normal.
3.   **Placenta:** Normal.
4.   **Measurement Data:** Normal.
5.   **When Detectable:** 13 weeks with the vaginal probe.

Pitfalls   In some examples of the limb body wall complex the thoracic anatomy may be so distorted that the defect may be overlooked.

Differential Diagnosis   Although associated abnormalities are commonly associated with ectopia cordis, the obstetric management issues are similar for all conditions with a displaced heart.

Where Else to Look   In the heart, there are numerous associated cardiac anomalies. Tetralogy of Fallot, ventricular septal defect, tricuspid atresia, Ebstein's anomaly, common atrium, atrioventricular canal, mitral atresia, total anomalous pulmonary venous return, single ventricle, pulmonary stenosis, pulmonary atresia, aortic stenosis, coarctation of the aorta, transposition of the great artery, left ventricular diverticulum, biventricular diverticulum, and persistent left superior vena cava (LSVC) have all been reported. Defects are common with the thoracoabdominal form. Omphalocele is common with both types. Ectopia cordis is a feature of the limb body wall complex, so there may be gastroschisis, missing limbs, caudal regression, and more.

PREGNANCY MANAGEMENT

Investigations and Consultations Required   Chromosome analysis is essential. Because of the association with neural tube defects, both amniotic fluid alpha-fetoprotein (AFP) and acetylcholinesterase studies should be done. Fetal echocardiography must be performed to delineate the precise cardiac defects. Pediatric surgery and pediatric cardiology consults should be obtained to assess prognosis and plan perinatal management.

Fetal Intervention   None is indicated.

Monitoring   The overall dismal prognosis for this disorder should preclude aggressive pregnancy intervention in most cases. If the structural cardiac malformation is relatively minor, then surgical correction may be successful, and standard obstetric management is appropriate.

Pregnancy Course   No specific obstetric complications are to be expected.

Pregnancy Termination Issues   Although an intact fetus will establish what the associated malformations are, it is unlikely to alter recurrence risk information. Therefore, the method of termination can be a destructive one.

Delivery   A nonaggressive approach without fetal monitoring should be considered. The site for delivery should be a tertiary center where an immediate evaluation of the neonate can be undertaken to assess whether surgical correction should be attempted.

NEONATOLOGY

Resuscitation Given the almost total lethality of this lesion, the decision to provide support following birth should be discussed with the family prior to delivery. When there is uncertainty regarding the prognosis it is appropriate to provide at least assisted ventilation pending full evaluation and determination of the prognosis.

Transport Immediate referral to a tertiary center with full pediatric cardiac diagnostic and surgical capabilities is essential, particularly for the infant with a minor or limited defect. The exposed viscera should be protected against trauma and contamination during transit with a warm, moist, sterile dressing.

Testing and Confirmation Careful physical examination, postnatal echocardiography, and abdominal ultrasonography will confirm the nature and severity of the lesions. If not obtained prenatally, chromosomal karyotyping is important.

Nursery Management Provision of respiratory support during the interval between birth and completion of the diagnostic evaluation is appropriate to allow time for parental adaptation and clarification of the feasibility of surgical correction.

SURGERY

Preoperative Assessment The initial goal of assessment is to determine the extent of the sternal defect and the severity of the associated anomalies, particularly cardiac, as the latter determine the survival prognosis. Ectopia cordia may also occur as a component of the limb-body wall complex.

Three categories of defects have been described: 1. cleft sternum—either a partial or complete cleft beginning superiorly and without associated anomalies; 2. ectopia cordis with the exposed heart presenting outside the chest wall through a cleft sternum and anterior chest wall of varying degrees; and 3. pentalogy of Cantrell—an association of defects, including cleft distal sternum, absent anterior crescent of the diaphragm, midline anterior abdominal-wall defect above the umbilicus (omphalocele), defect of the apical pericardium with communication into the peritoneum, and a cardiac anomaly, most commonly a VSD or left ventricular diverticulum.

Careful physical examination, echocardiography, chest radiography, and if necessary, cardiac catheterization may be used to define the anatomic and functional defects.

Operative Indications Experience has shown that surgical repair of the cleft sternum is best achieved in the newborn period while elasticity of the chest wall is such to allow approximation of the separated sternal bands. The presence of an omphalocele mandates immediate surgical intervention to place an appropriate prosthetic covering for prevention of infection and fluid losses. Use of such a prosthetic covering to protect the exposed heart in a true ectopia cordis has been reported as a temporizing measure to facilitate completion of the evaluation of the associated cardiac lesion. Staging of cardiac repair may be necessary in both the true ectopia and the pentalogy because of severe and unusual anatomic abnormalities.

Types of Procedures For the isolated cleft-sternal defect, usually a direct approximation of the sternal halves after appropriate excision or wedging to prevent buckling is done. If the thoracic volume is inadequate after approximation, sliding chondrotomy of several ribs on either side will provide further volume.

Return of the ectopic and exposed heart to the thoracic cavity and sternal closure, although technically possible, has not resulted in improved survival, usually because of the severity of the associated cardiac lesions. If a life-sustaining corrective or palliative procedure for the cardiac defect is possible in the newborn period, chest-wall closure, using prosthetic material to increase thoracic volume, is usually required.

Both primary and staged repair of the various defects present in the pentalogy of Cantrell have been reported. Small defects are more amenable to primary closure if the cardiac anomaly is limited to either a septal defect or ventricular diverticulum. The latter can be amputated during the primary procedure. For extensive defects, large omphaloceles, staged closure with an initial silastic silo may be necessary.

Surgical Results/Prognosis The prognosis is contingent primarily on the presence and severity of an accompanying cardiac defect. For an isolated cleft sternum repair, the prognosis for survival is very good though recurrence of the cleft has been reported. For the true ectopia cordis and for pentalogy of Cantrell, reported survival after surgical closure is poor, perhaps no more than 5% to 10%, with the underlying cardiac defect being the primary determinant of survival.

BIBLIOGRAPHY

Cantrell JR, Haller JA, Ravitch HH et al: A syndrome of congenital defects involving the abdominal wall, sternum, diaphragm, pericardium and heart. *Surg Gynecol Obstet* 1958; 107:602.

Carmi R, Boughman JA: Pentalogy of Cantrell and associated midline anomalies: a possible ventral midline developmental midline field. *Am J Med Genet* 1992; 42:90–95.

Jones AF, McGrath RL, Edwards SM et al: Immediate operation for ectopia cordis. *Ann Thora Surg* 1979; 28:484-486.

Khoury MJ, Cordero JF, Rasmussen S: Ectopia cordis, midline defects and chromosome abnormalities: an epidemiologic perspective. *Am J Med Genet* 1988; 30:811–817.

Ravitch MM: The chest wall. In Welch KJ, Randolph JG, Ravitch MM et al (editors): *Pediatric surgery*. ed 4. Chicago. Mosby–Year Book, 1986.

Ravitch MM: *Congenital deformities of the chest wall and their operative correction*. Philadelphia. WB Saunders, 1977.

Sabiston DC: Disorders of the sternum and the thoracic wall. In Sabiston, D.C., Spencer FC (ed.) *Gibbon's surgery of the chest*. Philadelphia. WB Saunders, 1990. p. 422-437

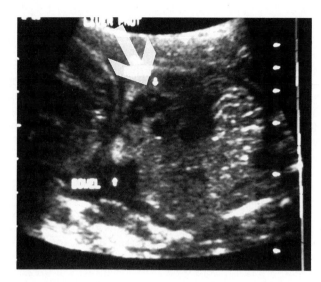

Cardiac chambers (*arrow*) are visualized here outside the thoracic cage. Bowel is also seen below the heart.

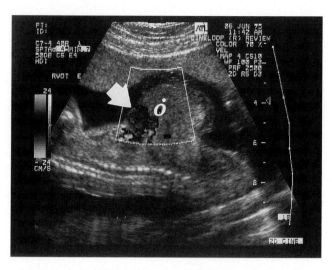

In addition to the omphalocele (*O*) the heart lies in the abdominal wall defect (*arrow*). Color flow Doppler shows flow in the heart.

3.7 ENDOCARDIAL CUSHION DEFECT
ATRIOVENTRICULAR CANAL (AV CANAL)

EPIDEMIOLOGY/GENETICS

Definition   Endocardial cushion defects (ECD) are a spectrum of heart defects that consist of an ostium primum ASD with associated VSDs, and abnormalities of the atrioventricular (AV) valves.

Epidemiology   0.36 out of 1,000 births. Endocardial cushion defects make up 2% of cases of congenital heart disease.

Embryology   Results from failure of the normal fusion process of the superior and inferior endocardial cushions. There is a strong association of endocardial cushion defects with Down syndrome.

Inheritance Patterns   Multifactorial when not associated with chromosomal abnormalities. Down syndrome accounts for 60% of the cases of ECD, and Ivemark's syndrome (asplenia/polysplenia) accounts for another 10% of cases. The recurrence risk is 3% if one sibling is affected and 10% if two siblings are affected.

Prognosis   The prognosis is related to the severity of the defect, associated abnormalities, and the presence of pulmonary vascular obstruction. Total correction in cases with favorable anatomy can be accomplished in the majority of cases.

SONOGRAPHY

Findings:
1. **Fetus:** In the complete form of endocardial cushion defect there is:
    a. Ostium primum ASD—The atrial septum will be deficient close to the mitral and tricuspid valves.
    b. Both mitral and tricuspid valves form a single AV valve.
    c. The ventricular septum adjacent to the mitral and tricuspid valves will be absent.
    d. There is frequently associated AV valve regurgitation by color flow Doppler.
    In the partial form of endocardial cushion defect there is:
    a. A primum ASD.
    b. A small inlet VSD.
    c. A cleft mitral valve or abnormal AV valve.
    Heart failure may develop, so fetal ascites, pleural effusion, and pericardial effusion may be seen.
2. **Amniotic Fluid:** Usually normal. If there is CHF or an associated rhythm abnormality there can be polyhydramnios.
3. **Placenta:** Usually normal, except in the presence of hydrops.

4. **Measurement Data:** Usually normal.
5. **When Detectable:** First detectable when cardiac structures can be well visualized: 12 to 14 weeks transvaginally and 16 to 18 weeks transabdominally.

Pitfalls
1. A small VSD may be difficult to visualize.
2. Mitral valve clefts may be difficult to visualize. Mitral regurgitation may be the only clue that they exist.
3. If all the outflow tracts are not well visualized or if there is a question of discrepancy in ventricular size, a repeat study should be performed because these factors greatly influence surgical options and prognosis.

Differential Diagnosis
1. Large isolated VSD.
2. Large isolated ostium primum ASD.

Where Else to Look
1. Associated cardiac defects are right or left ventricular hypoplasia and right or left outflow-tract obstruction.
2. Look for evidence of hydrops (pleural and pericardial effusion, scalp edema, ascites, skin thickening, etc.) if a rhythm abnormality is seen or severe AV regurgitation is present.
3. Associated noncardiac abnormalities are usually related to Down syndrome (e.g, duodenal atresia and omphalocele). Look for a spleen, to exclude Ivemark's syndrome.

PREGNANCY MANAGMENT

Investigations and Consultations Required   Chromosome evaluation is essential given the strong association with trisomy 21. Referral should be made to a pediatric cardiologist to discuss prognosis and neonatal management.

Pregnancy Monitoring   The frequency of follow-up investigations will depend partially upon the time of diagnosis and associated findings. Any patient with polyhydramnios or complete heart block associated with an ECD should receive frequent follow-up to be certain that hydrops is not developing or worsening.

Pregnancy Course   For isolated ECD no specific obstetric complications should be expected.

Pregnancy Termination Issues   If the chromosome studies are normal, the method of termination should result in an intact fetus for confirmation of the cardiac malformation and to exclude genetic syndromes that may have ECD as a component.

Delivery   If there is no evidence of outflow-tract obstruction, the site of delivery need not be changed. If the outflow tracts have not been well visualized or there is known obstruction, delivery should be at a center where pediatric cardiology is immediately available.

NEONATOLOGY

Resuscitation   Assistance with the onset of breathing is usually not required.

Transport   Immediate referral following birth to a tertiary center with full pediatric cardiac diagnostic and surgical capabilities is indicated if the infant has evidence of CHF, cyanosis, or decreased perfusion (decreased pulses or low systolic pressures). Consultation with a pediatric cardiologist prior to transport is recommended to plan care during transport.

Testing and Confirmation   Echocardiography will confirm both anatomical and functional abnormalities.

Nursery Management   Endocardial cushion defect is initially well tolerated. As the pulmonary vascular resistance falls, the infant will develop pulmonary overcirculation with associated tachypnea and tachycardia (usually by 4 to 6 weeks). Initial therapy should be with diuretics. If unexplained cyanosis or decreased perfusion develops, the infant should be started on PGE1 therapy and be reevaluated by pediatric cardiology.

SURGERY

Preoperative Assessment   An echocardiogram defines the diagnosis and screens for other lesions that might complicate surgical repair, such as persistent LSVC, other VSD, outflow-tract obstructions, and more.

Operative Indications   All patients require surgery. Complete AV canal is repaired within the first year of life to prevent CHF and pulmonary vascular disease. Medically refractory heart failure mandates urgent repair. Simple primum ASDs without symptoms can be deferred until 3 to 5 years of age for repair.

Types of Procedures   Open heart surgical repair of complete AV canal entails closure of the VSD with a Dacron patch and ASD closure with a piece of pericardium to septate the heart completely. Left AV valve incompetence may necessitate valve repair or later replacement. Ostium primum ASDs are closed with a patch of pericardium.

Surgical Results/Prognosis   Operative mortality for complete AV canal is approximately 5%; for primum ASD it is 1%. Long-term results are good, though late problems with the mitral valve and the LV outflow tract may appear. Quality of life is good after successful repair. The presence of Down syndrome may affect early and late risks.

BIBLIOGRAPHY

Bitarati S, Lev M: The spectrum of common atrioventricular orifice (canal). *Am Heart J* 1973; 86:553-556.

Machado MVL, Crawford DC, Anderson RN et al: Atrioventricular septal defect in prenatal life. *Br Heart J* 1988; 59:352-355.

Van Mifrhop LHS, Alley RD, Kansel HW et al: The anatomy and embryology of endocardial cushion defects. *J Thorac Cardiovasc Surg* 1962; 43:71.

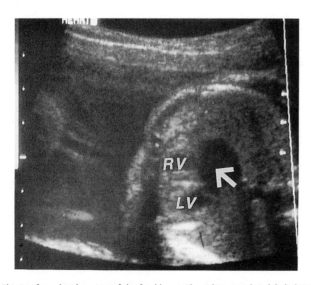

This is a four-chamber view of the fetal heart. The right ventricle is labeled RV and the left ventricle is labeled LV. Notice the absence of the crux of the heart with a single atrioventricular (AV) valve. This is an illustration of a complete AV valve defect.

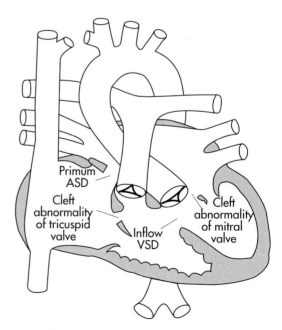

Diagram showing the abnormality seen with endocardial cushion defect. *Used with permission from Mullins CE, Mayer DC:* Congenital heart disease: a diagnostic atlas. *New York. Wiley-Liss, 1988.*

3.8 HYPOPLASTIC LEFT-HEART SYNDROME (HLHS)

EPIDEMIOLOGY/GENETICS

Definition   Hypoplasia of the left ventricle associated with atresia or severe stenosis of aortic and mitral valves and hypoplasia of the aortic arch.

Epidemiology   1 out of 10,000 (M2:F1). Hypoplastic left-heart syndrome (HLHS) syndrome accounts for up to 4% of all congenital heart disease.

Embryology   Most often sporadic. Hypoplastic left-heart syndrome has been associated with situs inversus and renal agenesis. Associated chromosomal anomalies are Turner's syndrome and duplication of chromosome 12p.

Inheritance Patterns   The inheritance pattern is not clearly defined. It is thought that left–sided obstructive lesions occur more frequently in first degree relatives of patients with hypoplastic left heart. For siblings there is a 5% recurrence of HLHS.

Teratogens   Vitamin A, maternal diabetes.

Prognosis   Untreated HLHS is lethal. With the Norwood procedure there are survival rate claims, with some eventual cardiac impairment (between 5% and 80%).

SONOGRAPHY

Findings
1. **Fetus**
   a. Small obliterated LV cavity is present frequently with a dilated right ventricular cavity. The left ventricle ends more proximally than the right ventricle.
   b. There is a normal or large tricuspid valve with a hypoplastic mitral valve.
   c. Severe hypoplasia of the aorta and aortic annulus is present. The aortic arch is frequently filled retrograde through the ductus arteriosus.
   d. The descending aorta is normal size because it is filled by the ductus arteriosus.
   e. There is a small left atrium with the interatrial septum bowing left to right.
2. **Amniotic Fluid:** Normal.
3. **Placenta:** Normal.
4. **Measurement Data:** Normal.
5. **When Detectable:** Hypoplastic left-heart syndrome can be detected at 13 weeks, using an endovaginal approach, or 16 to 17 weeks using a transabdominal approach. In some instances, typical features do not develop until the early third trimester.

Pitfalls
1. The aorta may be difficult to identify.
2. It may be difficult to distinguish HLHS from other lesions causing obliteration of the LV cavity (i.e., cardiac masses, critical aortic stenosis).
3. The LV cavity may be so small that a single ventricle may be diagnosed.

Differential Diagnosis   Other lesions causing obliteration of the left ventricular cavity:
1. Cardiac masses
2. Critical aortic stenosis
3. Single ventricle

Where Else to Look
1. There are occasional reports of associated omphalocele, diaphragmatic hernia, or hypospadias. Twenty-nine percent have been found to have minor or major CNS malformations at autopsy including microcephaly, immature cortical mantle formation, holoprosencephaly, and agenesis of the corpus callosum.
2. Look for stigmata of associated chromosomal anomalies—Turner's syndrome, trisomy 13, 18, and 21.
3. Look for evidence of hydrops—pleural effusion, ascites, and pericardial effusion.

PREGNANCY MANAGEMENT

Investigations and Consultations Required   Chromosome studies are essential, as is a careful sonographic evaluation for extracardiac abnormalities. A pediatric cardiologist should be consulted to discuss prognosis with the family and to plan perinatal management.

Fetal Intervention   No treatment is presently available. Balloon dilatation of the aortic valve has been attempted and may become available in the future.

Pregnancy Monitoring/Course   No change in standard obstetric care is necessary. The development of fetal hydrops, although rare, should prompt a reassessment of the obstetric plan. The extremely poor prognosis for the infant with structural heart disease with hydrops and the overall prognosis for surgical correction of uncomplicated HLHS may be an indication for a nonaggressive management of the fetus.

Pregnancy Termination Issues   Hypoplastic left-heart syndrome remains a difficult lesion to treat postnatally with a high mortality rate. For this reason any fetus diagnosed early in gestation should be offered the choice of termination.

Delivery   Delivery should be at an institution where a pediatric cardiologist is available at delivery and prostaglandin infusions can be immediately begun. Hypoplastic left-heart syndrome is well tolerated in utero and there is no contraindication to vaginal delivery. No specialized approach to the management of labor and delivery is necessary.

NEONATOLOGY

Resuscitation   Assistance with the onset of respiration is usually not required. If there is a delay in the spontaneous onset of breathing, oxygen supplementation may be provided. This should be held to a 40% to 60% level and given only for the time needed to establish adequate color because of the danger of closure of the ductus. Infants should be immediately transported to the neonatal intensive care unit and PGE1 infusion begun.

Transport   Immediate transport to a tertiary center with full pediatric cardiac diagnostic and surgical capabilities is essential. During transport the infant should receive continuous infusion of PGE1 to maintain patency of the ductus arteriosus. As apnea is a frequent side effect of prostaglandin infusion, intubation and assisted ventilation may be necessary. Supplemental oxygen should not be given.

Testing and Confirmation   The diagnosis should be confirmed by echocardiography. Special attention should be paid to the patency of the ductus arteriosus, the size of the ASD and the presence or absence of tricuspid regurgitation. Cardiac catherization is rarely needed and should be avoided if possible.

Nursery Management   The goal of initial neonatal management is to achieve and sustain a balance between pulmonary and systemic blood flow by maintaining patency of the ductus and a pulmonary to systemic shunt across the ductus to provide adequate perfusion to the vital organs. As supplemental oxygen may decrease pulmonary resistance and alter the direction and magnitude of ductal shunting, it should be avoided. Acidosis should be treated aggressively. Dopamine infusion may be needed to improve cardiac output and renal perfusion. The other body organ systems should be functioning normally before any surgery is undertaken.

SURGERY

Operative Indications   A detailed postnatal echocardiogram should confirm the diagnosis. All patients die without surgical intervention. However, the risk associated with surgical palliation and uncertainty over long-term results leads many parents to choose compassionate care without surgical intervention.

Types of Procedures   There are two surgical options available to these patients.
1. Norwood procedure—This is a 3-stage procedure. The first stage is performed in the neonatal period and consists of dividing the main pulmonary artery from the proximal stump to the descending aorta and closing the distal main pulmonary artery. A right-sided shunt is then formed to maintain pulmonary blood flow. The atrial septum is also excised at this point to maintain adequate intraatrial mixing. A 2-stage Fontan procedure follows. The first part consists of a superior vena cava to pulmonary artery anastomosis. The final stage is an inferior vena cava to pulmonary anastomosis. In the most experienced hands the mortality remains high with about a 75% survival rate.
2. Neonatal cardiac transplant—After being listed for a cardiac transplant the patient stands a 28% chance of cardiac difficulties before a transplant becomes available. If a cardiac transplant is not available, referral for a Norwood procedure is often performed. Survival with a cardiac transplant is above 80% at this time. There are no good data on long-term survival.

Surgical Results/Prognosis   At most centers, the Norwood staged approach carries a high combined operative mortality (greater than 50%). At low-risk centers, stage 1 mortality is 15%, and subsequent stages are 5% each. However, a significant percentage of children cannot proceed through the entire program because of right ventricular failure or tricuspid valve insufficiency. Even after a successfully completed Fontan, 10-year survival is likely to be less than 70%. Cardiac transplantation can be performed with lower initial operative risk (15%), but the quality of life may not be as good. Multiple medications, constant medical follow-up, and vigilance are essential to good long-term survival. A paucity of donors limits this approach.

BIBLIOGRAPHY

Chang AC, Huhta JC, Yoon GY et al: Diagnosis, transport and outcome in fetuses with left ventricular outflow tract obstruction. *J Thorac Cardiovasc Surg* 1991; 102:841.

Freed MD, Heymann MA, Lewis AB et al: Prostaglandin E1 in infants with ductus arteriosus-dependent congenital heart disease. *Circulation* 1981; 64:899-905.

Leoni F, Huhta JC, Douglas J et al: Effect of prostaglandin on early surgical mortality in obstructive lesions of the systemic circulation. *Br Heart J* 1984; 52:654-659.

Maxwell D, Allan L, Tynan MJ: Balloon dilatation of the aortic valve in the fetus: a report of two cases. *Br Heart J* 1991; 65:256.

Nora JJ, Nora AH: *Genetics and genetic counseling in cardiovascular diseases.* Springfield, IL. Charles C. Thomas, 1978.

Norwood WI, Lang P, Castaneda AR et al: Experience with operations for hypoplastic left heart syndrome. *J Thorac Cardiovasc Surg* 1981; 82:511.

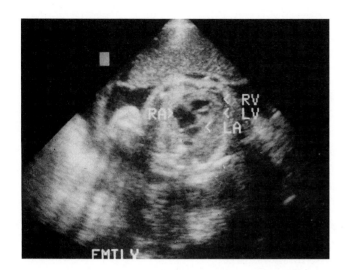

Four-chamber view of a fetal heart with hypoplastic left heart syndrome. The chambers are labeled appropriately with the right atrium labeled *RA*, left atrium labeled *LA*, right ventricle labeled *RV*, left ventricle labeled *LV*. Notice the small size of the left atrium and the left ventricle.

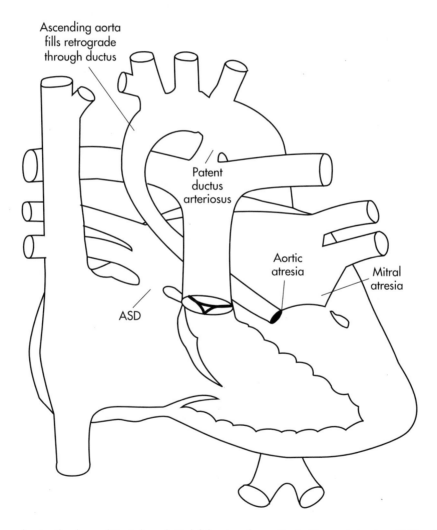

Diagram showing the abnormalities in hypoplastic left-heart syndrome. *Used with permission from Mullins CE, Mayer DC:* Congenital heart disease: a diagnostic atlas. *New York. Wiley-Liss, 1988.*

3.9 PREMATURE ATRIAL CONTRACTIONS
"DROPPED BEATS"

EPIDEMIOLOGY/GENETICS

Definition   A premature atrial contraction is an atrial contraction that occurs more than 8 ms prior to the expected atrial beat. They usually arise from ectopic focuses in the atria rather than from the sinus node.

Epidemiology   Incidence is unknown, but this is a relatively common entity in the early third trimester fetus.

Embryology   Unknown. It may represent developmental immaturity of the autonomic nervous system and its control on the conducting system. It has also been associated with large foraminal flaps.

Inheritance Patterns   Sporadic.

Teratogens   None. Some reports suggest an association with maternal caffeine intake.

Prognosis   Excellent. It usually resolves with advancing gestational age or within the first several weeks postnatally. One percent will develop supraventricular tachycardia (SVT).

SONOGRAPHY

Findings
1. Fetus: Two-dimensional
   a. A large "wind sock" foraminal flap may be seen bulging into the left atrium.
   b. A definitive diagnosis can be made with m-mode if a cursor line is placed through the atrial wall and the aortic valve or ventricular wall at the same time. There will be an early atrial contraction that will either be conducted or blocked. If conducted, it will be followed by a ventricular contraction. If blocked, there will be a dropped beat.
2. **Amniotic Fluid:** Normal.
3. **Placenta:** Normal.
4. **Measurement Data:** Normal.
5. **When Detectable:** Detectable at 18 weeks. Most common in the third trimester.

Pitfalls   It may be difficult to detect atrial contractions if the fetal heart is in an inconvenient position.

Differential Diagnosis   Premature atrial contraction (PACs) should be differentiated from premature ventricular contractions. This can be accomplished by M-mode echocardiography. Atrial contractions will precede ventricular contractions if PACs are present.

Where Else to Look   If bradycardia is unrecognized, signs of fetal hydrops may be present.

PREGNANCY MANAGEMENT

Investigations and Consultations Required   Fetal echocardiography is required to establish the diagnosis.

Pregnancy/Monitoring Course   The fetal heart rate should be checked one or two times a week until delivery or the arrhythmia resolves.

Delivery   There is no need for delivery to be in a tertiary center.

NEONATOLOGY

Resuscitation   No specific resuscitation measures are indicated.

Transport   Referral to a tertiary center is not necessary unless the diagnosis of the arrhythmia type is unclear on a postnatal electrocardiogram.

Testing and Confirmation   A 12-lead electrocardiogram will confirm the source of the irregular heart rate.

Nursery Management   If ectopy is frequent, electrolyte testing should be considered (especially Mg+, Ca+).

SURGERY

Preoperative Assessment   Most cases of premature atrial contractions are of little physiologic significance. Echocardiography is performed to rule out structural heart disease.

Operative Indications   None in the absence of structural heart disease.

Types of Procedures   Monitor for other rhythm disturbances.

BIBLIOGRAPHY
Bernstine RL, Wincer JE, Callagan DA: Fetal bigeminy and tachycardia. *Am J Obstet Gynecol* 1968; 101:856.
Kendall B: Abnormal fetal heart rates and rhythms prior to labor. *Am J Obstet Gynecol* 1967; 99:71.
Kleinman LS, Copel JA, Weinstein EM et al: In utero diagnosis and treatment of fetal supraventricular tachycardia. *Semin Perinatol* 1985; 9:113.
Southall DP, Richard J, Mitchell P et al: Study of cardiac rhythm in healthy newborn infants. *Br Heart J* 1980; 43:14-20.

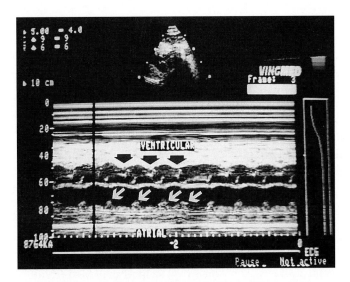

M-mode through a four-chamber view of the fetal heart. The ventricular contractions are illustrated with the thick, black arrows and the atrial contractions are illustrated with the thin, white arrows. The first three beats illustrate normal sinus rhythm. The fourth white arrow points to a premature atrial contraction that is blocked, resulting in a skipped ventricular contraction.

3.10 TACHYCARDIAS

EPIDEMIOLOGY/GENETICS

Definition   Sustained fetal heart rate greater than 180 bpm.

Epidemiology   0.5% to 1% incidence (SVT). Atrial flutter is less common, and sinus tachycardia is rare.

Embryology   Unknown.

Inheritance Patterns   Sporadic.

Teratogens   None known.

Prognosis   Incessant SVT or atrial flutter will go on to congestive failure, usually in less than 48 hours.
1. Atrial flutter—If the abnormal rhythm is controlled, the prognosis is good. However, there is a higher mortality rate when atrial flutter is complicated by hydrops.
2. SVT—If the abnormal rhythm is controlled, the prognosis is good. There is a higher mortality rate with associated hydrops.
3. Sinus tachycardia—Overall the prognosis is good if this is an isolated finding. There are rare reports of ventricular dysfunction if there is incessant sinus tachycardia.
4. Ventricular tachycardia—The prognosis is good. The rhythm is usually intermittent, not rapid, and well tolerated.

SONOGRAPHY

Findings
1. **Fetus:** Simultaneous M-mode echocardiography through the atrial wall and the aortic valve or ventricular wall will show similar rapid atrial and ventricular rates or a divergence in rate with a more rapid atrial beat. Findings vary based on underlying rhythm.
   a. Atrial flutter—The atrial rate is frequently monotonous at 400 to 460 bpm. There is a variable block, frequently 2 to 1, resulting in a ventricular rate of 200 bpm. Rates can be as high as 300 bpm. Uncontrolled atrial flutter will result in hydrops with possible mortality. If the rhythm is controlled, the prognosis is good.
   b. Supraventricular tachycardia—1 to 1 atrial ventricular conduction with heart rates of 180 to 200 depending on the underlying mechanism (e.g., reentrant versus ectopic); may be incessant or intermittent. Uncontrolled SVT will result in hydrops with possible mortality.
   c. Sinus tachycardia—1 to 1 conduction with a sustained heart rate of 180 to 190 bpm with very little variability. There are rare reports of ventricu-

lar dysfunction if there is incessant sinus tachycardia.
   d. Ventricular tachycardia—There is a normal atrial rate with a faster ventricular rate. The rate is usually just slightly above sinus rate, well tolerated, and as a rule, self-limited.
2. **Amniotic Fluid:** Normal, except with concurrent hydrops.
3. **Placenta:** Normal, except with concurrent hydrops.
4. **Measurement Data:** Normal.
5. **When Detectable:** May develop at any point in pregnancy.

Pitfalls   Without careful examination of the M-mode strip, it may be difficult to determine the type of tachycardia. Ventricular tachycardia may be mistaken for SVT; giving digoxin with SVT may precipitate ventricular fibrillation.

Differential Diagnosis   Supraventricular tachycardias should be differentiated from sinus tachycardia, which may be on the basis of amnionitis, maternal fever, or drug administration. Supraventricular tachycardia usually starts and stops abruptly. Sinus tachycardia usually has gradual changes in rate.

Where Else to Look
1. Look for signs of hydrops (i.e., skin edema, ascites, pleural effusions, pericardial effusion).
2. Rule out underlying cardiac structural abnormalities especially Ebstein's anomaly, rhabdomyoma, and corrected transposition. There is a higher incidence of Wolf-Parkinson-White (WPW) with these diagnoses and abnormal septal motion has been described as evidence of preexcitation.

PREGNANCY MANAGEMENT

Investigations and Consultations Required   The management of these pregnancies should be a joint effort involving a perinatologist and a pediatric cardiologist. A fetal echocardiogram should be done to exclude structural malformations.

Fetal Intervention   Fetal tachycardia is a medical emergency that should be treated aggressively. Administration transplacentally of a variety of antiarrhythmia medications has been successful in restoring normal sinus rhythm. Agents used have included digoxin, propranolol, procainamide, verapamil, and flecainide acetate. Digoxin remains the drug of choice despite concerns regarding its ability to cross the placenta. Direct intravenous or intramuscular therapy should be reserved for the hydropic fetus that does not respond to aggressive transplacental therapy. Drug therapy for fetal arrhythmias must be tailored to the degree of hydrops and the suspected underlying rhythm mechanism (e.g. ectopic reentrant, AV reentrant, flutter, etc.). Treatment should be in consultation with a person familiar with antiarrhythmic medications and their effects on fetus and newborn. Therapy may need to be altered secondary to maternal side effects.

1. Atrial flutter—Treatment is always indicated if the tachycardia is incessant. Intermittent tachycardia may or may not require therapy. Digoxin or verapamil may increase AV block resulting in a slower ventricular response rate. There is a need to control the atrial rate for hydrops to resolve or be prevented. Consider type I antiarrhythmic agents such as quinidine, procainamide, flecainide. Never use these substances before controlling ventricular response.
2. SVT—Incessant SVT should always be treated. Intermittent SVT may or may not require treatment. The medication chosen and the mode of delivery (maternal, umbilical vein, intramuscular) depend on the degree of hydrops, suspected mode of SVT, gestational age, and lung maturity. Frequently first-line therapy will be digoxin followed by verapamil, propranolol, or flecainide, if single drug therapy is unsuccessful.
3. Sinus tachycardia—Evaluate for causes of fetal anemia. No treatment is required if ventricular function is preserved and there are no signs of hydrops. The mother should be evaluated for thyroid disease.
4. Ventricular tachycardia—No treatment is required if the rhythm abnormality is intermittent and there are no signs of hydrops.

Monitoring The frequency of monitoring in fetuses with tachycardia will depend on the degree of hydrops and arrhythmia control. Any fetus with uncontrolled SVT or atrial flutter should be reevaluated at least twice a week for signs of fetal hydrops. Patients on therapy will need to be monitored for drug levels as well as maternal side effects. Patients with sinus tachycardia and ventricular tachycardia should be evaluated weekly for signs of hydrops.

Pregnancy Termination Issues The timing of onset of these conditions and the potential for successful therapy precludes termination as an option.

Delivery Delivery should occur in a tertiary center with immediate availability of a pediatric cardiologist. Every attempt should be made to maintain the pregnancy until lung maturity is reached. For the preterm infant with hydrops transplacental conversion is preferable to early delivery and neonatal therapy. Vaginal delivery is not contraindicated. Heart rate must be monitored closely with a low threshold for cesarean section if signs of fetal distress develop.

NEONATOLOGY

Resuscitation In the absence of hydrops, assistance with the onset of breathing usually is not required. (See Chapter 12 for details of management.)

Transport Immediate referral to a tertiary center with pediatric cardiac diagnostic capabilities is essential. Consultation with a pediatric cardiologist prior to transport is helpful in deciding medication to be administered during transport. In general, maintenance of adequate tissue perfusion and correction of acidosis are the primary issues. If hydrops is present ventilatory support is almost always required.

Testing and Confirmation Electrocardiography to establish the electrophysiologic abnormality and echocardiography to determine intracardiac anatomy are the confirming diagnostic procedures.

Nursery Management The need for continued postnatal drug therapy depends on underlying rhythm abnormality and degree of prenatal arrhythmia control. Patients treated prenatally do not always require postnatal drug therapy.

Adenosine 50 mcg to 350 mcg/kg is given intravenously to infants with sustained SVT. Serum concentration of any drug administered prenatally should be obtained prior to initiating postnatal therapy.

SURGERY

Preoperative Assessment See "Testing and Confirmation" above.

Operative Indications Life-threatening arrhythmias require specific diagnosis and identification of abnormal conduction pathways or activation foci, if present. If medical management is inadequate to control these arrhythmias, surgical or catheter ablation of accessory pathways or irritable foci may be required. Antitachycardiac pacemakers are available for older children.

Types of Procedures
1. Catheter ablation of foci or accessory pathways.
2. Surgical ablation of foci or accessory pathways.
3. Pacemaker therapy.

Surgical Results/Prognosis Ablation of accessory pathways has been very successful and has been performed at low risk.

BIBLIOGRAPHY
Kleinman CS: Prenatal diagnosis and management of intrauterine arrhythmias. *Fetal Ther* 1986; 1:92.

Kleinman CS, Copel JA, Weinstein EM et al: In utero diagnosis and treatment of fetal supraventricular tachycardia. *Semin Perinatol* 1985; 9:113.

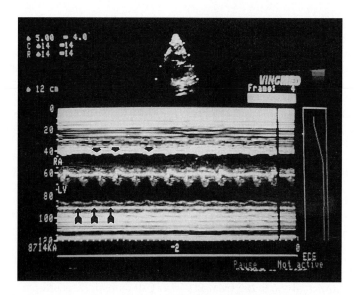

M-mode through a four-chamber view of the fetal heart. The short, thick black arrows point to the atrial contractions. The thinner black arrows point to the ventricular contractions. The ventricular rate exceeds the atrial rate, consistent with ventricular tachycardia.

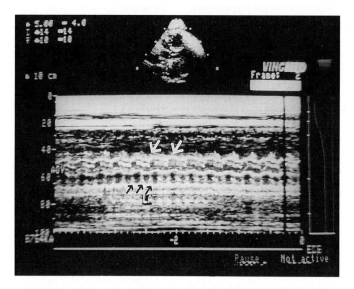

Four-chamber view through the long axis of the fetal heart. The small, black arrows point to the atrial wall motion and the larger, white arrows point to the opening of the aortic valve, consistent with the beginning of systole. Notice there are three atrial wall contractions for each opening of the aortic valve. The fluttering motion of the atrium can also be seen on the closed aortic valve leaflet. This is an example of atrial flutter.

3.11 TETRALOGY OF FALLOT

EPIDEMIOLOGY/GENETICS

Definition   This entity consists of four abnormalities: (1) VSD; (2) pulmonary stenosis at the infundibular level with or without associated valve stenosis; (3) right ventricular hypertrophy; and (4) an aorta that overrides the ventricular septal defect.

Epidemiology   5 out of 10,000 births. The defect accounts for between 6% and 10% of all CHFs.

Embryology   Teralogy of Fallot (TOF) results from unequal division of the conotruncus resulting in a large aorta and a small right ventricular outflow tract. The aorta subsequently overrides the intraventricular septum, resulting in an associated VSD.

Inheritance Pattern   Tetralogy of Fallot is usually a sporadic, isolated malformation, although autosomal dominant inheritance has been reported in rare families. The recurrence risk with one affected sibling is approximately 2.5% and there is an 8% recurrence risk if two siblings are affected. Common malformation syndrome associations include the DiGeorge/velocardiofacial syndrome; the coloboma, heart disease, atresia choanae, retarded growth and retarded development and/or central nervous system anomalies, genital hypoplasia, and ear anomalies and/or deafness (CHARGE) association; and Goldenhar's or hemifacial microsomia syndrome. When combined with other abnormalities, chromosome syndromes should be considered.

Teratogens   Vitamin A, thalidomide, alcohol, trimethadione, sex hormones.

Prognosis   Prognosis for isolated tetralogy of Fallot without complete pulmonary atresia is generally good. Essentially all children will require surgical repair.

SONOGRAPHY

Findings
1. **Fetus**
   a. There is a large subaortic VSD seen along the course of the aorta.
   b. The right ventricle is slightly larger than the left.
   c. The aorta is large and overrides the interventricular septum.
   d. The pulmonary artery is small. There is frequently infundibular stenosis below the pulmonary valve as well as a small pulmonary valve.
   e. There may be an associated ASD.
   f. Doppler flow may show increased velocities and turbulence across the right ventricular outflow tract.

2. **Amniotic Fluid:** Mild polyhydramnios is common.
3. **Placenta:** Normal.
4. **Measurement Data:** Normal.
5. **When Detectable:** 13 weeks with vaginal probe; 19 to 20 weeks with a transabdominal approach.

Pitfalls   The abnormality may be missed on a screening four-chamber view, depending on the VSD location.

Differential Diagnosis
1. Isolated malaligned VSD.
2. Truncal arteriosus may be difficult to differentiate from TOF with pulmonary atresia.

Where Else to Look
1. There is a 16% association with extracardiac anomalies. Although TOF is not an essential component of any syndromes, it is frequently associated with malformation groups (i.e., cardiofacial, CHARGE, VACTERL [vertebral abnormalities, anal atresia, cardiac abnormalities, tracheoesophageal fistula and esophageal atresia, renal agenesis and dysplasia, and limb defects]) and has been described in the de Lange, Goldenhar's, and Klippel-Feil syndromes. Look for: a. facial, orbital, and hypotelorism assymetry; b. hemivertebra, caudal regression, and short cervical spine; c. gut obstruction; d. IUGR; and e. genital hypoplasia in males.
2. It is associated with chromosomal anomalies such as trisomy 18, trisomy 13, and trisomy 21, therefore, a complete fetal assessment is indicated.

PREGNANCY MANAGEMENT

Investigations and Consultations Required   Chromosome studies are essential, as is consultation with a pediatric cardiologist.

Fetal Intervention   None available at this time.

Monitoring   In the absence of fetal hydrops there is no indication to alter standard obstetric management. In cases with an absent pulmonary valve, serial sonograms to detect early fetal hydrops are appropriate.

Pregnancy Course   Mild polyhydramnios is a common associated finding. In rare cases with absence of the pulmonary valve, fetal hydrops may develop. Tetralogy of Fallot is well tolerated in utero because only 11% of fetal cardiac output goes to the fetal lungs.

Pregnancy Termination Issues   An intact fetus should be delivered in order to confirm the sonographic diagnosis. Because TOF can be successfully surgically corrected in the absence of any extra cardiac abnormalities or chromosomal abnormalities, termination is not usually an issue. This is not the case for patients with TOF with associated pulmonary atresia where the prognosis is dismal.

Delivery   All cases should be delivered in a tertiary center where a pediatric cardiologist is immediately available to assess the need for prostaglandin therapy and urgent surgical intervention as the ductus arteriosus undergoes closure after delivery. For patients in whom fetal hydrops is present, delivery once fetal lung maturity is documented may be the best approach. The mode of delivery should be based on obstetric indications. There is no contraindication to vaginal delivery.

NEONATOLOGY

Resuscitation   Assistance with onset of respiration is usually not required. However, if there is evidence of fetal distress prior to delivery or delay in spontaneous onset of breathing, assisted breaths should be given with 40% to 60% oxygen to avoid stimulating early ductal closure with the concomitant effect of decreasing oxygenation.

Transport   Immediate referral to a tertiary center with full pediatric cardiac diagnostic and surgical capability is imperative once a diagnosis of cyanotic congenital heart disease is suspected. If cyanosis is present, a prostaglandin infusion should be started prior to transport. Even in the absence of cyanosis, a PGE1 infusion should be prepared at the bedside. Because prostaglandin may cause apnea, intubation should be considered prior to transport.

Testing and Confirmation   When cyanotic congenital heart disease is suspected after birth the initial screening procedures beyond a careful physical examination of the cardiac and respiratory systems include chest radiograph, twelve-lead electrocardiogram, and a hyperoxia test. Cyanosis secondary to an anatomic shunt will not resolve by increasing the inspired oxygen concentration.

Definitive confirmation of the anatomy is by postnatal echocardiography. Cardiac catheterization is needed frequently to assess the coronary arteries, the flow through the pulmonary outflow tract, the main and branch pulmonary arteries, and the anatomy of the ventricular septum. Infants who can undergo primary repair can be separated from those who will need a palliative shunt procedure initially.

Nursery Management   Once the diagnosis and anatomy are confirmed further management is dependent upon the magnitude of the oxygenation deficit and the planned surgery. Oxygen saturation will depend on the adequacy of antegrade pulmonary blood flow and determines initial management. If the oxygen saturation is less than 65% or if there is significant metabolic acidosis, continuous infusion of PGE1 should be instituted, and buffer given. Assisted ventilation without supple-

mental oxygen may be needed. If these steps are unsuccessful in raising the P_{O_2}, either a palliative shunt or complete repair will be necessary. If the initial oxygen saturation is adequate, further intervention is delayed until spontaneous closure of the ductus arteriosus. If the saturation continues to be adequate at that point, elective surgical repair is usually delayed until later in the first year of life.

SURGERY

Preoperative Assessment   Preoperative assessment for tetralogy of Fallot is by echocardiography and cardiac catheterization. Echocardiography can identify the size of the pulmonary arteries, as well as whether or not they are confluent. In addition, the anatomy of the pulmonary valve can be identified. Echocardiography may demonstrate additional VSDs and can frequently define the origin and course of the proximal right and left coronary arteries.

Operative Indications   All tetralogy of Fallot patients require surgical repair. Frequently the repair is needed during the first year of life because of increasing cyanosis. Due to the success of tetralogy repair at an early age, the age of elective repair has been steadily decreasing.

Types of Procedures   Repair consists of closure of the VSD with a Dacron patch, as well as enlargement of the infundibulum of the right ventricle, the pulmonary valve, and the main pulmonary artery. If pulmonary valve leaflets are thickened and dysplastic, they are frequently excised. Likewise, if there is narrowing of the branches of either of the pulmonary arteries, the incision is extended to these vessels. In patients who are not candidates for complete repair, but have persistent cyanosis, a Blalock-Taussig shunt is used as a temporizing measure until complete repair can be attempted.

Surgical Results/Prognosis   Survival for repair of tetralogy of Fallot with pulmonary stenosis is dependent upon the age of repair, as well as the underlying anatomy. Surgical survival ranges between 93% and 98%. Quality of life is usually excellent postoperatively. There is a small risk of reoperation, most commonly for residual right ventricular outflow tract obstruction. Other indications have been development or aortopulmonary collaterals and residual VSDs. There is a small incidence of late cardiac death, most likely secondary to arrhythmias. Prognosis and survival for tetralogy of Fallot with pulmonary atresia is changing rapidly.

BIBLIOGRAPHY
Casta-neda AR, Jonas RA: Neonatal repair of tetralogy of Fallot. In: Long WA (ed): *Fetal and neonatal cardiology*. Philadelphia. WB Saunders, 1990; pp. 774-779.
Freed MD, Heymann MA, Lewis AB et al: Prostaglandin E1 in infants with ductus arteriosus-dependent congenital heart disease. *Circulation* 1981; 64:899-905.

Kirklin JW et al: Surgical results and protocols in the spectrum of tetralogy of Fallot. *Ann Surg* 1983; 198:251.

Morris DC, Felner JM, Schlant RC et al: Echocardiographic diagnosis of tetralogy of Fallot. *Am J Cardiol* 1975; 36:908.

Neches WH, Park SC, Ettedgui: Tetralogy of Fallot and tetralogy of Fallot with pulmonary atresia. In: Garson Jr A, Bricker JT, McNamara DG (eds): *The science and practice of pediatric cardiology.* 1st edition. Philadelphia. Lea & Febiger, 1990.

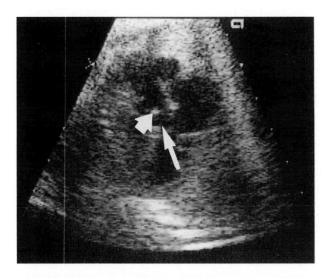

This is a fetal echocardiogram at 34 weeks gestation in the infant of a mother with tetralogy of Fallot. The infant also has tetralogy of Fallot. The aorta (short arrow) can be seen overriding an interventricular septal defect (long arrow), and there is equal size of the left and right ventricles.

Diagram showing the abnormality with tetralogy of Fallot. *Used with permission from Mullins CE, Mayer DC: Congenital heart disease: a diagnostic atlas. New York. Wiley-Liss, 1988.*

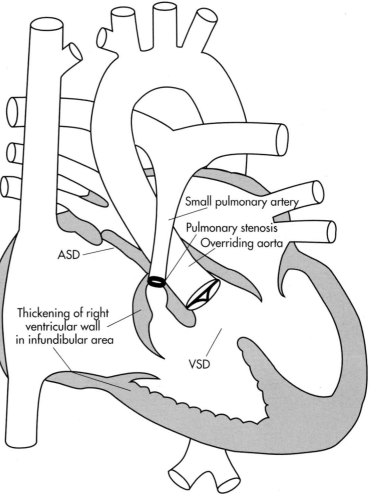

3.12 TRANSPOSITION OF THE GREAT ARTERIES
D-TRANSPOSITION OR SIMPLE TRANSPOSITION

EPIDEMIOLOGY/GENETICS

Definition   The aorta arises from the right ventricle and is located anteriorly and to the right of the pulmonary artery. The pulmonary artery arises from the posterior left ventricle resulting in complete separation of the circulations and profound hypoxia without mixing of the two circulations.

Epidemiology   1 out of 2,000 (M2:F1). Transposition accounts for 5% of all congenital heart defects.

Embryology   Initially this entity was thought to be a result of faulty spiraling of the aortopulmonary septum. More recent theories propose that it results from abnormalities in the differential growth rates of the subaortic and subpulmonary conal musculature. Only rarely does it occur in association with genetic syndromes, but can be found with situs inversus.

Inheritance Patterns   Multifactorial. The recurrence risk is low (1% or less).

Teratogens   Vitamin A, amphetamines, trimethadione, sex hormones.

Prognosis   Good with surgical intervention. Most often an isolated, nonsyndromic abnormality.

SONOGRAPHY

Findings
1.   **Fetus:** The hallmark of transposition of the great arteries is ventricular/arterial disconcordance. A posterior pulmonary artery is seen arising from the posterior left ventricle, which is the ventricle located closest to the spine of the fetus. The anterior aorta arises parallel to the pulmonary artery from the anterior right ventricle. There is frequently an associated ASD or stretched foramen ovale and a VSD is present in 40% of the cases. If a VSD is present, pulmonary stenosis occurs in 30% to 35% of cases. Left ventricular outflow-tract obstruction is more common in the patients without the VSD. A dynamic left ventricular outflow obstruction occurs in 20% of these patients.
2.   **Amniotic Fluid:** Normal.
3.   **Placenta:** Normal.
4.   **Measurement Data:** Normal.
5.   **When Detectable:** 19 to 20 weeks. 13 weeks transvaginally.

Pitfalls
1.   It is important to differentiate the pulmonary artery from the aortic arch. The aortic arch is identified by

the head and neck vessels arising from it. The pulmonary artery arises and joins the ductus arteriosus that is of the same caliber and then enters the descending aorta. Frequently in utero the branch pulmonary arteries are not well visualized.

Differential Diagnosis   Double outlet right ventricle. Both major vessels will arise from the anterior ventricle.

Where Else to Look   Simple transposition is rarely associated with other noncardiac malformations. Associated cardiac abnormalities are frequent. Look for evidence of congestive failure—pleural effusion and ascites.

PREGNANCY MANAGEMENT

Investigations and Consultations Required   Chromosome analysis should be performed, although chromosome abnormalities or extracardiac abnormalities are rare with simple transposition. Consultation with a pediatric cardiologist is essential.

Fetal Intervention   None is indicated.

Monitoring   No change in standard obstetric care is indicated. Serial ultrasound evaluations should be performed to detect signs of congestive failure, if there are associated obstructive lesions.

Pregnancy Course   Transposition of the great arteries is well tolerated in utero because both ventricles are pumping into the systemic circulation.

Pregnancy Termination Issues   An intact fetus should be delivered in order to confirm the sonographic diagnosis. This is not often a consideration given the high degree of success with surgical repair.

Delivery   The site for delivery should be a tertiary center where a pediatric cardiologist is immediately available. The mode of delivery should be based on obstetric indications. There is no need to change the mode of delivery based on the presence of transposition of the great arteries.

NEONATOLOGY

Resuscitation   Assistance with onset of respiration is usually not required. However, if there is evidence of fetal distress prior to delivery or delay in spontaneous onset of breathing, assisted breaths should be given with 40% to 60% oxygen to avoid stimulating early ductal closure with the concomitant effect of decreasing oxygenation.

Transport   Immediate referral to a tertiary center with full pediatric cardiac diagnostic and surgical capability is imperative once a diagnosis of cyanotic congenital heart disease is suspected. Consultation with a pediatric cardiologist prior to transport is recommended to determine the need for initiation of a prostaglandin (PGE1) infusion.

Testing and Confirmation   Definitive confirmation of the anatomy is by postnatal echocardiography. When cyanotic congenital heart disease is suspected after birth the initial screening procedures beyond a careful physical examination of the cardiac and respiratory systems include: chest radiograph, twelve-lead electrocardiogram, and a hyperoxia test. Cyanosis secondary to an anatomic shunt will not resolve by increasing the inspired oxygen concentration.

Nursery Management   Once the diagnosis and anatomy are confirmed, further management is dependent upon the magnitude of the oxygenation deficit and the planned surgery. If the oxygen saturation is less than 65% or there is significant metabolic acidosis, continuous infusion of PGE1 should be instituted, and a buffer given. Assisted ventilation without supplemental oxygen may be needed. If this is unsuccessful in raising the Po_2, a balloon atrial septostomy or definitive surgery should be performed on an emergency basis. If there is adequate mixing with an acceptable oxygen saturation, no intervention prior to definitive surgery is usually needed.

SURGERY

Preoperative Assessment   Echocardiography reliably identifies the anatomy with simple transposition of the great vessels. It is imperative that the origin and pathway of the coronary arteries be identified preoperatively. The outflow tract also needs to be evaluated to make sure there is no left or right ventricular obstruction. Infants with intractable cyanosis and a small ASD may require balloon atrial septostomy prior to their surgical procedure. Cardiac catheterization may be required if the anatomy is unclear.

Operative Indications   All patients with simple transposition of the great arteries require surgical intervention. In uncomplicated transposition, this should be undertaken within the first 2 weeks of life.

Types of Procedures   The arterial switch operation is the treatment of choice for patients with simple transposition of the great vessels. This is the only surgical intervention that results in an anatomic repair. The pulmonary artery is divided proximal to its bifurcation and the aorta is divided distal to the origin of the coronary arteries. The coronary artery ostia are then isolated and transferred to the native proximal pulmonary artery followed by the anastomosis of the distal aorta to that site. Likewise, the distal pulmonary artery is anastomosed to the native proximal aorta. Anatomical switch procedure is substituted in patients with poorly placed coronary arteries or outflow tract obstruction. The atrial switch requires using the pericardial or synthetic baffle and redirecting pulmonary venous return to a tricuspid valve and systemic venous return to the mitral valve. It results in a physiologic correction but not an anatomic correction, as the right ventricle continues to pump into the system circulation. Patients who have not had their switch repair done in the neonatal period because of other complicating factors undergo a two-stage procedure with banding of the pulmonary artery in order to condition the left ventricle for a subsequent arterial switch procedure.

Surgical Results/Prognosis   The overall mortality rate for the arterial switch procedure is about 5%. This number is considerably higher in patients with complicating factors such as multiple VSDs, outflow tract obstruction, or abnormal coronary arteries. Likewise, in patients with simple transposition, the mortality rate is considerably lower. Long-term survival appears to be excellent. However, the procedure has been the operation of choice for less than 2 decades and it will need to be reevaluated as time goes on. Operative mortality for the atrial switch procedure is also low. However, over time, these patients have a high incidence of atrial dysrhythmias as well as a low incidence of right ventricular or systemic ventricular failure.

BIBLIOGRAPHY

Bass NM, Roche AHG, Brandt PWT et al: Echocardiography in assesssment of infants with complete d-transposition of the great arteries. *Br Heart J* 1978; 40:1165.

Castaneda AR, Norwood WI, Jonas RA et al: Transposition of the great arteries and intact ventricular septum: anatomic repair in the neonate. *Ann Thorac Surg* 1984; 38:438-443.

Freed MD, Heymann MA, Lewis AB et al: Prostaglandin E1 in infants with ductus arteriosus-dependent congenital heart disease. *Circulation* 1981; 64:899-905.

Graham TP: Hemodynamic residua and sequellae following intraatrial repair of transposition of the great arteries: a review. *Pediatr Cardiol* 1982; 2:203-213.

Neches WH, Park SC, Ettedgui JA: Transposition of the great arteries. In: Garson Jr A, Bricker JT, McNamara DG (eds): *The science and practice of pediatric cardiology*. 1st edition. Philadelphia. Lea & Febiger, 1990.

Paul MH: Transposition of the great arteries. In: Adams FH, Emmanouloides GC (eds): *Heart disease in infants, children and adolescents*. 3rd edition. Baltimore. Williams & Wilkins, 1983; pp. 296-333.

Quaegebeur JM, Rohmer J, Ottenkamp B et al: The arterial switch: an eight year experience. *J Thorac Cardiovasc Surg* 1986; 92:361-384.

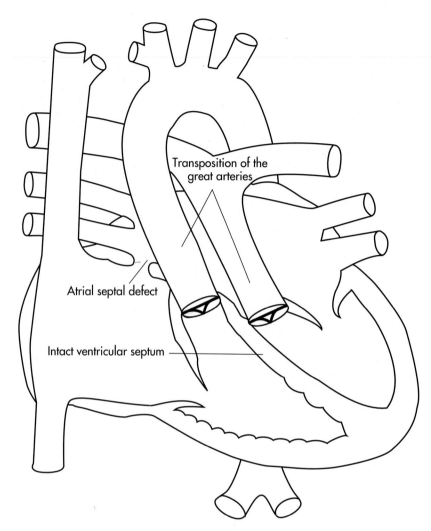

Diagram showing the appearance of transposition of the great arteries. *Used with permission from Mullins CE, Mayer DC:* Congenital heart disease: a diagnostic atlas. *New York. Wiley-Liss, 1988.*

3.13 Ventricular Septal Defect

EPIDEMIOLOGY/GENETICS

Definition   Absence of part or all of the interventricular septum.

Epidemiology   1 out of 400 live births (M1:F1). Twenty percent to 30% of congenital heart disease.

Embryology   Muscular defects are thought to be due to excessive excavation during ventricular growth. Inlet, outlet, and membranous defects are thought to be due to a failure of fusion.

Inheritance Patterns   The majority of VSDs are sporadic. However, over 100 genetic and chromosomal syndromes have been described with VSD as an abnormality. The recurrence risk for fetuses with one affected sibling is approximately 3%.

Teratogens   Alcohol, hydantoin, valproic acid.

Prognosis   Prognosis is frequently dependent upon associated abnormalities or syndrome diagnosis. Small isolated defects frequently undergo spontaneous closure particularly in the muscular septum. Most other VSDs are amenable to surgical repair. Because a VSD is difficult to identify in utero, those that are discovered usually represent the severe end of the spectrum. Complete absence of the interventricular septum is difficult to repair.

SONOGRAPHY

Findings:
1. **Fetus:** The ventricular septum should be viewed from multiple positions including four-chamber, long-axis, and multiple short axis views. The defect will appear as dropout of the septum and may only be visible in one view depending on the size and shape of the defect and the portion of the septum involved. Color flow Doppler may show flow across the defect. Frequently, in utero, the flow is bidirectional and can be confirmed by pulsed Doppler. If the ventricular pressures are equal, no flow will be appreciated.
2. **Amniotic Fluid:** Normal.
3. **Placenta:** Normal.
4. **Measurement Data:** Normal.
5. **When Detectable:** Usually undetectable before 17 to 18 weeks.

Pitfalls
1. Small defects are difficult to visualize.
2. There is frequently false dropout of the subaortic area. It is important to visualize this area from multiple views. Pseudodropout is most likely to occur

when the transducer is aimed along the axis of the ventricle, rather than from a lateral position.

Where Else to Look   Ventricular septal defects are associated with chromosomal anomalies, so the remainder of the fetus should be studied for signs of chromosomal anomalies.

PREGNANCY MANAGEMENT

Investigations and Consultations Required   Ventricular septal defects have been described with most chromosomal abnormalities with an incidence of 10% to 15%. Chromosomal analysis should be offered.

Pregnancy Monitoring/Course   Well tolerated in utero. No change in standard obstetric management is indicated.

Pregnancy Termination Issues   Should be considered only in the presence of chromosomal abnormalities or other major associated malformations. An intact fetus should be delivered for complete morphologic and pathologic evaluation.

Delivery   Mode should not be altered based on cardiac defect. If the defect is isolated delivery need not be in a tertiary care center but the infant should be evaluated by a pediatriac cardiologist at the time of hospital discharge.

NEONATOLOGY

Resuscitation   An isolated VSD will not be symptomatic in the delivery room and standard resuscitation should be used.

Transport   Rarely necessary with an isolated defect. Should an infant with the prenatal diagnosis become symptomatic in the early neonatal period, pediatric cardiology consultation or immediate referral to a tertiary center is indicated as the presence of symptoms early suggests the likelihood of additional unrecognized cardiac lesions.

Testing and Confirmation   The anatomy should be confirmed by postnatal echocardiography.

Nursery Management   Small, muscular VSDs usually remain asymptomatic whereas moderate to large and membraneous defects become progressively more symptomatic as pulmonary vascular resistance falls in the first 4 to 6 weeks of life. Sodium and fluid restriction and diuretic therapy are used to control congestive heart failure. High-calorie formulas and tube feedings may be needed to sustain adequate growth.

SURGERY

Preoperative Assessment   Preoperative assessment in VSDs is predominantly by two-dimensional echocardiography. If it is uncertain whether or not the VSD is significant or whether there is irreversible pulmonary vascular disease, cardiac catheterization will also be required preoperatively.

Operative Indications   Because the majority of membranous and muscular VSDs tend to close spontaneously, surgical closure is indicated ony if the infant has failed aggressive medical management with digitalis and diuretics. Failure of medical management is usually indicated by intractable CHF and failure to thrive. Approximately 30% of infants with symptomatic VSDs in the first year of life will require surgical repair. Repair in older children should be dictated by pulmonary vascular resistance as well as the shunt through the VSD. Early closure of VSDs will prevent irreversible pulmonary disease from developing.

Types of Procedures   The majority of VSDs can be approached through the tricuspid valve and a Dacron patch can be sewn in place. Ventricular septal defects that are difficult to reach or complicated by other CHFs may require pulmonary artery banding to control pulmonary blood flow with a subsequent repair at a later date.

Surgical Results/Prognosis   The prognosis for an infant who undergoes VSD repair in the first year of life is excellent. These patients should have a normal life span and normal standard of living. There is a small risk of complete heart block during surgery.

BIBLIOGRAPHY

Allan LD, Crawford DC, Anderson RH et al: Echocardiographic and anatomical correlations in fetal congenital heart disease. *Br Heart J* 1984; 52:542.

Baraitser M, Winter RM: *The London dysmorphology database.* Oxford Medical Press. New York, 1993.

Dickenson DF, Arnold R, Wilkinson JL: Ventricular septal defect in children born in Liverpool 1960-1969: evaluation of natural course and surgical implications in an unselected population. *Br Heart J* 1981b: 46-47-54.

Gumbiner C, Takao A: Ventricular septal defect. In: Garson Jr A, Bricker JT, McNamara DG (eds): *The science and practice of pediatric cardiology.* 1st edition. Philadelphia. Lea & Febiger, 1990.

Somerville J: Changing form and function in one ventricle hearts. *Herz* 1979; 4:206-212.

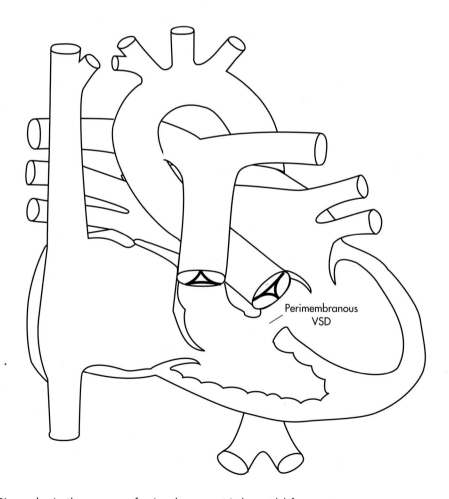

Diagram showing the appearance of perimembranous ventricular septal defect. *Used with permission from Mullins CE, Mayer DC: Congenital heart disease: a diagnostic atlas. New York. Wiley-Liss, 1988.*

4 The Genitourinary Tract

4.1 ADRENAL HEMATOMA

EPIDEMIOLOGY/GENETICS

Definition   An adrenal hematoma is the result of extravasation of blood from the vascular system into the tissue of the adrenal gland resulting in an extravascular collection of blood. Large bleeds may result in fetal hypotension and death. Smaller bleeds may be asymptomatic and present as incidental calcification in the adrenal gland.

Epidemiology   Unknown, but rare.

Embryology   It has been suggested that ischemia, resulting from hypotension, vascular abnormalities, occlusion, emboli, or antenatal infection, is the most likely cause of adrenal hematomas.

Inheritance Patterns   Sporadic.

Teratogens   Antenatal infections.

Prognosis   Prognosis is dependent on the size of the bleed and ranges from lethal, for large bleeds, to asymptomatic, for smaller bleeds.

SONOGRAPHY

Findings
1. **Fetus:** A mass is present, superior to the kidney, involving all or part of the adrenal gland. The mass may be echogenic or cystic with rapid changes in sonographic appearance on sequential studies. The process may be one-sided or bilateral.
2. **Amniotic Fluid:** Normal.
3. **Placenta:** Normal.
4. **Measurement Data:** Usually large babies.
5. **When Detectable:** This is a third trimester finding, usually seen close to delivery.

Pitfalls   The hematoma may be technically difficult to find due to fetal position.

Differential Diagnosis
1. Neuroblastoma may occur in the same location prior to delivery. Neuroblastoma does not change rapidly in appearance, unless there is associated hemorrhage.
2. A hydronephrotic second collecting system may be confused with an adrenal hematoma, but will not change internal acoustic appearance with time.
3. Liver mass—rare and should be visibly located in the liver.
   No specific changes in obstetric management are entailed by the other disorders in the differential diagnosis of suprarenal masses.

Where Else to Look   Renal vein thrombosis is associated. Look for renal enlargement with prominent sinus echoes. The veins may become calcified.

PREGNANCY MANAGEMENT

Investigations and Consultations Required   In the absence of other abnormalities on sonographic evaluation, no further diagnostic evaluation is necessary. A neonatology consult should be obtained to plan perinatal management.

Monitoring   A sonogram should be performed every 2 weeks because neuroblastoma is hard to exclude before birth.

Pregnancy Course   There are no obstetric complications associated with this fetal malformation.

Pregnancy Termination Issues   A diagnosis of fetal adrenal hematoma should not influence decisions about pregnancy termination.

Delivery   The rare occurrence of unexplained shock with large hemorrhages requires that delivery occur in a location where personnel and facilities are available to manage this complication.

NEONATOLOGY

Resuscitation   If the diagnosis is made prior to onset of labor and the lesion is small, no resuscitation should be required on the basis of the hematoma. Acute adrenal hemorrhage occurs as a complication of a traumatic delivery or severe perinatal asphyxia. Rapid volume expansion, to support perfusion, may be needed in such a situation.

Transport   Referral to a tertiary care center, on the basis of a prenatal diagnosis, is probably not indicated, unless the hemorrhage was massive and there is concern for adrenal insufficiency.

Testing and Confirmation   Postnatal radiographic studies may detect an acute hematoma or adrenal calcification from an earlier bleed.

Nursery Management   No specific intervention is required for a prenatally diagnosed lesion. If the hematoma was massive or bilateral, the infant should be monitored closely for evidence of adrenal insufficiency (i.e., salt wasting, hypoglycemia, hypotension, or failure to thrive).

BIBLIOGRAPHY

Eklof O, Grotte G, Jorulf H et al: Perinatal haemorrhagic necrosis of the adrenal gland. *Pediatr Radiol* 1975; 24:31-36.

Hata K, Hata T, Kitao M: Ultrasonographic identification and measurement of the human fetal adrenal gland in utero: clinical application. *Gynecol Obstet Invest* 1988; 25:16-22.

Morganti VJ, Anderson NG: Simple adrenal cysts in fetus, resolving spontaneously in neonate. *J Ultrasound Med* 1991; 10:521-524.

Romero R et al (eds): *Normal anatomy of the adrenal gland.* In: *Prenatal diagnosis of congenital anomalies.* Appleton and Lange, Norwalk, CT. pp. 295-296.

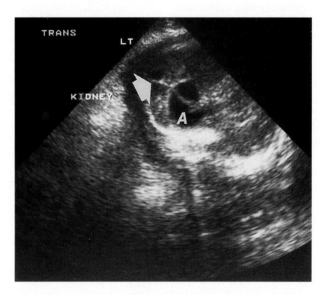

Transverse view of an adrenal hematoma (*A*). In this instance, the hematoma is cystic apart from a septum. Some adrenal hematomas can appear echogenic and can change appearance rapidly, almost on a daily basis. The kidney (*arrow*) can be seen alongside the hematoma.

4.2 Exstrophy of the Bladder

EPIDEMIOLOGY/GENETICS

Definition Bladder exstrophy is a failure of closure of the bladder, lower urinary tract, overlying symphysis pubis, rectus muscles, and skin.

Epidemiology Occurs in 1 out of 30,000 births (M3:F1).

Embryology Bladder exstrophy is thought to be due to a defect in the development of the cloacal membrane, preventing medial migration of mesenchyme. Only rarely are there associated malformations outside of the genitourinary tract.

Inheritance Patterns Most cases are sporadic. There are rare familial case reports of affected siblings.

Teratogens None known.

Screening Maternal serum alpha-fetoprotein is elevated in most cases of bladder extrophy.

Prognosis Surgical correction is difficult, but in experienced hands, approximately 60% to 80% of patients will eventually have continence. In unrepaired cases from the older literature, there was an 8% risk of malignancy, probably related to mucosal exposure and chronic infection.

SONOGRAPHY

Findings
1. **Fetus**
   a. The bladder is absent. A sagittal anterior view will show a mound on the anterior aspect of the abdomen.
   b. Male genitalia will lie anterior and superior to the usual location. The umbilical cord insertion site is at a low level.
2. **Amniotic Fluid:** Normal.
3. **Placenta:** Normal.
4. **Measurement Data:** Appropriate.
5. **When Detectable:** At about 16 weeks.

Pitfalls
1. A sagittal anterior view is the only view that will show the diagnostic mass on the anterior abdomen.
2. The fetal bladder occasionally empties completely when the fetus voids. Apparent absence of the bladder may be a transient normal finding. In patients with severe oligohydramnios, of renal origin, the bladder may be very small.

Differential Diagnosis
1) Sacrococcygeal teratoma—The mass will displace the bladder anteriorly and superiorly and will be in the posterior aspect of the pelvis.

2) Omphalocele—The cord exits through the center of an omphalocele and it lies at a higher level.

Where Else to Look Occasionally, there is secondary hydroureter and hydronephrosis.

PREGNANCY MANAGEMENT

Investigations and Consultations Required Associated abnormalities are rare in bladder exstrophy. In patients planning to continue the pregnancy, fetal echocardiography may be appropriate to exclude cardiac defects before deciding on the site for delivery. A pediatric urologist should be consulted to discuss management with the family. Although chromosome abnormalities are not associated with bladder exstrophy, confirmation of fetal sex may be useful in defining prognosis for surgical repair.

Monitoring No alteration in standard obstetric care is indicated.

Pregnancy Course No obstetric complications are associated with this disorder.

Pregnancy Termination Issues An intact fetus should be delivered to allow confirmation of the sonographic diagnosis.

Delivery There is no evidence that cesarean delivery improves prognosis. Delivery at a tertiary center is not required. It is more important that the infant be transferred to an institution with individuals experienced in the repair of this rare condition.

NEONATOLOGY

Resuscitation Respiratory difficulty is not expected with this lesion.

Transport Referral to a tertiary center is always indicated for early surgical intervention.

Testing and Confirmation The bladder and lower urinary tract are open anteriorly from the urethral meatus to the umbilicus. There is wide separation of the pubic symphysis and rectus muscles. In males, the scrotum is broad, frequently with undescended testes and a short, broad penis without canalization. In females, the clitoris and labia are widely separated with occasional vaginal stenosis. Upper tract anomalies are rare with this lesion, in contrast with hypospadius lesions. A screening abdominal sonogram is adequate to confirm upper tract anatomy.

Nursery Management The exposed viscera should be covered with warm, moist, sterile dressing to limit heat and water loss and contamination. Administration of antibiotics should be considered to reduce the risk of infection.

SURGERY

Preoperative Assessment   Imaging of the upper urinary tracts to make sure there are normal kidneys by ultrasound or nuclear medicine is helpful.

Operative Indications   Surgery is indicated if the bladder is opened to the surface of the abdomen. Surgery is not feasible if the bladder plate is too small to close.

Types of Procedures   The bladder and posterior urethra are reapproximated to form a new bladder. Augmentation of the bladder with a portion of ilium may be necessary. An iliac osteotomy is required so that the pubic symphysis can be reapproximated. An epispadias repair with the creation of a satisfactory penis is also needed.

Surgical Results/Prognosis   The prognosis is dependent upon any associated renal anomalies, but there is a sur-vival rate of more than 90%. Secondary surgical procedures are frequently required at approximately age 4 to 5 to achieve urinary continence and functioning genitalia. An epispadias repair may be performed as early as 2 to 3 years of age. Possible surgical complications include wound dehiscence and infection.

BIBLIOGRAPHY

Barth RA, Filly RA, Sondheimer FK: Prenatal sonographic findings in bladder exstrophy. *J Ultrasound Med* 1990; 9:359-361.

Canning DA, Gearhart JP: *Exstrophy of the bladder* In: Ashcraft KM, Holder TM (eds): *Pediatric Surgery*, WB Saunders, Philadelphia, 1993. pp. 678-693.

De la Hunt MN, O'Donnell B: Current management of bladder exstrophy: a BAPS collective review from eight centers of 81 patients born between 1975 and 1985. *J Pediatr Surg* 1989; 24:584-585.

Jaffee R, Schoenfeld A, Ovadia J: Sonographic findings in the prenatal diagnosis of bladder exstrophy. *Am J Obstet Gynecol* 1990; 162:675–678.

Jeffs RD: Exstrophy, epispadias, and cloacal and urogenital sinus abnormalities. *Pediatr Clin North Am* 1987; 34:1233-1257.

Mirk P, Calisti A, Fileni A: Prenatal sonographic diagnosis of bladder extrophy. *J Ultrasound Med* 1986; 5:291-293.

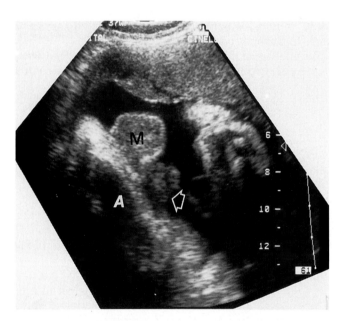

Bladder exstrophy. Sagittal midline view. A large bulge can be seen related to the exstrophy (*M*). The cord insertion (*arrow*) is directly superior to the mass. *A*, abdomen.

4.3 HYDRONEPHROSIS
URETEROPELVIC JUNCTION OBSTRUCTION AND REFLUX

EPIDEMIOLOGY/GENETICS

Definition   Distention of the pelvis and calyces of the kidney, with urine, as a result of ureteral obstruction.

Epidemiology   1 to 5 out of 1,000 births (ureteropelvic junction obstruction (UPJ) M4:F1; ureterovesicular junction obstruction M>F).

Embryology   Hydronephrosis accounts for 75% of prenatally diagnosed fetal renal abnormalities. Many cases of unilateral, and even bilateral, hydronephrosis resolve spontaneously after birth. Ureteropelvic junction obstruction is the most common cause of hydronephrosis and is unilateral in 70% of cases. Vesicoureteric reflux is a common cause of renal pelvicalyceal dilation particularly in males. Rare cases of hydronephrosis are due to ureteral stenosis or other lower urinary tract obstructions. Thirty percent of cases have other associated urinary tract abnormalities and 20% of cases are part of a multiple malformation syndrome. Over 70 genetic, chromosomal, and sporadic multiple malformation syndromes have been described with hydronephrosis.

Inheritance Patterns   Sporadic, unless part of a recognizable syndrome such as the urofacial syndrome (autosomal recessive [AR]) that combines a distinctive grimacing face with bilateral hydronephrosis.

Teratogens   Thalidomide, maternal diabetes, cocaine, and benzodiazepine.

Prognosis   At least 40% of antenatally diagnosed cases of ureteropelvic junction obstruction resolve spontaneously in the neonatal period. Many patients with hydronephrosis will have good renal function because the ureters can absorb increased pressure by dilating. Oligohydramnios, however, suggests a poor prognosis. Untreated reflux, especially of infected urine, is thought to cause permanent renal damage that may lead to renal failure. Most cases can be treated either medically or surgically with excellent results.

SONOGRAPHY

Findings
1. **Fetus:** There is dilation of the pelvis and sometimes the calyces that is graded by severity: grade 1—renal pelvis only; grade 2—renal pelvis and a few calyces; grade 3—renal pelvis and all calyces; and grade 4—renal pelvis, calyceal dilation, and parenchymal thinning.
   a. Ureteropelvic junction obstruction—One or both renal pelves are distended. The distension is asymmetrical, if the condition is bilateral. In severe cases, the calyces are also dilated. No ureteric or bladder distension is seen, if there is UPJ. Dysplastic changes in the kidneys are very rare. Urinoma may develop. A fluid-filled sac will be seen generally posterior to the obstructed kidney, which will be decompressed. The decompressed kidney is usually dysplastic.
   b. Ureterovesical Junction Obstruction—In this rare entity the kidney and ureter are dilated down to a normal bladder. The condition can be bilateral.
   c. Reflux—There is a dilated renal pelvis and ureter that may be unilateral or bilateral and may vary in size over the course of the examination. The dilated pelvis can usually be traced into the ureter. Peristalsis is often visible within the ureter. The bladder may be enlarged and empty ineffectively because much of the urine returns up the ureter. The variant of reflux in which the bladder and ureters are persistently dilated, due to reflux, is termed the megacystis megaureter syndrome. Reflux is much more common in males in utero, although females are much more likely to suffer long-term complications.
   d. For ureterocele, see Section 4.10.
   e. For posterior urethral valves, see Section 4.7.
2. **Amniotic fluid:** Oligohydramnios is unusual. Polyhydramnios occurs if the left renal pelvis is much enlarged and compresses the stomach or small bowel.
3. **Placenta:** Normal.
4. **Measurement Data:** With severe unilateral or bilateral UPJs, the abdomen may be widened to a size that prevents delivery.
5. **When Detectable:** Renal obstruction may develop at any stage of pregnancy, but is usually seen by 20 weeks. Lesser degrees of pelvic dilatation carry more significance if they are seen before 18 weeks. Reflux is usually detectable by 22 weeks. It may only become apparent that the cause of renal pelvic dilatation is reflux when marked variations in renal pelvic size are seen on follow-up exams.

Pitfalls
1. An extrarenal pelvis, with measurements of under 1.5 cm, may simulate a mild UPJ.
2. Renal pelvic measurements of 5 to 10 mm should be considered as, most likely, a normal variant, unless the calyces are distended. However, the patient should be followed with serial studies. Renal pelvic dilatation of less than 5 mm after 20 weeks is considered a normal variant not requiring follow-up.
3. Reflux may simulate other types of renal obstruction. There will be an inconsistent renal pelvic diameter. Reflux is easily confused with normal variant renal pelvic dilatation and UPJ. Variability in pelvic and ureteric size is the diagnostic key.

4. Large renal veins can be mistaken for mild renal pelvic dilatation. Color flow Doppler will show the distinction.

Where Else to Look   Look for stigmata of trisomy 13, 18, and 21. Look at the other kidney for reflux. Reflux has no known associations.

PREGNANCY MANAGEMENT

Investigations and Consultations Required   Chromosome evaluation should be done in all cases of true UPJ, as the incidence of aneuploidy approaches 5%. Fetal echocardiography should be performed as heart defects are the most commonly associated abnormality. Consultation with a pediatric urologist is necessary to develop a prenatal and postnatal management plan.

Fetal Intervention   Because of the significant risk of in utero manipulation, fetal intervention for unilateral lesions usually is not indicated. In the rare case resulting in bowel obstruction and polyhydramnios, intervention might be considered, if preterm labor became a significant problem. In cases with bilateral disease and with normal amniotic fluid, no intervention is appropriate. Decrease in amniotic fluid volume may be an indication for early delivery, if the gestation is 32 weeks or greater. In utero intervention should be considered before this gestational age in circumstances where bilateral obstruction and oligohydramnios are present. Any attempt at intervention should be preceded by an evaluation of renal function.

Monitoring   No change in standard obstetric management is necessary for unilateral disease or reflux. Depending on the severity, ultrasound examination should be performed every 2 to 4 weeks in cases with bilateral UPJ. Serial ultrasound examinations should be performed approximately monthly for reflux to assess amniotic fluid status in the event a misdiagnosis has been made.

Pregnancy Course   No specific obstetric complications should be expected for unilateral disease, although there have been rare reports of polyhydramnios resulting from bowel obstruction by a left-sided lesion.

Pregnancy Termination Issues   The method of termination should provide an intact fetus for pathologic confirmation of the sonographic diagnosis. Isolated reflux would not be an indication for pregnancy termination.

Delivery   When there is severe obstruction, the need for neonatal evaluation and treatment requires that delivery occur in a tertiary center with a pediatric urologist available. Even severe obstruction should not result in dystocia and no change in standard obstetric care is necessary.

NEONATOLOGY

Resuscitation   Usually not an issue. Onset of effective respiration may be impeded by abdominal distension secondary to renal enlargement. Intubation and ventilation may be required, at least initially.

Transport   Indicated with bilateral lesions for full confirmation of diagnosis and establishment of care plan, including surgical intervention. Infants with isolated unilateral lesions and normal renal function, as indicated by serum creatinine, can be referred for outpatient evaluation and management.

Testing and Confirmation   Careful physical examination and abdominal ultrasound will confirm the diagnosis. Diuretic renal nuclear scan is the best technique to assess renal function and drainage.

Nursery Management   Support respiration as necessary to maintain adequate gas exchange. Avoid fluid and protein loading initially until urinary tract patency and renal function have been determined. Subsequent procedures will be contingent upon specific lesion suspected or discovered.

SURGERY

Preoperative Assessment   If the obstruction is considered, with the aid of prenatal sonograms, to be of a severity that may warrant surgery, careful, staged evaluation of renal function and structure by urine production, urinalysis, blood and urine chemistries, and abdominal sonogram is appropriate. If the infant is minimally symptomatic and immediate relief of obstruction is not necessary, imaging can be delayed for several days for better visualization. If the anatomy is not clearly defined prenatally, or immediate relief of obstruction is required, ultrasound imaging should be obtained immediately. Subsequent procedures will be needed to further delineate the site of obstruction, status of reflux, and renal function (e.g., cystogram, renal scan with and without diuretic stimulation, and excretory urography).

Operative Indications   The surgical goal is to perform any needed decompression or pyeloplasty procedure, prior to hypertrophy of the contralateral kidney. Poor renal function can frequently be improved by a decompression pyelostomy or ureterostomy. After 2 to 3 months of decompression, the renal scintigraphy is repeated. If the kidney demonstrates at least 10% of total renal function, a pyeloplasty is indicated.

Types of Procedures   Decompression versus primary repair is dependent on the amount of ipsilateral renal function. Early, neonatal pyeloplasty is very successful with a low recurrence rate.

Surgical Results/Prognosis Ultimate prognosis is dependent upon the amount of remaining renal function and the degree of associated lung hypoplasia. It is excellent for unilateral or mild bilateral hydronephrosis. Repeat pyeloplasties are uncommon even when the initial procedure is done in early infancy (1.5%). Prognosis for infants treated with intrauterine decompression techniques have been poor.

BIBLIOGRAPHY

Anderson PA, Rickwood AM: Features of primary vesicoureteric reflux detected by prenatal sonography. *Br J Urol* 1991; 67:267-271.

Arger PH, Coleman BG, Mintz MC: Routine fetal genitourinary tract screening. *Radiology* 1985; 156:485-489.

Betz BW, Hertzberg BS, Carroll BA et al: Mild fetal renal pelviectasis: Differentiation from hilar vascularity using color Doppler sonography. *J Ultrasound Med* 1991; 10:243-245.

Brock WA, Kaplan G: *Abnormalities of the lower tract.* In: Edelmann CM Jr (ed): *Pediatric kidney disease.* Boston. Little, Brown, 1992. p. 2037.

Caione P, Zaccara A, Capozza N: How prenatal ultrasound can affect the treatment of ureterocele in neonates and children. *Eur Urol* 1989; 16:195-199.

Chapman CJ, Bailey RR, Janus ED et al: Vesicoureteric reflux: Segregation analysis. *Am J Med Genet* 1985; 20:577-584.

Chevalier RL: *Renal physiology and function.* In: Kelalis PP, King LR, Belman AB (eds): *Clinical pediatric urology.* Philadelphia. WB Saunders, 1992. pp. 1106-1120.

Dunn V, Glasier CM: Ultrasonographic antenatal demonstration of primary megaureters. *J Ultrasound Med* 1985; 4:101-103.

Fernbach SK, Maizels M, Conway JJ: Ultrasound grading of hydronephrosis: Introduction to the system used by the Society for Fetal Urology. *Pediatr Radiol* 1993; 23:478-480.

Flushner SC, King LR: *Ureteropelvic obstruction.* In: Kelais PP, King LR, Belman AB (eds): *Clinical pediatric urology.* Philadelphia. WB Saunders, 1992. pp. 693-725.

Grignon A, Filiatrault D, Homsy Y et al: Ureteropelvic junction stenosis: antenatal ultrasonographic diagnosis, postnatal investigation, and follow-up. *Radiology* 1986; 160:649-651.

Grignon A, Filion R, Filiatrault D et al: Urinary tract dilatation in utero: classification and clinical applications. *Radiology* 1986; 160:645-647.

Guys JM, Borella F, Monfort G: Ureteropelvic junction obstructions: prenatal diagnosis and neonatal surgery in 47 cases. *J Pediatr Surg* 1988; 23:156-158.

Hoddick WK, Filly RA, Mahony BS et al: Minimal fetal renal pyelectasis. *J Ultrasound Med* 1985; 4:85-89.

Kass EJ, Bloom D: *Anomalies of the upper urinary tract.* In: Edelmann CM Jr (ed): *Pediatric kidney disease.* Boston. Little, Brown, 1992. p. 2023.

King LR, Hatcher PA: Natural history of fetal and neonatal hydronephrosis. *Pediatr Urol* 1990; 35:433-438.

Kleiner B, Callen PW, Filly RA: Sonographic analysis of the fetus with ureteropelvic junction obstruction. *Am J Roentgenol* 1987; 148:359-363.

Koff SA, Campbell K: Non-operative management of unilateral neonatal hydronephrosis. *J Urol* 1992; 148:525-531.

Lyon RP, Marshall SK, Scott MP: Treatment of vesicoureteral reflux: point system based on twenty years of experience. *Urology* 1980; 16:38-46.

Mandell MD et al: Current concepts in the perinatal diagnosis and management of hydronephrosis. *Urol Clin North Am* 1990; 17:247-261.

Mann CM Jr, Ellis DG: *Ureteropelvic junction obstruction.* In: Ashcraft KW, Holder TM (eds): *Pediatric surgery,* WB Saunders, Philadelphia, pp. 582-587, 1993.

Patten RM, Mack LA, Wang KY et al: The fetal genitourinary tract. *Radiol Clin North Am* 1990; 28:115-130.

Persutte W, Lenke RR: Ultrasonographic standards for measuring renal collecting system dilation. *Am J Obstet Gynecol* 1992; 167:858-860.

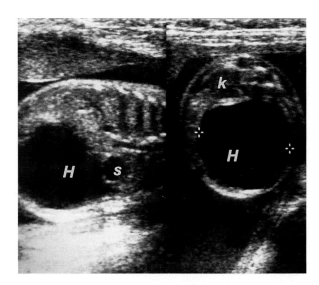

Severe renal pelvic dilatation due to ureteropelvic junction obstruction (*between x's*). The dilatation is so severe that all calyces have been effaced. There was polyhydramnios.

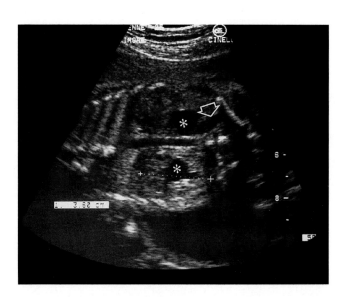

Urinoma due to hydronephrosis (*U*). The kidney (*right K*) is displaced anteriorly by the urinoma. The normal kidney (*left K*) can be seen lateral to the spine.

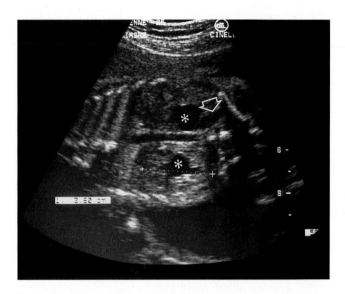

Renal pelvic dilation (*) due to reflux. Calyces arising from the renal pelvis are dilated, consistent with grade 3, and both ureters can be seen (*arrow*). The ureters varied in size during the real-time study.

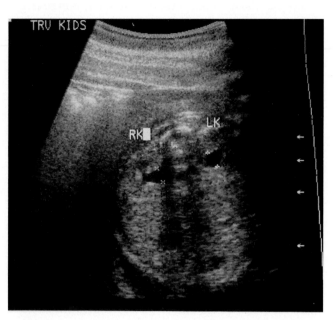

Mild bilateral renal pelvic dilatation to 6 mm (*x's*). This form of mild renal pelvic dilatation has an excellent prognosis and is usually without long-term consequences. There is a low-grade association with Down syndrome.

4.4 INFANTILE POLYCYSTIC KIDNEY DISEASE

EPIDEMIOLOGY/GENETICS

Definition   An autosomal recessive genetic disorder characterized by the replacement of normal renal tissue with dilated collecting tubules, resulting in symmetric renal enlargement and renal failure.

Epidemiology   1 out of 20,000 to 50,000 births (M1:F1).

Embryology   Infantile polycystic kidney disease (IPKD) causes both renal and hepatic cysts. The pathophysiology and genetic defects in this condition are unknown.

Inheritance Patterns   Autosomal recessive. Whereas the gene for IPKD has not been localized, the gene for autosomal dominant adult polycystic disease (APKD) has been mapped and DNA diagnosis is available.

Teratogens   None.

Prognosis   Many fetuses with IPKD, diagnosed in utero, will be stillborn. Only a rare patient survives the first year of life, when the condition is diagnosed in utero. Of these, about 50% will reach adolescence and all will ultimately need renal transplantation.

SONOGRAPHY

Findings
1.   **Fetus:** Both kidneys are large and well above the 90th percentile for length. The renal parenchyma is very echogenic, particularly in the medullary areas. No cysts are visible in most cases. The cortex may be less echogenic. The bladder size is small, but some urine will be present. The liver appearances are normal, despite the presence of cysts and fibrosis.
2.   **Amniotic Fluid:** Oligohydramnios is often severe, but fluid volume can be normal.
3.   **Placenta:** Normal.
4.   **Measurement Data:** A large abdominal circumference measurement is due to the massive kidney enlargement. Remaining fetal measurements are normal or small.
5.   **When Detectable:** Oligohydramnios does not develop until 15 to 18 weeks at the earliest. Kidney findings may not develop until the late second or third trimester, but have been seen at 18 weeks.

Differential Diagnosis
1.   Meckel-Gruber syndrome (look for polydactyly and encephalocele). Renal cysts in this condition are visible.
2.   Benign glomerulosclerosis—large echogenic kidneys, but pyramids are echopenic and the amniotic fluid is normal or mildly increased.
3.   APKD—Large kidneys that may not be symmetrically enlarged. Cysts may be visible and the kidneys are often echogenic. A positive family history can be obtained. An sonographic appearance identical to IPKD can be seen.
4.   Trisomy 13—The kidneys may be slightly enlarged and are echogenic with cysts. Numerous other pathological findings, such as holoprosencephaly, will be seen.

Where Else to Look
1.   Look at paternal and maternal kidneys to exclude APKD.
2.   Look at the feet and hands for polydactyly and the skull for encephalocele (Meckel-Gruber).
3.   Look for stigma of trisomy 13.
4.   Look at the cervix to exclude premature rupture of membranes as a cause of oligohydramnios.

PREGNANCY MANAGEMENT

Investigations and Consultations Required   If there is no family history of IPKD the following investigations are appropriate.
1.   Chromosome evaluation.
2.   Fetal echocardiography, to exclude other conditions that present with polycystic kidneys (trisomy 13 and Meckel-Gruber syndrome).
3.   Consultation with a pediatric nephrologist should be arranged to develop a management plan and to discuss the implication of this diagnosis with the family.

Monitoring   In recurrent cases or new cases with oligohydramnios, fetal assessment/monitoring is contraindicated. There should be no electronic monitoring in labor.

Pregnancy Course   Most cases will develop oligohydramnios by the third trimester.

Pregnancy Termination Issues   A precise pathologic diagnosis is essential for counseling the family regarding the risk of recurrence. An intact fetus should be delivered for complete external and internal examination.

Delivery   Unless a precise diagnosis has been established prenatally (cases with a previous affected child), delivery should occur at a tertiary center where an immediate evaluation can be performed to establish a diagnosis and to determine prognosis. Dystocia from extremely large abdominal circumference may be an indication for elective cesarean section, in very rare cases.

NEONATOLOGY

Resuscitation   Infants may present with respiratory distress at delivery, either from oligohydramnios leading to pulmonary hypoplasia or from severe abdominal distension from renal enlargement. Use positive pressure ventilation with caution, as pneumothorax is a high risk situation.

A decision to withhold resuscitation should be considered when a prenatal diagnosis of a lethal entity is certain. If limited renal function is possible, but not certain, initial support is indicated until the prognosis can be determined.

Transport   Indicated for full confirmation of diagnosis and prognosis, if an infant demonstrates survival potential initially.

Testing and Confirmation   Ninety percent of IPKD patients present with bilateral abdominal masses at birth. Careful, staged evaluation of renal function and structure by urine production, urinalysis, blood and urine chemistries, and an abdominal sonogram is appropriate. If the infant is minimally symptomatic, imaging can be delayed for 24 to 36 hours for better visualization. If the anatomy is not clearly defined prenatally, ultrasound imaging should be obtained immediately. Subsequent procedures may be necessary to define renal function and survival potential (e.g., renal scan with and without diuretic stimulation).

Nursery Management   Support respiration as necessary to maintain adequate gas exchange. Avoid fluid and protein loading initially until renal function has been determined.

BIBLIOGRAPHY

Bernstein J, Slovis TJ: *Polycystic diseases of the kidney*. In: Edelmann CM Jr (ed): *Pediatric kidney disease*. Boston. Little, Brown, 1992. p. 1139.

Fong KW Rahmani MR, Rose TH et al: Fetal renal cystic disease: sonographic-pathologic correlation. *Am J Roentgenol* 1986; 146:767-773.

Gillerot Y, Koulischer L: Major malformations of the urinary tract. Anatomic and genetic aspects. *Biol Neonate* 1988; 53:186-196.

Kaplan BS, Fay J, Shah V et al: Autosomal recessive polycystic kidney disease. *Pediatr Nephrol* 1989; 3:43-49.

Mahony BS, Callen PW, Filly RA et al: Progression of infantile polycystic kidney disease in early pregnancy. *J Ultrasound Med* 1984; 3:277-279.

Pretorius DH, Lee ME, Manco-Johnson ML et al: Diagnosis of autosomal dominant polycystic kidney disease in utero and in the young infant. *J Ultrasound Med* 1987; 6:249-255.

Reuss A, Wladimiroff JW, Niermeyer MF: Sonographic, clinical and genetic aspects of prenatal diagnosis of cystic kidney disease. *Ultrasound Med Biol* 1991; 17:687-694.

Romero R, Cullen M, Jeanty P et al: The diagnosis of congenital renal anomalies with ultrasound. II. Infantile polycystic disease. *Am J Obstet Gynecol* 1984; 150:259-262.

Zerres K, Volpel MC, Weiss H: Cystic kidneys: genetics, pathologic anatomy, clinical picture and prenatal diagnosis. *Hum Genet* 1984; 68:104-135.

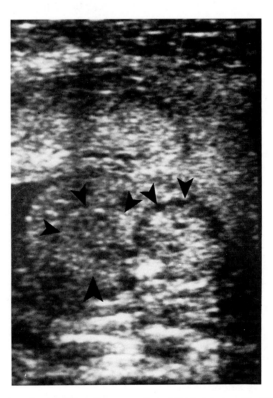

Infantile polycystic kidney. Transverse view of fetal abdomen. The kidneys (*arrowheads*) have almost the same echogenicity as the remainder of the abdomen. Notice that they occupy more than half of the anteroposterior diameter of the abdomen.

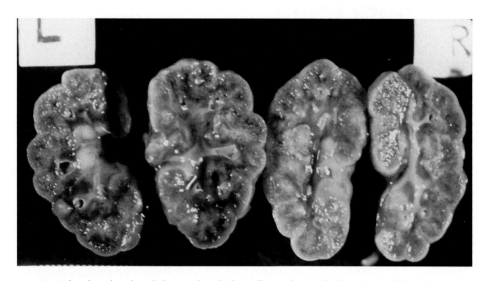

Massively enlarged newborn kidneys with multiple small cysts due to infantile polycystic kidney disease.

4.5 MULTICYSTIC DYSPLASTIC KIDNEY

EPIDEMIOLOGY/GENETICS

Definition   Multicystic dysplastic kidney is a congenital dysplasia of the kidneys that is characterized by large nonhomogeneous dilations of the collecting tubules. It may occur unilaterally or bilaterally.

Epidemiology   1 out of 1,000 to 5,000 births. (M>F). This is the most common cystic renal abnormality noted in the newborn.

Embryology   Multicystic dysplastic kidney disease is a renal abnormality with severely disorganized tubules, glomeruli, ducts, and cortical cystic lesions of the collecting tubules. Although the pathogenesis is unknown, it is thought to be due to an early error in development of the mesonephric blastema or early obstructive uropathy. Ninety percent of cases are associated with urinary obstruction or other renal abnormalities. Eighty percent of cases are unilateral. Associated nonrenal malformations include anencephaly, hydrocephalus, spina bifida, cleft palate, microphthalmia, duodenal stenosis, tracheoesophageal fistula, and imperforate anus. Over 35 genetic, chromosomal, and sporadic syndromes have been described with dysplastic kidneys.

Inheritance Patterns   As an isolated abnormality, it is usually sporadic, but families with autosomal dominant inheritance have been described whose defects range from bilateral renal agenesis to double ureter, renal cysts, or hydronephrosis. It can occur as part of the Meckel-Gruber syndrome (autosomal recessive [AR]), short rib polydactyly syndromes (AR), the Zellweger syndrome (AR), Roberts' syndrome (AR), Fryn's syndrome (AR), the Smith-Lemli-Opitz syndrome (AR), Apert's syndrome (autosomal dominant [AD]), and the brachio-oto-renal syndrome (AD).

Teratogens   Maternal diabetes.

Prognosis   Unilateral and isolated abnormalities may be asymptomatic and go undetected. Unilateral multicystic kidney disease spontaneously regresses with time and by age 2 the mass has often disappeared. Alternatively, a small bag of cysts with a calcified rim is seen at the site where the kidney lay. Bilateral severe defects are lethal. Partial dysplastic involvement of both kidneys leads eventually to renal function impairment.

SONOGRAPHY

Findings
1. **Fetus**
   a. Cysts—There are multiple varied size cysts that start at the periphery of the kidney. Initially, they are small, but they enlarge with time and may develop in the renal hilum. Eventually, the cysts will start to decrease in size, but this may not be until after birth.
   b. Parenchymal echogenicity—Echogenic renal parenchyma may lie between the cysts. In early cases, echogenic parenchyma is the initial feature. Some normal, or partially normal, renal parenchyma may be interspersed with echogenic dysplastic areas.
   c. Kidney size—The overall kidney mass may be too small or too large. Large kidneys filled with large cysts occur when dysplastic kidney is due to a high (UPJ) obstruction. More distal obstructions, for example, posterior urethral valve, result in small dysplastic kidneys with few and small cysts.
   d. Bilateral—Bilateral multicystic kidneys may occur. The bladder may contain urine even if the condition is bilateral, because decreased renal function worsens progressively.
   e. Contralateral kidney—Compensatory hypertrophy and enlargement of the contralateral kidney will occur if the condition is unilateral. Mild hydronephrosis of the contralateral kidney is common.
2. **Amniotic Fluid:** If bilateral, there will be no amniotic fluid after 15 to 18 weeks. If unilateral, amniotic fluid volume will be normal.
3. **Placenta:** Normal.
4. **Measurement Data:** There may be a large abdominal circumference due to the kidney mass that can impede delivery with very large multicystic kidneys.
5. **When Detectable:** Usually first detectable at 15 to 20 weeks. There is progressive enlargement of the cysts as pregnancy continues.

Pitfalls   Echogenic parenchyma may occur normally. In the absence of cysts, distinguishing a dysplastic kidney from normal, on the basis of coarse texture and increased echogenicity, is difficult and ultrasound system-dependent. This is particularly a problem with posterior urethral valve kidneys.

Differential Diagnosis
1. APKD—The cysts are randomly distributed, instead of being grouped at the periphery as they are in early multicystic dysplastic kidney.
2. Meckel-Gruber syndrome—The cysts are all the same size, are relatively small, and are scattered throughout the kidney.
3. IPKD—As a rule, no cysts are visible and the kidneys are greatly enlarged.
4. Trisomy 13 kidneys—The kidneys are enlarged and echogenic. Randomly dispersed small cysts are present.
5. Severe hydronephrosis with no remaining parenchyma—This entity may be indistinguishable from the hydronephrotic form of multicystic kidney.

Where Else to Look Parents should have a renal ultrasound to look for unilateral renal agenesis or other renal abnormalities that may suggest AD inheritance. Look for stigmata of chromosomal disorders.

PREGNANCY MANAGEMENT

Investigations and Consultations Required The incidence of chromosome abnormalities is quite low in isolated unilateral multicystic dysplastic kidney (MCDK), but amniocentesis should be performed to exclude this possibility before establishing a management plan. Fetal echocardiography should be performed to rule out an associated heart defect. A pediatric urologist should be consulted to discuss the neonatal evaluation and management of unilateral MCDK with the family. The presence of bilateral MCDK is a lethal condition and a neonatologist should be consulted to assist in the development of a noninterventional perinatal management plan.

Fetal Intervention There is an increased incidence of contralateral renal malformation when unilateral MCDK is present. If UPJ obstruction is present in the opposite kidney, it is possible that either early delivery or in utero placement of a shunt may be necessary, in rare cases.

Monitoring No changes in obstetric management should be necessary for unilateral MCDK. Monthly ultrasound examinations should be performed to monitor the status of the normal kidney. In bilateral MCDK no intervention for fetal indications should be performed. Electronic fetal monitoring in labor is contraindicated once this diagnosis has been established.

Pregnancy Course No specific obstetric complications are to be expected.

Pregnancy Termination Issues Pathologic confirmation is essential because of the similar sonographic appearance of MCDK and other forms of renal dysplasia, especially the infantile presentation of APKD. Termination should be done by a nondestructive procedure, unless done in an institution with special expertise in suction evacuation and retrieval of the fetal organs.

Delivery For unilateral disease, no special considerations for delivery are necessary. In cases of bilateral MCDK, the site should be one where the staff is comfortable with a noninterventional approach to labor management.

NEONATOLOGY

Resuscitation With bilateral MCDK, respiratory distress is usually present from delivery secondary to pulmonary hypoplasia with significant oligohydramnios. Use positive pressure ventilation cautiously when pulmonary hypoplasia is suspected because of the high risk for pneumothorax. Onset of effective respiration may be impeded by abdominal distension from renal enlargement, particularly with bilateral involvement.

A decision to withhold resuscitation should be considered when prenatal diagnosis of a lethal prognosis is certain as with bilateral involvement and severe oligohydramnios. If limited renal function is possible, but not certain, initial support is indicated until the prognosis can be determined.

Transport Indicated for bilateral lesions for full confirmation of diagnosis if the infant demonstrates survival potential after resuscitation. Infants with isolated unilateral lesions and normal renal function, as indicated by serum creatinine, can be referred for outpatient evaluation and management.

Testing and Confirmation Careful, staged evaluation of renal function and structure by urine production, urinalysis, blood and urine chemistries, and an abdominal sonogram is recommended. If the infant is minimally symptomatic, imaging can be delayed for 24 to 36 hours for better visualization. If the anatomy is not clearly defined prenatally, ultrasound imaging should be obtained immediately. Subsequent procedures may be needed to further delineate renal function (i.e., renal scan with and without diuretic stimulation).

Nursery Management Support respiration as necessary to maintain adequate gas exchange. Avoid fluid and protein loading initially until renal function has been determined.

With adequate upper tract development (ureters) renal transplant may be possible in early childhood for bilateral lesions with limited function at birth.

BIBLIOGRAPHY

Avni EF, Thoua Y, Lalmand B et al: Multicystic dysplastic kidney: evolving concepts. In utero diagnosis and post-natal follow-up by ultrasound. *Ann Radiol* 1986; 29:663-668.

Bernstein J: *Renal hypoplasia and dysplasia*. In: Edelmann CM Jr (ed): *Pediatric kidney disease*. Boston. Little, Brown, 1992. p. 1121.

D'Alton M, Romero R, Grannum P et al: Antenatal diagnosis of renal anomalies with ultrasound. IV. bilateral multicystic kidney disease. *Am J Obstet Gynecol* 1986; 154:532-537.

Gillerot Y, Koulischer L: Major malformations of the urinary tract. anatomic and genetic aspects. *Biol Neonate* 1988; 53:186-196.

Hashimoto BE, Filly RA, Callen PW: Multicystic dysplastic kidney in utero: changing appearance on ultrasound. *Radiology* 1986; 159:107-109.

Kleiner B, Filly RA, Mack L et al: Multicystic dysplastic kidney: observations of the contralateral disease in the fetal population. *Radiology* 1986; 161:27-29.

Sanders RC, Nussbaum AR, Solez K: Renal dysplasia: sonographic findings. *Radiology* 1988; 167: 623-626.

Wackman J et al: Report of multicystic kidney registry: preliminary findings. *J Urol* 1993; 150:1870-1872.

Zerres K, Volpel MC, Weiss H: Cystic kidneys: Genetics, pathologic anatomy, clinical picture and prenatal diagnosis. *Hum Genet* 1984; 68:104-135.

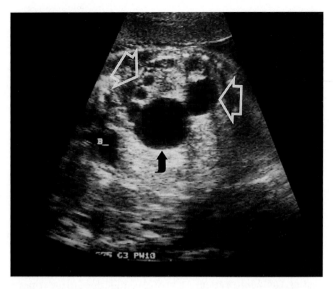

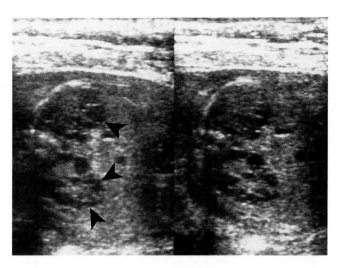

Unilateral multicystic dysplastic kidney disease. Some of the kidney mass (*between the black and white arrows*) is occupied by cysts of varying sizes. The echogenic area elsewhere within the kidney is filled with tiny cysts. These cysts are too small for the ultrasound system to show the individual cysts, but large enough to cause echoes.

Bilateral multicystic kidney disease. There is no amniotic fluid. Both kidneys (*arrows*) have multiple small cysts around the periphery in a typical location. As the disease progresses, these cysts will enlarge and apparently lie more in the center.

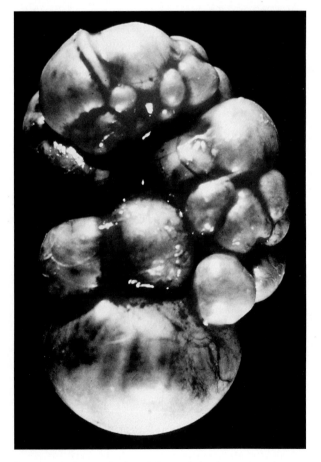

Left newborn multicystic dysplastic kidney with abundant cysts varying in size.

4.6 OVARIAN CYSTS

EPIDEMIOLOGY/GENETICS

Definition   Ovarian cysts are fluid-filled ovarian tumors.

Epidemiology   Unknown. Although ovarian cysts are rarely detected in infants, they are slightly more common on fetal ultrasound (M0:F1).

Embryology   Almost all ovarian cysts are benign corpus luteal cysts of germinal or graafian tissue origin. The fetal ovaries respond to maternal hormonal stimulus.

Inheritance Patterns   Most cases are sporadic, except for very rare genetic syndromes like the McKusick-Kaufman syndrome (AR) with congenital heart disease, polydactyly and hydrometrocolpos.

Teratogens   None.

Prognosis   Generally excellent. Most spontaneously resolve without postnatal treatment. Very large cysts can cause lethal complications like ovarian torsion and bleeding.

SONOGRAPHY

Findings
1.   **Fetus:** A cyst is present in the fetal abdomen in the mesentery, not related to the kidneys or gut. This entity only occurs in females. The cysts are usually echo-free, but if torsed, may contain internal echoes or a crescent-shaped mass. On rare occasions, very large cysts may cause gut obstruction. Because the broad ligament in utero is very stretchable, they can be located anywhere in the abdomen.
2.   **Amniotic Fluid:** Normal, unless there is gut obstruction in which case polyhydramnios may develop.
3.   **Placenta:** Normal.
4.   **Measurement Data:** Normal.
5.   **When Detectable:** Ovarian cysts do not develop before about 23 weeks as they are related to maternal hormonal influence on the maturing fetal ovaries.

Pitfalls
1.   An extrarenal pelvis with a UPJ can appear intramesenteric.
2.   Ovarian cysts can lie in the upper abdomen because all fetal ligaments are so weak.

Differential Diagnosis
1.   Duplication cysts are usually associated with gut dilatation and may occur in males.
2.   A mesenteric cyst may have a similar appearance to an ovarian cyst, but is less common and may occur in males.

3.   Liver cysts appear on the right and are related to the liver.
4.   A choledochal cyst is related to, and partially within, the right lobe of the liver. A dilated bile duct entering a choledochal cyst is often seen.

Where Else to Look   Make sure the fetus is a female.

PREGNANCY MANAGEMENT

Investigations and Consultations Required   Because the diagnosis is often one of exclusion, chromosome studies and fetal echocardiography may be appropriate before making this presumptive diagnosis. Pediatric surgical consultations should be obtained in the event that neonatal complications require surgical intervention.

Fetal Intervention   None. Aspiration of the cysts is contraindicated because of the high incidence of spontaneous resolution, the significant risk of misdiagnosis, and the theoretical concerns of spillage of an irritant (contents of a dermoid cyst) or malignant cells into the peritoneal cavity.

Monitoring   No alterations in obstetric care are necessary. Those cases complicated by polyhydramnios should be monitored for evidence of preterm labor. Follow-up at monthly intervals, with sonography, to check for ovarian cyst size, polyhydramnios, and gut dilatation, is helpful.

Pregnancy Course   Polyhydramnios may develop secondary to extrinsic bowel obstruction.

Pregnancy Termination Issues   Termination of pregnancy is not indicated if major associated malformations have been excluded.

Delivery   In rare instances of large cysts that could result in dystocia, cesarean section may be indicated.

NEONATOLOGY

Resuscitation   Rarely is there an issue with the onset of respiration. Giant-sized cysts may create such severe abdominal distension that they inhibit efficient breathing.

Transport   Neonatal transport to a tertiary facility with a pediatric surgeon is always indicated for an abdominal mass in the female infant.

Testing and Confirmation   Obtain an abdominal ultrasound to confirm the prenatal diagnosis. Additional contrast studies of the gastrointestinal (GI) and urinary tracts may be necessary for a very large mass.

Nursery Management   Support respiration mechanically if abdominal distension is severe.

SURGERY

Preoperative Assessment   Repeat postnatal sonography is indicated to determine if the cyst is still present, as well as its characteristics.

Operative Indications

1. Cyst greater than 6 cm in diameter
2. Evidence of hemorrhage or torsion
3. Failure of regression after several months' observation or obstruction of alimentary or genitourinary tracts.

Types of Procedures   If the mass is uniformly echogenic (i.e., no "layering" or loculations of cyst contents), and it is relatively small, less than 6 cm in a full-term infant, then it can be observed for spontaneous resolution. Repeat sonography at monthly intervals will allow appropriate monitoring. If the cyst enlarges or signs of GI or urinary tract obstruction appear, then excision should be performed.

Careful dissection during surgical excision will frequently result in preservation of all or a part of the ovary. Careful preservation of both ovary and fallopian tube vascularity is imperative. A multiloculated or layered ovarian cyst should encourage an abdominal exploration because this is a frequent finding with an intrauterine torsed ovary or ovarian necrosis. Early removal of the dead tissue prevents subsequent sepsis.

The fallopian tube can be involved and also requires excision. Pexis of the contralateral ovary is a controversial addition to the procedure.

Surgical Results/Prognosis   Excellent prognosis. Future reproduction is facilitated by retention of the involved ovary but sterility is not a significant problem even if the ipsilateral ovary is removed.

BIBLIOGRAPHY

Adelman S, Benson CD, Hertzler JH: Surgical lesions of the ovary in infancy and childhood. *Surg Gynecol Obstet* 1975; 141:219-226.

Ikeda K, Suita S, Nakano H: Management of ovarian cyst detected antenatally. *J Pediatr Surg* 1988; 23:432-435.

Jafri SZ, Bree RL, Silver TM et al: Fetal ovarian cysts: sonographic detection and association with hypothyroidism. *Radiology* 1984; 150:809-812.

Nicolaides KH, Campbell S: Ultrasound diagnosis of congenital abnormalities. In: Harrison MR, Golbus MS, Filly RA (eds): *The unborn patient, antenatal diagnosis and treatment.* Philadelphia. WB Saunders, 1991. p 595-648.

Nussbaum AR, Sanders RC, Benator RM et al: Spontaneous resolution of neonatal ovarian cysts. *Am J Roentgenol* 1987; 148:175-176.

Nussbaum AR, Sanders RC, Hartman DS et al: Neonatal ovarian cysts: sonographic-pathologic correlation. *Radiology* 1988; 168:817-821.

Patten RM: The fetal genitourinary tract. *Radiol Clin North Am* 1990; 28:115-130.

Rizzo N, Gabrielli S, Perolo A et al: Prenatal diagnosis and management of fetal ovarian cysts. *Prenat Diagn* 1989; 9:97-103.

Woo JS, Li DF, Wan MC et al: Intrauterine cystocentesis: a simple procedure to relieve anatomic and physiologic dysfunction in the fetus. *J Clin Ultrasound* 1986; 14:474-477.

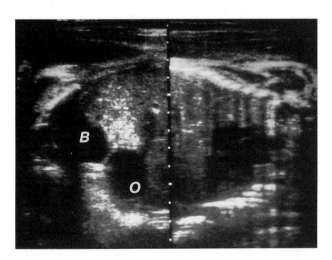

Coronal view of a female fetus with a cystic mass in the abdomen. Adjacent to the bladder (*B*) is a cyst (*O*). This echo-free cyst was treated conservatively after birth and disappeared spontaneously.

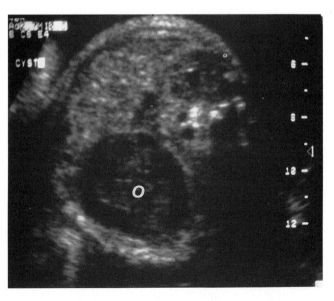

Transverse view of a fetus with a cyst (*O*) anterior to the kidney. This cyst contains echogenic material. The fetus was a female and long-term follow-up failed to show any resolution of the cyst, which, at surgery, proved to be a torsed ovarian cyst.

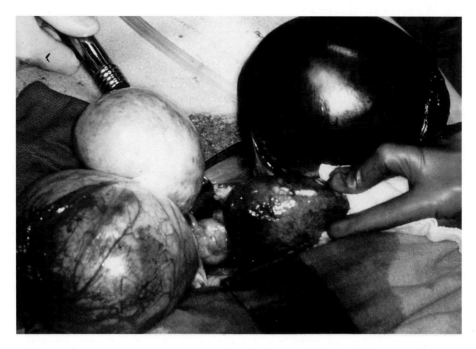

Newborn girl with massive ovarian bilateral cysts. Cyst on right side had torsion of the stalk and hemorrhagic necrosis.

4.7 POSTERIOR URETHRAL VALVES

EPIDEMIOLOGY/GENETICS

Definition   Membrane-like valvular structures in the posterior urethra in a male infant that can result in urinary tract obstruction.

Epidemiology   Undetermined, but rare. Unknown in females.

Embryology   Posterior urethral valves (PUV) are structures that normally develop in the prostatic urethra between 6 and 8 weeks of gestation. Hypertrophy of these valves causes proximal urethral distention, a thick-walled distended bladder, reflux, and hydronephrosis. Chromosome abnormalities, including trisomies 13, 18, and 21, have been reported in up to 20% of cases.

Inheritance Patterns   Sporadic. Rare reports of familial recurrence.

Teratogens   None.

Prognosis   The prognosis is dependent on renal function. Whereas the overall mortality rate for antenatally diagnosed cases is 50%, it is 95% for those cases with oligohydramnios. Forty percent of neonatal survivors develop chronic renal failure.

SONOGRAPHY

Findings
1.   **Fetus:** Only males are affected. There is a dilated, thick-walled bladder with "keyhole" posterior urethral expansion. There are three sonographic forms:
   a. The bladder occupies the entire abdomen and pushes up the diaphragm. The renal pelves may be only slightly distended. Signs of dysplastic kidney may be seen with echogenic parenchyma and possibly small cysts. No amniotic fluid is usual with this lethal form.
   b. Ascites may be present without other features of hydrops. With this form, the bladder may not be greatly enlarged because it may have burst. There is usually moderate ureteropelvicalyceal dilatation, sometimes with findings of dysplasia. No amniotic fluid is usual with this form.
   c. Moderate bladder dilatation with dilated pelvicalyceal systems and tortuous ureters is the most common form. Obvious dysplastic changes (echogenic renal parenchyma with peripherally placed cysts) indicate a hopeless prognosis.
2.   **Amniotic Fluid:** As the disease progresses, amniotic fluid decreases. No fluid is almost always associated with pulmonary hypoplasia.
3.   **Placenta:** Normal.

4.   **Measurement Data:** A large abdomen, due to kidney enlargement and ascites, may be seen.
5.   **When Detectable:** Posterior urethral valves have been detected as early as 11 weeks using the vaginal probe. The disease usually presents at 18 to 22 weeks.

Pitfalls
1.   Bilateral ureteropelvic junction obstruction or fullness with "full" bladder. The fetal bladder may not empty until the baby is born. This is a normal variant.
2.   Be very cautious in the diagnosis of dysplasia if there are no cysts present. It is easy to overdiagnose echogenic parenchyma.
3.   Dilated renal pelves, ureters, and a thick-walled bladder with a "keyhole" notch may not relate to current obstruction. It is possible that urethral valves may have burst and left secondary obstructive consequences. This situation may be the origin of the Eagle-Barrett (prune-belly) syndrome.

Differential Diagnosis
1.   Megacystis megaureter syndrome—also most often seen in males. This process is due to severe reflux. The bladder is enlarged, but thin-walled with no keyhole urethra. The renal pelves vary in size and the ureter shows much peristalsis.
2.   Megacystis microcolon syndrome—similar appearances to posterior urethral valves, but polyhydramnios occurs. This very rare entity is more frequent in females.

Where Else to Look   Look for signs of trisomy 13, 18, and 21.

PREGNANCY MANAGEMENT

Investigations and Consultations Required   Chromosome abnormalities are found in up to 20% of cases. Therefore, fetal karyotyping is essential. Fetal echocardiography should be performed to exclude associated heart defects. Pediatric urologic consultation is required to plan prenatal management.

Fetal Intervention   Significant experience has been gained in this area. Generally, no intervention is appropriate if amniotic fluid volume remains normal. In pregnancies of 32 weeks' gestation or greater, decreasing amniotic fluid volume should prompt early delivery for ex utero drainage. In cases less than 32 weeks' gestation, assessment of fetal renal function, by aspiration of bladder urine, should be performed. The analysis of urinary sodium, chloride, osmolality, and beta 2 microglobulin should be done on "fresh" urine. An initial drainage of the fetal bladder should be followed in 3 to 7 days by a repeat aspiration. The criteria outlined by Crombleholme et al should be used to ascertain those fetuses with a "good prognosis" who may benefit from intervention, either by catheter drainage or open fetal surgery.

Monitoring Ultrasound evaluation every 2 to 3 weeks should be performed to monitor amniotic fluid volume.

Pregnancy Course Many examples of posterior urethral valves are recognizable as being so severe that the fetus cannot survive when the first sonogram is performed. In others a steady reduction in amniotic fluid with the development of dysplastic kidneys makes it apparent that the condition is lethal. In yet others apparently normal kidneys with decreasing amniotic fluid compel drainage or early delivery. In some the condition is mild and amniotic fluid volume is maintained.

Pregnancy Termination Issues Confirmation of the sonographic diagnosis should be done and requires pathologic examination of the intact fetus.

Delivery The need for immediate neonatal evaluation and treatment and the potential for respiratory complications in cases with oligohydramnios require that delivery occur in a tertiary center.

NEONATOLOGY

Resuscitation Respiratory distress is usually present secondary to pulmonary hypoplasia in infants with significant oligohydramnios. Positive pressure ventilation should be used cautiously when pulmonary hypoplasia is suspected because of high risk for pneumothorax. Onset of effective respiration may be impeded from abdominal distension secondary to bladder enlargement as well as renal enlargement.

Transport Indicated for full confirmation of diagnosis and prognosis if infant demonstrates survival potential.

Testing and Confirmation Neonatal presentation depends on the severity and timing of the urethral obstruction. Very early and severe obstruction causes an oligohydramnios sequence with pulmonary hypoplasia and death. Severe early obstruction, that is later relieved, may cause a "prune belly." Milder or later obstruction is compatible with survival to birth. Presentations in the newborn period and early infancy include decreased urinary stream (25%), distended bladder (67%), urinary infection (50%), abdominal distension (30%), renal failure (33%), palpable kidneys (50%), and failure to thrive (50%).

Careful evaluation of renal function and structure by urine production, urinalysis, blood and urine chemistries, and an abdominal sonogram is appropriate. Voiding cystourethrogram, cystoscopy, and renal scan with and without diuretic stimulation may also be useful in confirming the diagnosis and in assessing renal function.

Nursery Management Support respiration, as necessary, to maintain adequate gas exchange. Avoid fluid and protein loading initially until urinary tract patency and renal function have been determined.

SURGERY

Preoperative Assessment See Testing and Confirmation in opposite column.

Operative Indications Surgical management is based on adequate resuscitation of the patient and decompression of the chronically obstructed bilateral upper urinary tracts and bladder. If the urethra is patent, early temporary catheter drainage is feasible. Surgical repair is needed for bladder and upper tract decompression with prevention of further renal parenchymal damage.

Types of Procedures Drainage is best accomplished by vesicostomy, temporary loop cutaneous ureterostomies, or pyelostomy. These procedures are usually planned dependent upon the degree of lung hypoplasia and potential for pulmonary function. Milder forms of PUV can be successfully treated by transurethral or open vesicostomy repair of the lesion.

Surgical Results/Prognosis The degree of renal function is difficult to determine by radiographic contrast examination and is best assessed by nuclear renal scan technique. Potential renal function may appear to be insufficient, but early poor function can improve significantly after adequate decompression. Some patients have borderline renal function that becomes insufficient with subsequent skeletal growth and the need for dialysis or renal transplantation becomes apparent. Urethral bladder dysfunction, associated with PUV, can have an adverse effect on the success of renal transplantation. Posterior urethral valves can be associated with prune-belly syndrome with marginal early renal function. Incontinence occurs in approximately 14% to 38% of surviving patients.

BIBLIOGRAPHY

Brock WA, Kaplan GW: Abnormalities of the lower tract. In Edelmann CM Jr (ed): *Pediatric kidney disease*. Boston. Little, Brown, 1992. p. 2037.

Clinical outcome of fetal uropathy. I. Predictive value of prenatal echography positive for obstructive uropathy. *J Urol* 1991; 146:1094-1096.

Clinical outcome of fetal uropathy. II. Sensitivity of echography for prenatal detection of obstructive pathology. *J Urol* 1991; 146:1097-1098.

Crombleholme TM, Harrison MR, Golbus MS et al: Fetal intervention in obstructive uropathy: prognostic indicators and efficacy of intervention. *Am J Obstet Gynecol* 1990; 162:1239-1244.

Glazer GM, Filly RA, Callen PW: The varied sonographic appearance of the urinary tract in the fetus and newborn with urethral obstruction. *Radiology* 1982; 144:563-568.

Henneberry MO, Stephens FD: Renal hypoplasia and dysplasia in infants with posterior urethral valves. *J Urol* 1980; 123:912-915.

Hulbert WC, Duckett JW: Current views on posterior urethral valves. *Pediatr Ann* 1988; 17:31-36.

Kaplan CW, Scherg HC: Intravesical obstruction. In Kelalis PP, King LR, Belman BA (eds): *Clinical pediatric urology.* Philadelphia. WB Saunders, 1992 pp. 835-849.

Mahony BS: Fetal urethral obstruction: US evaluation. *Radiology* 1985; 157:221-224.

Meizner I: Prenatal ultrasonic diagnosis of the extreme form of prune belly syndrome. *J Clin Ultrasound* 1985; 13:581-583.

Prune belly syndrome with ultrasound demonstration of reduction of megacystis in utero. *Br J Radiol* 1985; 58:374-376.

Reinburg Y, Gongalez R, Fryd D et al: The outcome of renal transplantation in children with posterior urethral valves. *J Urol* 1988; 140:1491-1493.

Washaw BL et al: Prognostic features in infants with obstructive uropathy due to posterior urethral valves. *J Urol* 1985; 133:240-242.

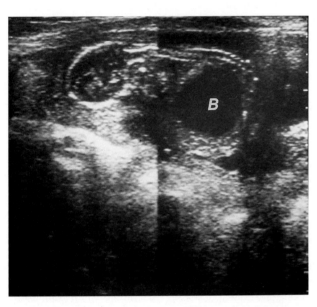

Sagittal view of fetus with a huge bladder (*B*). The bladder is so large it compresses the chest. There is no amniotic fluid present. This type of posterior urethral valves is fatal.

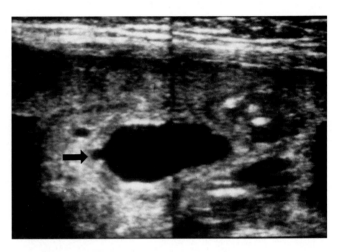

Sagittal view of lower fetal abdomen. There is a dilated bladder with a thick wall. A dilated proximal urethra can be seen, obstructed by posterior urethral valves (*arrow*). The kidneys and ureters were also dilated.

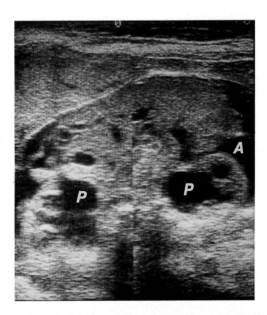

Transverse view of fetal abdomen. Both renal pelves (*P*) are markedly dilated as are the calyces. The renal parenchyma is echogenic. There is fetal ascites (*A*) present within the fetal abdomen. No amniotic fluid is present between the fetal trunk and the placenta. Posterior urethral valves were found at autopsy.

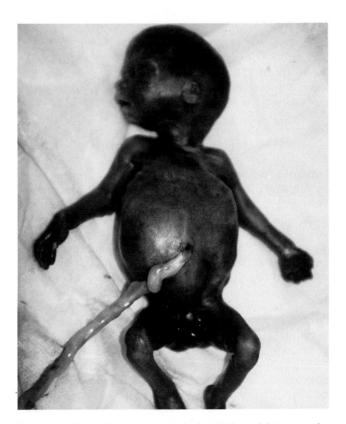

22-week male fetus with posterior urethral valves. Abdominal distension is due to massive hydronephrosis.

4.8 RENAL AGENESIS

EPIDEMIOLOGY/GENETICS

Definition   Bilateral or unilateral absence of the kidneys.

Epidemiology   Unilateral renal agenesis occurs in 1 out of 1000 births (M1:F1), whereas bilateral renal agenesis occurs in 12 out of 100,000 births (M2.5:F1).

Embryology   The pathophysiology of this abnormality is unknown. Some cases of bilateral renal agenesis may represent the severe expression of an autosomal dominant gene the effects of which range from unilateral renal agenesis to double ureter, renal cysts, or hydronephrosis. Renal agenesis is associated with other genitourinary, gastrointestinal, and cardiac abnormalities, and is part of more than 50 multiple malformation syndromes. Two birth defect associations, the vertebral abnormalities, anal atresia, cardiac abnormalities, tracheoesophageal fistula or esophageal atresia, renal agenesis and dysplasia, and limb defects (VACTERL) association and the mullerian duct, renal and cervical somite (MURCS) association, have a high incidence of renal abnormalities, including renal agenesis.

Inheritance Patterns   Generally sporadic. Some cases may represent a highly variable autosomal dominant gene. Parents should have renal ultrasounds looking for unilateral renal agenesis or other renal abnormalities that may suggest autosomal dominant inheritance.

Teratogens   Warfarin, cocaine, and maternal diabetes.

Prognosis   Forty percent of infants with bilateral renal agenesis are stillborn and the remainder die shortly after birth from respiratory or renal insufficiency. Unilateral renal agenesis may be asymptomatic and compatible with a normal life span.

SONOGRAPHY

Findings
1.   **Fetus:** In bilateral renal agenesis, both kidneys are absent and the adrenals assume a discoid shape and move laterally and inferiorly. The bladder is apparently absent or is seen as an echopenic area.
2.   **Amniotic Fluid:** There is no amniotic fluid after 15 to 18 weeks.
3.   **Placenta:** Normal.
4.   **Measurement Data:** Because there are no kidneys, there is a small trunk circumference. Limbs and head measurements are normal. There may be IUGR.
5.   **When Detectable:** 15 to 18 weeks.

Pitfalls
1.   Absence of fluid makes the study difficult.

2.   Confusion between adrenals and hypoplastic kidneys has often occurred because in utero the adrenal glands are about one third the size of the kidneys and have an echogenic center.
3.   With unilateral renal agenesis, make sure a pelvic kidney is not present.

Where Else to Look
1.   Sirenomelia—Fused legs, with femur, tibia, and fibula alongside each other, is associated with renal agenesis.

PREGNANCY MANAGEMENT

Investigations and Consultations Required   Unilateral renal agenesis, if isolated, is not likely to be a marker for chromosome abnormalities. Fetal echocardiography should be performed to exclude associated congenital heart disease. Chromosomal analysis is appropriate for bilateral agenesis because the condition is associated with trisomy 18, but the analysis may best be done if termination is elected. In cases with either unilateral or bilateral renal agenesis, evaluation of parents' kidneys should be done to detect the families with autosomal dominant inheritance.

Fetal Intervention   An amnioinfusion procedure may be helpful in establishing the diagnosis. Dextrose Ringer's solution injection (150 to 250 ml) into the amniotic space will improve fetal visualization and may show renal function. The fetus will start to drink, the stomach will fill, and bladder visualization with ultrasound may occur. Concomitant injection of indigo carmine may allow detection of premature rupture of membranes (PROM). A vaginal tampax will be stained blue. A false positive diagnosis of PROM can occur if solution is placed in the extraamniotic space.

Monitoring   No change in obstetric care is indicated for unilateral renal agenesis. For the pregnancy in which the fetus has bilateral renal agenesis, no further fetal assessment or monitoring is appropriate. Supportive care of the family should be provided.

Pregnancy Course   No specific obstetric complications are to be expected with unilateral lesions.

Pregnancy Termination Issues   Bilateral renal agenesis may be a component of multiple malformation syndromes. Therefore, a complete evaluation of an intact fetus should be done.

Delivery   No special precautions are necessary for the fetus with unilateral disease. For bilateral renal agenesis, vaginal delivery without electronic fetal monitoring in labor is appropriate.

NEONATOLOGY

Resuscitation   The majority of newborns with renal agenesis manifest severe respiratory distress from birth secondary to associated severe pulmonary hypoplasia. Use positive pressure cautiously as the risk for pneumothorax is high. Early cessation of resuscitative efforts should be discussed with the parents prior to delivery as this is a uniformly lethal condition.

Transport   Rarely an issue as survival time is usually limited to hours, even with ventilatory support. In the occasional infant with mixed agenesis/dysplasia the respiratory insufficiency may be adequately controlled with ventilatory assistance. In that circumstance transport is indicated for confirmation of diagnosis and prognosis.

Testing and Confirmation   A postnatal ultrasound will confirm the absence of kidneys.

Nursery Management   Continuing ventilatory support, even with severe respiratory failure, until diagnostic confirmation, determination of associated abnormalities, and parental counselling have been completed, is appropriate. At present, there is no palliative or curative treatment for complete renal agenesis. Prolonged renal dialysis has not been successful.

BIBLIOGRAPHY

Bernstein J: Renal hypoplasis and dysplasia. In: Edelmann CM Jr (ed): *Pediatric kidney disease.* Boston. Little Brown, 1992. p. 1121.

Dubbins PA, Kurtz AB, Wapner RJ et al: Renal agenesis: spectrum of in utero findings. *J Clin Ultrasound* 1981; 9:189-193.

Gillerot Y, Koulischer L: Major malformations of the urinary tract. Anatomic and genetic aspects. *Biol Neonate* 1988; 53:186-196.

Hoffman CK, Filly RA, Callen PW: The "lying down" adrenal sign: a sonographic indicator of renal agenesis or ectopia in fetuses and neonates. *J Ultrasound Med* 1992; 11:533-536.

Potter EL: Bilateral absence of ureters and kidneys: a report of 50 cases. *Obstet Gynecol* 1965; 25:3-12.

Romero R, Cullen M, Grannum P et al: Antenatal diagnosis of renal anomalies with ultrasound. III. bilateral renal agenesis. *Am J Obstet Gynecol* 1985; 151:38-43.

Roodhooft AM, Birnholz JC, Holmes LB: Familial nature of congenital absence and severe dysgenesis of both kidneys. *N Engl J Med* 1984; 310:1341-1345.

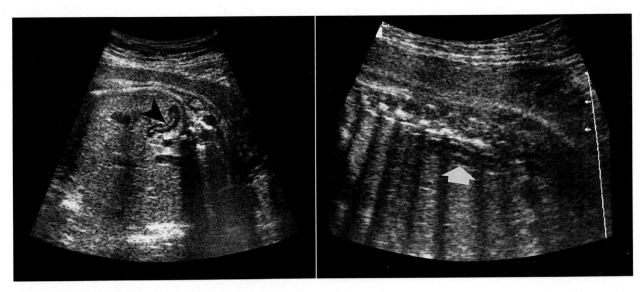

Transverse (*A*) and longitudinal (*B*) views of a sonogram of renal agenesis. There is no amniotic fluid. The adrenal (*arrows*) has assumed a discoid shape and moved laterally. Because, at this stage of life, the adrenal has an echogenic center, it can be mistaken for a small kidney.

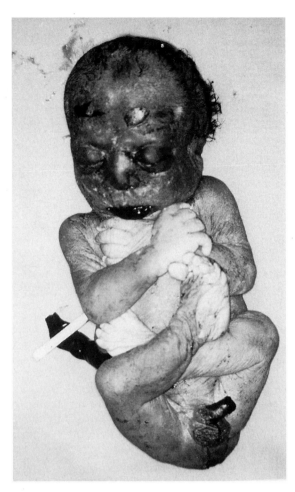

34-week fetus with severe oligohydramnios deformities due to bilateral renal agenesis.

4.9 SACROCOCCYGEAL TERATOMA

EPIDEMIOLOGY/GENETICS

Definition   Teratomas are tumors that are derived from totipotent cells and include embryonic ectodermal, endodermal, and mesodermal tissue derivatives. Commonly gastrointestinal, respiratory, and nervous system tissue elements are present.

Epidemiology   1 out of 40,000 births (M1:F3).

Embryology   Teratomas occur most often in a paraaxial, gonadal, or midline location from the brain to the sacral area. Primary sites in infants and children include sacrococcyx (60%), gonads (20%) and chest and abdomen (15%). Sacrococcygeal teratoma (SCT) are the most common tumors presenting at birth. Forty-seven percent of the tumors are external, 34% external with a significant presacral component, and 19% are predominantly, or completely, presacral.

Inheritance Patterns   Generally sporadic. Rare families with autosomal dominant presacral teratomas and sacral dysgenesis have been reported.

Teratogens   None.

Prognosis   Two thirds of the tumors present in the first 2 months of life, as a perineal mixed solid and cystic mass with only a 10% incidence of malignancy. After 2 months of age, the tumors usually present with bowel or bladder dysfunction and 92% of the tumors are malignant. Calcification occurs in one third of benign tumors. Some patients have associated neural tube defects or genitourinary malformations as a result of tumor distortion of developing structures. Nine percent of patients have nonspecific, noncontiguous associated malformations. The cure rate following complete excision of benign teratomas is 100%, but recurrence with incomplete excision can be as high as 30%. Two thirds of patients with malignant teratomas die within 1 year.

SONOGRAPHY

Findings
1. **Fetus**
   a. There is a mass arising from the distal spine and rump area that may be cystic or solid or a mixture of both. Calcification is often present. There is almost always a large external component and there may be an intrapelvic component. The mass may grow to a huge size; it may be larger than the fetal trunk.
   b. Secondary hydronephrosis and ureterectasis often develop if there is an intrapelvic component. The bladder is elevated by the intrapelvic component. Secondary gut dilatation may also occur.
   c. Considerable arteriovenous shunting occurs through the mass and occasionally there may be secondary hydrops with ascites and skin thickening
2. **Amniotic Fluid:** Severe polyhydramnios is virtually always present and may be the presenting problem.
3. **Placenta:** Normal.
4. **Measurement Data:** Intrauterine growth retardation may develop.
5. **When Detectable:** The mass is usually visible by 18 weeks, but it may present later.

Pitfalls
1. The mass develops first between the legs, so it may be missed when it is small.
2. The teratoma may have a similar texture to a fibroid with which it has been confused.

Differential Diagnosis   Anterior and posterior myelomeningoceles widen the spine, whereas teratomas destroy the spine.

Where Else to Look   Secondary bladder and kidney dilatation, due to obstruction, may occur and may result in renal dysplasia. Arteriovenous shunts within the teratoma may cause heart failure and fetal hydrops.

PREGNANCY MANAGEMENT

Investigations and Consultations Required   No specific associated abnormalities are known, but the high likelihood that intervention may be necessary mandates that other life-threatening abnormalities be excluded. Chromosome analysis and fetal echocardiography should be performed. It should be noted that the amniotic fluid alpha-fetoprotein (AFP) may be elevated and acetylcholinesterase may be present in cases of SCT. Amniotic fluid analysis will not help differentiate SCT from myelomeningocele.

Fetal Intervention   In rare cases, the development of fetal hydrops prior to 32 weeks will raise the issue of in utero tumor resection. Although successful resection has been reported, the benefits of this approach have not been established. Intervention, at this late stage, may not reverse the pathophysiology. At 32 weeks gestation or greater, delivery, when early signs of hydrops are present, may improve prognosis.

Monitoring   Serial ultrasounds every 1 to 4 weeks, depending on the size of the lesion, may be appropriate. Follow: 1) the mass for size increase, which may be very rapid; 2) kidneys and bladder for renal obstruction, which may be severe; 3) gut for evidence of obstruction; 4) fluid for evidence of polyhydramnios, which may be massive; and 5) look for development of hydrops with high output failure.

The presence of polyhydramnios may increase the risk of preterm labor, and regular assessment is necessary.

Pregnancy Course Large lesions with predominantly solid components are associated with an increased risk for fetal hydrops, preeclampsia, and polyhydramnios.

Pregnancy Termination Issues A precise diagnosis is essential for counseling regarding recurrence risk. Therefore, the method of termination should result in an intact fetus for a complete pathologic examination.

Delivery The significant risk of maternal and neonatal complications necessitates delivery in a tertiary center. Because of the significant risk of hemorrhage, moderate (greater than 4.5 cm) and large size lesions should prompt cesarean delivery to avoid dystocia. The section should be performed when fetal lung maturity is present or sooner if early evidence of hydrops is present. There appears to be no benefit from in utero decompression of cystic components of the mass to facilitate vaginal delivery.

NEONATOLOGY

Resuscitation Assistance with onset of respiration is usually not required, unless the infant is premature or fetal hydrops is present. Extreme care must be taken with the tumor mass as tears of surface vessels can result in life-threatening hemorrhage. Support the mass to avoid torsion if there is a "stalk." Cover the mass with a warm, moist sterile dressing to minimize heat and water loss if the surface is thin and membraneous.

Transport Transfer to a tertiary care center is always indicated. Extreme care must be taken to avoid trauma to the mass, insensible water loss, and surface contamination. Reliable venous access should be established and adequate blood pressure documented before beginning transport.

Testing and Confirmation Postnatally an elevated serum AFP is highly correlated with malignancy. Diagnostic evaluation should include imaging (computed tomography [CT] scan or magnetic resonance imaging [MRI]) to determine, preoperatively, the extent of the lesion internally. Bedside sonography may be helpful in outlining the extent of the tumor and its relationship to other pelvic structures and associated involvement of the genitourinary structures.

Nursery Management Maintain thermal balance. Maintain perfusion with volume expanders, packed red blood cells (RBCs), and fluid and electrolytes. Parenteral nutrition may be required for protracted periods if the mass involves the distal alimentary tract or the course is complicated. Systemic antibiotics may be indicated, preoperatively, and, through the early recovery period, after surgical excision.

SURGERY

Preoperative Assessment Acute management includes evaluation of the extent of the intraperitoneal presacral portion of the tumor. Diagnostic studies should include serum levels of alpha-fetoprotein for a possible malignant component and sonography to determine the degree of presacral and intraperitoneal extension. A decision is then made whether or not to use an abdominal approach to obtain control of the primary feeding vessels of the tumor, the middle sacral arteries, before attempting a perineal excision.

The acute preoperative complications of a large SCT are cardiac failure due to arteriovenous shunting in the tumor, renal failure due to bilateral ureteral obstruction, and hemorrhage secondary to intraperitoneal, retroperitoneal, or surface necrotic tumor with bleeding. Delayed excision can also predispose to sepsis because of the necrotic tumor.

Operative Indications Surgical excision is always required, but can be delayed to complete the diagnostic evaluation unless serious hemorrhaging is present.

Types of Procedures Most tumors can be excised from the perineal approach but blood loss can be large and preparations for adequate replacement are essential. Careful dissection and preservation of the thinned gluteal muscles over the tumor, excision of the coccyx, and reconstruction of the levator sling are very important to a good functional outcome. Extension into the dural space is rare, but can occur.

Surgical Results/Prognosis Survival after successful excision is excellent. Intraoperative mortality can approach 5% to 10% depending on tumor and patient size. A malignancy occurs in approximately 10% of the newborn infants with SCTs and can be totally excised in most patients. Secondary operations for retained benign teratoma are uncommon if a total coccygectomy is performed. The malignant germ cell tumors that commonly occur in sacrococcygeal teratomas are usually responsive to new chemotherapy modalities. A major long-term disability is stool and urinary incontinence in patients who have had neurologic impairment due to the pressure of very large sacrococcygeal teratomas. This is as high as 25% in some series.

BIBLIOGRAPHY

Altman RP, Randolph JG, Lilly JR: Sacrococcygeal teratoma: American Academy of Pediatrics surgical section survey— 1973. *J Pediatr Surg* 1974; 9:389-398.

Billmire DF, Grosfeld JL: Teratomas in childhood: analysis of 142 cases. *J Pediatr Surg* 1986; 21:548-551.

Chervenak FA, Isaacson G, Touloukian R et al: Diagnosis and management of fetal teratomas. *Obstet Gynecol* 1985; 66:666-671.

Gross SJ, Benzie RJ, Sermer M et al: Sacrococcygeal teratoma: pre-
    natal diagnosis and management. *Am J Obstet Gynecol* 1987;
    156:393-396.

Holzgreve W, Mahony BS, Glick PL et al: Sonographic demonstra-
    tion of fetal sacrococcygeal teratoma. *Prenat Diagn* 1985;
    5:245-257.

Irving IM: Sacrococcygeal teratoma. In Lister J, Irving IM (eds)
    Neonatal surgery, 3rd ed. London. Butterworths', 1990. pp.
    142-151.

Langer JC, Harrison MR, Schmidt KG et al: Fetal hydrops and
    death from sacrococcygeal teratoma: rationale for fetal surgery.
    Am J Obstet Gynecol 1989; 160:1145-1150.

Lockwood C, Ghidini A, Romero R et al: Fetal bowel perforation
    simulating sacrococcygeal teratoma. *J Ultrasound Med* 1988;
    7:227-229.

Milan DF et al: Urologic manifestations of sacrococcygeal ter-
    atoma. *J Urol* 1993; 149:574-576.

Mintz MC, Mennuti M, Fishman M: Prenatal aspiration of sacro-
    coccygeal teratoma. *Am J Roentgenol* 1983; 141:367-368.

Sheth S, Nussbaum AR, Sanders RC et al: Prenatal diagnosis of
    sacrococcygeal teratoma: sonographic-pathologic correlation.
    Radiology 1988; 169:131-136.

Teal LN, Angtuaco TL, Jimenez JF et al: Fetal teratomas: antenatal
    diagnosis and clinical management. *J Clin Ultrasound* 1988;
    16:329-336.

Woolley MM: Teratomas. In Ashcraft K, Holder T (eds): *Pediatric
    surgery*. Philadelphia. WB Saunders, 1993. pp. 847-862.

Yates VD, Wilroy RS, Whitington GL et al: Anterior sacral defects:
    an autosomal dominantly inherited condition. *J Pediatr* 1983;
    102:239-242.

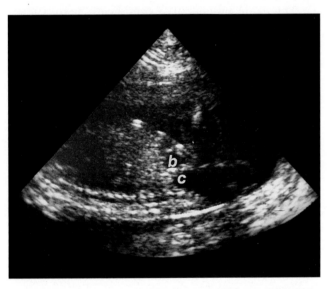

Small mostly cystic teratoma (*c*) elevating the bladder (*b*). Although the baby
was premature, the mass was successfully removed. The child was left with
fecal incontinence.

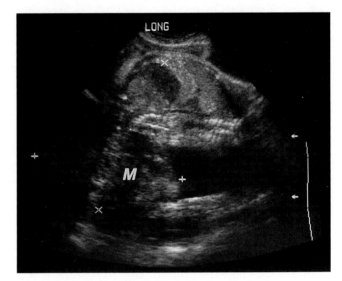

Large sacrococcygeal teratoma with intrapelvic and extraabdominal components (*between x's*). The entire mass (*M*) is solid. The fetus was stillborn and
premature.

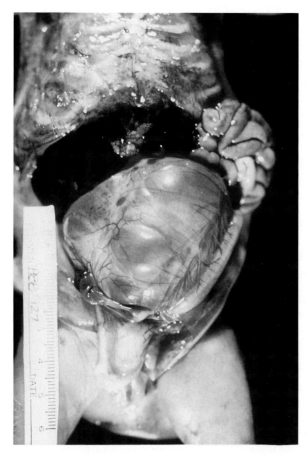

Newborn with large sacrococcygeal teratoma. Photograph shows massive intraabdominal portion of the tumor.

4.10 Ureterocele

EPIDEMIOLOGY/GENETICS

Definition   A ureterocele is a cystic dilatation of the intravesicular portion of the ureter.

Epidemiology   1 out of 5000 births (M1:F5).

Embryology   Ureteroceles are most frequently associated with the upper pole ureter in a duplicated collecting system. The portion of the kidney served by the accessory ureter is usually small and dysplastic, possibly as a result of obstruction. Approximately 10% to 20% of cases are bilateral.

Inheritance Patterns   Sporadic.

Teratogens   None.

Screening   None.

Prognosis   If found as an isolated defect with good renal function, the prognosis for surgical correction is excellent.

SONOGRAPHY

Findings
1. **Fetus**
   a. Kidney—If associated with a double collecting system (75% of cases) there will usually be a dilated upper pole collecting system. The lower pole of the kidneys may well be intermittently dilated due to reflux. With a simple ureterocele, there is unilateral hydronephrosis.
   b. Ureters—Ureteric dilatation is usual. The ureter may be very tortuous and is sometimes the most pronounced feature. The ureters may end alongside the bladder in an ectopic location rather than within the bladder as ureteroceles.
   c. Bladder—A crescent-shaped line will be seen at the base of the bladder. Two semicircles in the bladder are sometimes seen because there are often bilateral ureteroceles. The bladder may be large if the ureterocele interferes with voiding (a windsock ureterocele) and the contralateral renal unit may be secondarily obstructed.
2. **Amniotic Fluid:** Normal, unless renal function is so impaired resulting in oligohydramnios.
3. **Placenta:** Normal.
4. **Measurement Data:** Normal.
5. **When Detectable:** At about 15 weeks.

Pitfalls   The umbilical arteries, as they pass alongside of the bladder, can be mistaken for ureteroceles. Color flow Doppler will show the difference.

Differential Diagnosis
1. Posterior urethral valves—The typical "keyhole" dilated urethra, at the base of the bladder, will be seen.
2. Reflux—The ureters will vary in size. No ureterocele will be seen.

Where Else to Look   If a rectocele is seen in the bladder, look for a second collecting system.

PREGNANCY MANAGEMENT

Investigations and Consultations Required   The diagnosis will be made most commonly because of hydronephrosis. Therefore, the evaluation should include chromosome analysis and fetal echocardiography. Pediatric urologic consultation should be obtained.

Fetal Intervention   In the rare case where ureterocele mimics the picture of posterior urethral valves with oligohydramnios, bladder decompression may be indicated. A single-needle aspiration may be both diagnostic and therapeutic.

Monitoring   No change in obstetric care is indicated. Serial ultrasound examinations monthly may be helpful in detecting the rare case where the obstruction results in oligohydramnios.

Pregnancy Course   No obstetric complications should be expected.

Pregnancy Termination Issues   Ureterocele should not be an indication for pregnancy termination.

Delivery   In cases with significant obstruction there is a need for immediate neonatal evaluation to establish a diagnosis and delivery should be in a tertiary center

NEONATOLOGY

Resuscitation   Usually not an issue. Onset of effective respiration may be impeded by abdominal distension secondary to renal enlargement. Intubation and ventilation may be required, at least initially.

Transport   Indicated, if associated with renal enlargement, particularly bilateral, for confirmation of diagnosis, and establishment of care plan, including surgical intervention. Isolated unilateral lesions and normal renal function, as indicated by serum creatinine, can be referred for outpatient evaluation and management.

Testing and Confirmation   Ureteroceles usually present with urinary infection in infants and children. Very large ureteroceles can cause bladder neck obstruction and they are the most common cause of bladder obstruction in females. Large ureteroceles can also disrupt the anatomy of the contralateral ureter and cause reflux.

Careful, staged evaluation of renal function and structure by urine production, urinalysis, blood and urine chemistries, and an abdominal sonogram is appropriate. If infant is minimally symptomatic and immediate relief of obstruction is not required, imaging can be delayed for 24 to 36 hours for better visualization. If the anatomy is not clearly defined prenatally, or immediate relief of obstruction is required, ultrasound imaging should be obtained immediately. Subsequent procedures will be contingent upon the specific lesion suspected, that is, voiding cystourethrogram, cystoscopy, renal scan without and with diuretic stimulation, or abdominal computerized tomography.

Nursery Management   Support respiration as necessary to maintain adequate gas exchange. Avoid fluid and protein loading initially until urinary tract patency and renal function have been determined.

SURGERY

Preoperative Assessment   An ultrasound assessment of the dilated upper pole and ureter serving the ureterocele is essential. Also, a functional scan showing the function of the upper pole is helpful to assess whether the upper pole can be saved.

Operative Indications   A small ureterocele may not cause upper tract dilatation, but all those discovered in utero so far have caused significant urinary back up and have required drainage.

Type of Procedures   An upper pole nephrectomy with partial ureterectomy is effective in over 60% of cases. Lately, there has been a resurgence in interest in transurethral incision of the ureterocele followed by an interval to see if there is improvement in upper pole function.

Surgical Results/Prognosis   The surgical prognosis is good. Damage to the lower pole of the kidney following an upper pole heminephrectomy can occur. The small size of the renal units increases the technical difficulty of the surgery.

Possible Surgical Complications

1. Incontinence secondary to sphincter damage if the ureterocele is excised from the bladder-neck area.
2. Reflux secondary to transurethral incision of the ureterocele causing urinary tract infections may necessitate removal of the remaining renal unit.

BIBILIOGRAPHY

Brock WA, Kaplan GW: Abnormalities of the lower tract. In: Edelmann CM Jr (ed): *Pediatric kidney disease*. Boston. Little, Brown, 1992. p. 2037.

Caione P, Zaccara A, Capozza N et al: How prenatal ultrasound can affect the treatment of ureterocele in neonates and children. *Eur Urol* 1989; 16:195-199.

Patten RM: The fetal genitourinary tract. *Radiol Clin North Am* 1990; 28:115-130.

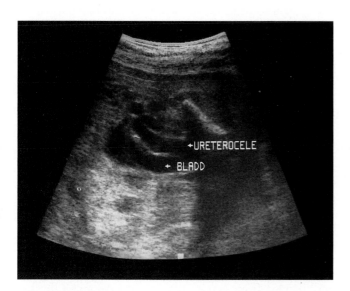

Sagittal view of the pelvic area of a prone fetus. A ureterocele can be seen impinging on the bladder.

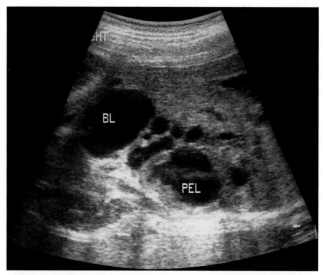

Sagittal sonographic view of the dilated renal pelvis (*PEL*) and the bladder (*BL*) in the same case. The cystic areas between the bladder and the pelvis represent portions of the tortuous dilated ureter.

5 The Chest

5.1 CYSTIC ADENOMATOID MALFORMATION OF THE LUNG

EPIDEMIOLOGY/GENETICS

Definition   Cystic adenomatoid malformations (CAMs) are benign hamartomatous or dysplastic lung tumors characterized by overgrowth of terminal bronchioles.

Epidemiology   Unknown, but presumed rare (M1:F1).

Embryology   Cystic adenomatoid malformations develop during the first 6 weeks of gestation. They are generally unilateral and classified into macrocystic forms (type I), mixed (type II), or microcystic (type III). There is a 26% incidence of associated malformations including pectus excavatum, hydrops, and renal agenesis.

Inheritance Patterns   Sporadic.

Teratogens   None.

Prognosis   Many patients, detected antenatally with microcystic disease, have associated hydrops and poly-hydramnios, and die. The macrocystic form is less likely to be associated with hydrops or compression of intrathoracic structures and has a 70% survival. About half of patients with cystic adenomatoid malformation, not antenatally diagnosed, present in the newborn period, and there is a 78% mortality rate.

SONOGRAPHY

Findings
1.   **Fetus:** A mass is present within the lung that is categorized by appearance into three types:
     Type 1 (macrocystic)—variably sized and shaped large cysts (2 to 10 cm) with thin intervening echogenic areas. There may be only one cyst.
     Type 2 (mixed)—small to moderate sized cysts with adjacent echogenic areas.
     Type 3 (microcystic)—echogenic areas in the fetal lungs. Fetal hydrops is more common with this form.
     All three types may displace the fetal heart or diaphragm. With more sizable masses, fetal ascites and hydrops may be seen.
2.   **Amniotic Fluid:** Polyhydramnios is seen often (65%).
3.   **Placenta:** Placentomegaly is usually present if hydrops occurs.

4.   **Measurement Data:** Normal growth is expected. Umbilical artery Doppler may be abnormal if hydrops occurs.
5.   **When Detectable:** First detectable between 12 and 18 weeks. If there is no hydrops the mass often regresses and may even disappear.

Pitfalls   Acoustic enhancement posterior to the heart can create the impression of a microcystic mass.

Differential Diagnosis
1.   Diaphragmatic hernia—Can look very similar, but no diaphragm will be visible and the stomach will usually be in the chest or shifted to the right.
2.   Bronchogenic and neuroenteric cysts—The single cystic form of cystic adenomatoid malformation can look similar. Neuroenteric cysts are central and posterior in location.

Where Else To Look   There is no association with chromosomal anomalies. Renal anomalies (e.g., renal agenesis) and gastrointestinal malformations (diaphragmatic hernia and bowel atresias) should be sought.

PREGNANCY MANAGEMENT

Investigations and Consultations Required   Invasive testing is not indicated if a precise diagnosis can be made by ultrasound. Cardiac status should be assessed by fetal echocardiography. Early consultation with a pediatric surgeon is warranted to establish a fetal management plan.

Fetal Intervention   In macrocystic lesions associated with fetal hydrops, placement of a shunt in the largest cyst has resulted in successful outcomes in a small number of cases. The successful in utero resection of cystic adenomatoid malformations also has been reported. Unfortunately, it is difficult to determine which cases may benefit from active intervention, as awaiting the development of hydrops may counter successful intervention. On the other hand, surgical procedures prior to clinical evidence of fetal compromise may be unnecessary in many fetuses because many cystadenoma regress. Further work is needed to develop criteria for fetal therapy.

Monitoring   The significant incidence of pregnancy complications requires that care is coordinated at a tertiary center. Ultrasound examinations at least every 3 to 4 weeks are appropriate to detect early evidence of hydrops or polyhydramnios. Careful maternal assessment for the development of preeclampsia is necessary in those cases with hydrops.

Pregnancy Course   Polyhydramnios may result in preterm labor. Fetal hydrops and resultant preeclampsia also may complicate obstetrical management. The presence of hydrops greatly worsens the prognosis. More mild examples may regress or disappear during pregnancy.

Pregnancy Termination Issues   A nondestructive procedure that provides both anatomic and microscopic evaluation is appropriate.

Delivery   In the absence of fetal hydrops, delivery should be at term. After 32 weeks gestation, any evidence of fetal compromise should prompt steroid administration to enhance fetal lung maturity and early delivery. Because immediate resuscitation may be necessary in any infant with cystic adenomatoid malformations, delivery should occur in a tertiary center.

NEONATOLOGY

Resuscitation   The two major issues affecting onset of respiration at birth are preterm delivery and the presence of fetal hydrops. Of the three histologic types, type III, microcystic, is most likely to be associated with both problems. Prompt intubation following delivery and assisted ventilation is indicated when the diagnosis is known prior to delivery, when one or both complicating factors are present or with any evidence of early onset of respiratory distress. Care should be taken to avoid malposition of the endotracheal tube as the malformed lung can become massively overdistended, compromising gas exchange in normal lung tissue.

Transport   Immediate transfer to a tertiary center with a pediatric surgeon is essential as the postnatal mortality rate is very high and the only successful treatment is prompt surgical excision. Maintenance of ventilatory support with avoidance of tube malposition is critical during transport. Positioning the infant with the involved side dependent may help to avoid overdistension.

Testing and Confirmation   Respiratory distress is the most frequent presentation in the newborn period. Older children may present with recurrent respiratory symptoms and some cases are detected incidentally.

If there is confusion regarding the diagnosis or the extent of the affected lung, a computed tomography (CT) scan of the thorax is useful. Echocardiography is useful to evaluate compromise of cardiac filling and myocardial contractility.

Nursery Management   Positive pressure ventilatory support should be maintained prior to surgery. When the area of lung involvement is small, surgery in a preterm infant may be delayed until co-existing respiratory distress syndrome can be abated with surfactant replacement therapy. As above, careful attention to tube position and to positioning the infant may reduce the overdistension of the involved segment.

If there is coexisting hydrops, restriction of fluid intake, pharmacologic diuresis, and administration of ionotropic infusions may help to mobilize the fluid from the interstitial space while sustaining adequate perfusion. Rapid infusion of albumin or plasma should be avoided as massive shifts of fluid into the intravascular space can compromise cardiac function.

SURGERY

Preoperative Assessment   Acute management includes evaluation of the degree of respiratory insufficiency and identification of major associated anomalies, most notably cardiac defects. Echocardiography is helpful for the latter evaluation.

Operative Indications   The need for immediate surgery is determined by the presence of respiratory distress requiring ventilatory support. In some patients, and particularly those with an early intrauterine diagnosis, the pulmonary symptoms are very severe and unresponsive to standard respiratory support. If there are no other apparent associated potentially lethal anomalies, then preoperative and/or postoperative extracorporeal membrane oxygenation (ECMO) support can be considered for the infant with evidence of severe respiratory insufficiency due to lung hypoplasia and pulmonary hypertension. Most patients will have unilateral disease with involvement of only one or at most two pulmonary lobes.

Types of Procedures   A posteriolateral thoracotomy with resection of the involved lobe is the standard therapy. An exception to this is the patient described above with pulmonary hypertension and mild pulmonary hypoplasia who may require preoperative or postoperative ECMO.

Surgical Results/Prognosis   The patient with macrocytic CAM responds dramatically to excision of the involved pulmonary lobe or lobes with an excellent (95+%) long-term prognosis. The mixed and microcystic varieties with a higher incidence of associated anomalies and fetal hydrops have a much lower survival rate and poorer long-term outcome with chronic respiratory insufficiency being the major complication. The presence of fetal hydrops is ominous with few survivors expected.

BIBLIOGRAPHY

Adzick NS: The fetus with cystic adenomatoid malformation. In: Harrison MR, Golbus MS, Filly RA (eds): *The unborn patient, antenatal diagnosis and treatment.* Philadelphia. WB Saunders, 1991. pp. 320-372.

Adzick NS, Harrison MR, Glick PL et al: Fetal cystic adenomatoid malformation: prenatal diagnosis and natural history. *J Pediatr Surg* 1985; 20:483-488.

Budorick NE, Pretorius DH, Leopold GR et al: Spontaneous improvement of intrathoracic masses diagnosed in utero. *J Ultrasound Med* 1992; 11:653-662.

Clark SL, Vitale DJ, Minton SD et al: Successful fetal therapy for cystic adenomatoid malformation associated with second-trimester hydrops. *Am J Obstet Gynecol* 1987; 157:294-295.

Graham D et al: Prenatal diagnosis of cystic adenomatoid malformation of the lung. *J Ultrasound Med* 1982; 1:9-12.

Haddon MJ, Bowen A: Bronchopulmonary and neurenteric forms of foregut anomalies: imaging for diagnosis and management. *Radiol Clin North Am* 1991; 29:241-254.

Johnson JA, Rumack CM, Johnson ML et al: Cystic adenomatoid malformation: antenatal diagnosis. *Am J Roentgenol* 1984; 142:483-484.

Neilson IR, Russo P, Laberge JM et al: Congenital adenomatoid malformation of the lung: current management and prognosis. *J Pediatr Surg* 1991; 26:975-980.

Othersen B Jr: Pulmonary and bronchial malformations. In: Ashcraft K, Holder T (eds): *Pediatric surgery.* Philadelphia. WB Saunders, 1993.

Roelofsen J, Oostendorp R, Volovics A et al: Prenatal diagnosis and fetal outcome of cystic adenomatoid malformation of the lung: case report and historical survey. *Ultrasound Obstet Gynecol* 1994; 4:78-82.

Saltzman DH, Adzick NS, Benacerraf BR: Fetal cystic adenomatoid malformation of the lung: apparent improvement in utero. *Obstet Gynecol* 1988; 71:1000-1002.

Stocker JT, Madewell JE, Drake RM: Congenital cystic adenomatoid malformation of the lung: classification and morphological spectrum. *Hum Pathol* 1977; 8:155-171.

Wesley JR, Heidelberger KP, DiPietro MA et al: Diagnosis and management of congenital cystic disease of the lung in children. *J Pediatr Surg* 1986; 21:202-207.

Wilson J, Maenner V: Congenital cystic adenomatoid malformation. *Neonatal Netw* 1993; 12:15-20.

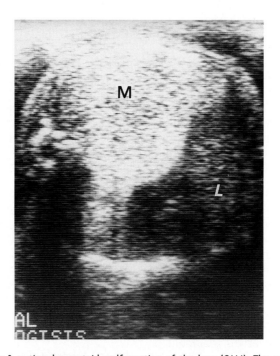

Type 3 cystic adenomatoid malformation of the lung (CAM). The more echogenic area of the lung (*M*) represents the CAM. Myriads of tiny cysts are present so no drainage procedure can be performed. This type has a worse prognosis. *L,* normal lung.

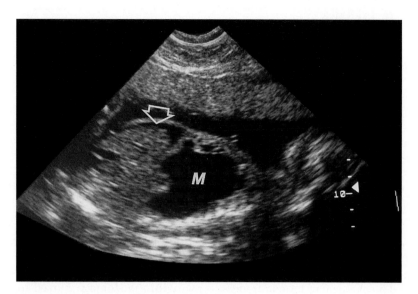

Type 1 cystic adenomatoid malformation. At least two cysts are present in the lungs (*M*). A drainage procedure is feasible. Note the presence of a small amount of ascites around the liver (*arrow*).

5.2 DIAPHRAGMATIC HERNIA

EPIDEMIOLOGY/GENETICS

Definition   A group of diaphragmatic defects in which some portion of the abdominal contents protrude into the chest cavity, most frequently through a posterolateral (foramen of Bochdalek hernia) or retrosternal (foramen of Morgagni hernia) defect.

Epidemiology   Posteriolateral hernia, 15 to 20 out of 100,000 births (M2:F1); retrosternal hernia, less than 1 out of 1,000,000 births.

Embryology   Diaphragmatic hernias probably develop between the sixth and tenth week of gestation when the gut is returning from the yolk sac and the diaphragm is developing. One proposed mechanism of formation proposes an imbalance in timing of these events with thoracic migration of the gut, resulting in failure of diaphragmatic closure. Frequently associated abnormalities include cardiac (20%) and central nervous system (CNS) malformations (30%), but renal anomalies, vertebral defects, pulmonary hypoplasia, and facial clefts have also been reported. Chromosome abnormalities including trisomies 18 and 21, as well as over 30 multiple malformation syndromes, including the Fryn's and Cornelia de Lange's syndromes, have been described with diaphragmatic hernias.

Inheritance Patterns   Generally sporadic. Less than 2 percent recurrence risk in siblings for isolated defects. Rare families have shown dominant and X-linked recessive inheritance for isolated diaphragmatic hernias.

Teratogens   None known.

Prognosis   The two primary factors determining survival are the degree of pulmonary hypoplasia and the coexistence of other anomalies. Mortality is particularly high in prenatally diagnosed cases (80% in Adzick's series). Diagnosis prior to 25 weeks gestation and the development of polyhydramnios has been associated with very low survival potential.

In liveborn infants, survival potential has been correlated with age at presentation and severity of gas exchange problems as markers for the degree of pulmonary hypoplasia. The Liverpool group reports mortality rates of less than 5% for those who are minimally affected to asymptomatic in the first 6 hours with near normal blood gases; approximately 30% in the group who are symptomatic early, but who can achieve normal blood gases with ventilatory support; and 100% in the most severe group, those who are symptomatic from birth and despite maximal support do not achieve normal blood gas values secondary to severe pulmonary hypoplasia and pulmonary hypertension.

SONOGRAPHY

Findings
1. **Fetus**
   Left-sided hernia—The heart is deviated to the right. Usually the stomach is in the chest alongside the heart so there is no stomach or gallbladder in the abdomen. Small bowel in the chest may have a slightly mottled pattern, but may look like lung. Peristalsis may be seen. The left diaphragm is not visible. The liver may be displaced.
   Right-sided hernia—There is liver in the chest so the heart is deviated to left. One may be able to see a liver-lung interface above the site of the normal diaphragm. The stomach alignment is abnormal with the stomach moved to the right and horizontally aligned. The liver alignment is changed in the abdomen. Portal vessels can be tracked within the liver into the chest.
2. **Amniotic Fluid:** Normal amniotic fluid volume, unless the bowel is obstructed, in which case there is polyhydramnios. The presence of polyhydramnios is correlated with pulmonary hypoplasia and, therefore, a worse prognosis.
3. **Placenta:** Normal.
4. **Measurement Data:** Small abdomen because much of the contents are in the chest. Overall small growth would favor a chromosomal disorder.
5. **When Detectable:** Usually detectable before 18 weeks, however the hernia may be in the chest intermittently.

Pitfalls
1. Lung changes are easily overlooked especially if the stomach is in the abdomen.
2. Often initially diagnosed as "dextrocardia" because the lung changes are subtle.
3. The heart may be very difficult to examine in the presence of diaphragmatic hernia.

Differential Diagnosis
1. Cystic adenomatoid malformation—The diaphragm is intact and no peristalsis is seen.
2. Lung tumor—Exceedingly rare, often with calcification.
3. Dextrocardia—The heart still points to the left in diaphragmatic hernia, although it is on the right side.

Where Else To Look   Associated with chromosomal disorders (trisomies 18 and 21), so look at the hands, feet, heart, and face. Approximately 20% have an anomaly elsewhere, even when chromosomally normal. Look at the cardiovascular, genitourinary, musculoskeletal, and gastrointestinal systems.

PREGNANCY MANAGEMENT

Investigations and Consultations Required Fetal chromosome evaluation and echocardiography are essential. Consultation with a pediatric surgeon and neonatologist to plan neonatal management is appropriate.

Fetal Intervention Cases of isolated diaphragmatic hernia presenting with polyhydramnios before 24 weeks may be candidates for open fetal surgery. Initial results with this approach have been disappointing. However, the newer approach of tracheal ligation holds promise. Untreated fetuses in this category have a dismal prognosis for survival.

Monitoring Prophylactic tocolysis, if polyhydramnios develops, may be appropriate in view of the poor results to be expected if prematurity complicates the surgical correction. Therefore, serial ultrasound examinations every 3 to 4 weeks and regular clinical assessment should be performed.

Pregnancy Course Polyhydramnios is a common complicating factor and may result in preterm labor. The presence of polyhydramnios is correlated with pulmonary hypoplasia and, therefore, a worse prognosis.

Pregnancy Termination Issues Diaphragmatic hernia is a component of a number of genetic syndromes. To provide appropriate counseling regarding recurrence, a complete external and internal pathologic examination of an intact fetus is required.

Delivery Immediate resuscitation is often necessary, therefore, delivery should be in a tertiary center. There are no fetal indications for early delivery or delivery by cesarean section.

NEONATOLOGY

Resuscitation An experienced team that is prepared to initiate full ventilatory and pharmacologic support is essential to maximize survival potential particularly for the more severely involved neonate. Rapid, atraumatic intubation and assisted ventilation, gastric decompression, and pharmacologic paralysis are recommended initially. Hypoplastic lungs are highly prone to develop air leaks and pneumothorax with positive pressure ventilation. The goal is to facilitate pulmonary vasodilatation and promote rapid and sustained transition from the fetal to the adult circulatory pattern. Prompt correction of acidosis is essential.

Transport Transfer to a tertiary center with pediatric surgeons is mandatory and should be done only by an experienced neonatal transport team as these infants have very labile courses.

Testing and Confirmation Diagnostic evaluation preoperatively should be limited to those studies that are essential to confirm the diagnosis and to exclude the presence of serious anomalies affecting long-term prognosis, that is, chromosomal abnormalities, cardiac, or CNS defects, if not done prenatally.

Nursery Management The initial care of the infant is directed toward maintaining adequate gas exchange by mechanical ventilation and the avoidance of reflex pulmonary vasoconstriction with reversion to right-to-left shunting by way of fetal pathways by limiting stressful handling.

The role of ECMO preoperatively and postoperatively in the treatment of infants with diaphragmatic hernia remains somewhat unclear. Improved early survival has been demonstrated in the group of infants previously shown to be nonsurvivors. However, overall survival remains low in this group because of late deaths secondary to severe respiratory failure. In addition, significant CNS injury related to intracranial hemorrhage and to ischemia has been observed following ECMO treatment.

Recent reports suggest that high frequency ventilation and surfactant replacement therapy are of benefit in improving survival rates.

SURGERY

Preoperative Assessment The acute pathophysiology of a congenital diaphragmatic hernia (CDH) postnatally results from a mechanical space-occupying lesion with accompanying lung hypoplasia, pulmonary vascular malformation, and decreased lung expansion with respiration. The hypoxemia is therefore the result of poor ventilation plus associated pulmonary hypertension.

Operative Indications Despite the use of sophisticated ventilatory support and pharmacologic therapy to produce pulmonary vasodilatation, some infants will have persistent hypoxemia. In a large percentage of these unresponsive infants, this is due to a degree of lung hypoplasia incompatible with survival. However, this severe hypoxemia can be the result of pulmonary hypertension unresponsive to ventilatory or pharmacologic manipulation but still potentially reversible using temporary pulmonary bypass, that is, the use of ECMO. Extracorporeal membrane oxygenation can be used as preoperative therapy with either CDH repair while on bypass or after cessation of bypass therapy. It can also be used after surgical repair of CDH in infants who have had the commonly occurring postoperative "honeymoon period," with temporarily improved hypoxemia and then subsequent acute irreversible respiratory failure. Extracorporeal membrane oxygenation is not applicable in small premature infants because of the need for anticoagulation, nor in patients who have complex, noncorrectable cardiac defects. There are significant potential acute and chronic complications of ECMO, but new access techniques (i.e., veno-venous circuits, heparin-bonded tubing, etc.) are improving these problems. Although ECMO is no longer considered experimental therapy for most forms of neonatal respiratory distress, it must be applied cautiously in CDH because clinical criteria for its successful application are still evolving and the mortality rate remains extremely high, 45+%.

The operative goals are reduction of the viscera from the thoracic cavity, closure of the diaphragmatic defect, and elimination of potential duodenal obstruction due to nonrotation of the intestine. Surgical options include abdominal versus thoracic repair. Left posterior lateral diaphragmatic lesions occur 75% to 80% of the time and most surgeons prefer an abdominal approach to accomplish the above goals. Some surgeons who prefer the thoracic approach do so particularly for the less frequent right posterior lateral CDH. This defect is associated with a higher incidence of hepatic herniation into the chest and may result in abnormal angulation of the suprahepatic inferior vena cava with more difficulty in reducing the liver back into the abdomen without occluding the lower body venous return. An abdominal approach for this problem is possible, but a thoracic approach improves surgical exposure and manipulation of the vessels. Rare anterior retrosternal CDH is repaired by way of the abdominal approach. Posterior lateral CDH is frequently associated with insufficient remaining diaphragmatic musculature and will not allow closure of the defect. Tailored nonabsorbable woven plastic prosthetic sheets are used to cover this defect and are attached to the surrounding musculature. The ipsilateral chest is not drained by a chest tube with applied suction because this tends to acutely shift the mobile infant mediastinum and produce hemodynamic instability.

Surgical Results/Prognosis   The overall survival rate is 65% to 75%. This has improved with the use of ECMO from 50%. Survival is directly related to the presence or absence of prematurity, polyhydramnios (extremely poor prognosis), and associated anomalies, most notably cardiac defects. A prenatal diagnosis made before 24 weeks gestation is associated with poor long-term results.

Morbidity can be related to the congenital defects, but can also be iatrogenic in nature. Chronic respiratory insufficiency can occur in survivors and may be related to barotrauma induced by the need for prolonged oxygenation and ventilation. These children have an increased incidence of pathologic gastroesophageal reflux that is frequently unresponsive to standard medical therapy and increases their respiratory and nutritional complications.

BIBLIOGRAPHY

Adzick NS, Harrison MR, Glick PL et al: Diaphragmatic hernia in the fetus: prenatal diagnosis and outcome in 94 cases. *J Pediatr Surg* 1985; 20:357-361.

Benacerraf BR, Greene MF: Fetal diaphragmatic hernia: ultrasound diagnosis prior to 22 weeks gestation. *Radiology* 1986; 158:809-810.

Bohn DJ, James I, Filler RM et al: The relationship between $PaCO_2$ and ventilation parameters in predicting survival in congenital diaphragmatic hernia. *J Pediatr Surg* 1984; 19:666-671.

Bohn D, Tamura M, Perrin D et al: Ventilatory predictors of pulmonary hypoplasia in congenital diaphragmatic hernia, confirmed by morphologic assessment. *J Pediatr* 1987; 111:423-431.

Breaux CW Jr, Rouse TM, Cain WS et al: Congenital diaphragmatic hernia in an era of delayed repair after medical and/or extracorporeal membrane oxygenation stabilization: a prognostic and management classification. *J Pediatr Surg* 1992; 27:1192-1196.

Crane JP: Familial congenital diaphragmatic hernia: prenatal diagnostic approach and analysis of twelve families. *Clin Genet* 1979; 16:244-252.

Cunniff C, Jones KL, Jones MC: Patterns of malformation in children with congenital diaphragmatic defects. *J Pediatr* 1990; 116:258-261.

DeLorimer AA: Diaphragmatic hernia. In: Aschcraft KW, Holder TM (eds): Pediatric surgery. Philadelphia. WB Saunders, 1993. pp. 204-217.

Haugen SE, Linker D, Eik-Nes S et al: Congenital diaphragmatic hernia: determination of the optimal time for operation by echocardiographic monitoring of the pulmonary arterial pressure. *J Pediatr Surg* 1991; 26:560-562.

Irving IM, Booker PD: Congenital diaphragmatic hernia and eventration of the diaphragm. In: Lister J, Irving IM (eds): *Neonatal surgery*. London. Butterworths, 1990. p. 199.

Langham MR, Krummel TM, Bartlett RH et al: Mortality with extracorporeal membrane oxygenation following repair of congenital diaphragmatic hernia in 93 Infants. *J Pediatr Surg* 1987; 22:1150.

Nakayama DK, Harrison MR, Chinn DH et al: Prenatal diagnosis and natural history of the fetus with a congenital diaphragmatic hernia: initial clinical experience. *J Pediatr Surg* 1985; 20:118-124.

Puri P, Gorman F: Lethal nonpulmonary anomalies associated with congenital diaphragmatic hernia: implications for early intrauterine surgery. *J Pediatr Surg* 1984; 19:29-32.

Steinhorn RH, Kriesmer PJ, Green TP et al: Congenital diaphragmatic hernia in Minnesota: impact of antenatal diagnosis on survival. *Arch Pediatr Adolesc Med* 1994; 148:626-631.

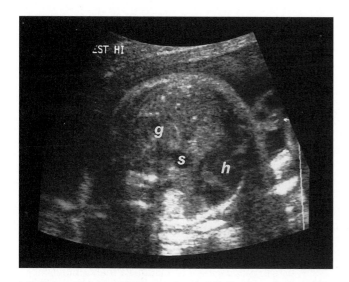 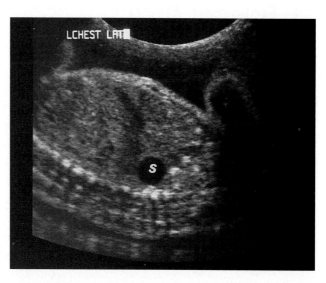

Left diaphragmatic hernia. Transverse view through the chest. The heart (*h*) is deviated to the right. The stomach (*s*) lies alongside the chest. A slight difference between the texture of the normal lung and the area that is gut-filled (*g*) can be seen.

Sagittal view. The stomach (*s*) is visible in the chest as a fluid-filled cystic structure. An irregular texture due to small bowel can be seen superior to the stomach.

5.3 Esophageal Atresia
Tracheal Atresia, Tracheoesophageal Fistula, TE Fistula (TEF)

EPIDEMIOLOGY/GENETICS

Definition   Esophageal atresia is a congenital lack of continuity of the esophagus resulting in a blind-ending esophageal pouch. There is frequently an associated tracheoesophageal fistula.

Epidemiology   1 out of 5,000 (M1:F1), 90% of patients have esophageal atresia with a distal tracheoesophageal fistula (TEF).

Embryology   Failure of the anterior foregut to divide into the anterior trachea and posterior esophagus around the fourth week of gestation results in various types of esophageal atresia and tracheoesophageal fistula. Fifty percent of patients have associated anomalies including cardiac (20%), gastrointestinal defects (10%), and imperforate anus (10%). The vertebral abnormalities, anal atresia, cardiac abnormalities, tracheoesophageal fistula and esophageal atresia, renal agenesis and dysplasia, and limb defects (VACTERL) association occurs in approximately 6% of cases. Over 25 genetic, chromosomal, and sporadic syndromes have been described with esophageal atresia or tracheoesophageal fistula. Two to three percent of cases have trisomy 21.

Inheritance Patterns   Sporadic.

Teratogens   Retinoic acid, alcohol.

Prognosis   Survival and prognosis are determined by the etiology and associated malformations. Greater than 95% of patients with isolated TEF fistula survive with a functional repair.

SONOGRAPHY

Findings
1. **Fetus**
   a. Nonvisualization of the stomach is seen in the form of esophageal atresia and TEF in which there is no connection between the pharynx and the stomach. A narrow connection through the lungs between the esophagus and stomach may result in a small stomach. Many other examples of TEF are not diagnosable with ultrasound because there is a large connection between the esophagus and stomach by way of the lungs.
   b. A fluid-filled proximal esophagus or a fluid-filled distal esophageal segment and fetal regurgitation after swallowing may be seen.
2. **Amniotic Fluid:** There is massive polyhydramnios with an amniotic fluid index that is often over 40 cm in the third trimester.
3. **Placenta:** Normal.

4. **Measurement Data:** Normal unless the fetus is chromosomally abnormal or the VACTERL syndrome is present.
5. **When Detectable:** Usually detectable only after 24 weeks, because before this point in gestation, fetal swallowing plays only a limited role in amniotic fluid dynamics.

Pitfalls
1. Nonvisualization of the stomach may be a transient normal finding.
2. Technical problems such as maternal obesity may result in an inability to visualize the stomach.
3. Brain malformations may prevent swallowing and cause nonvisualization of the stomach.
4. The stomach may be in the chest or abnormally positioned as with diaphragmatic hernia and, therefore, not seen.
5. In many examples of TEF a connection to the stomach through the lungs exists. Consequently, the stomach will be seen and the amniotic fluid volume is normal.

Differential Diagnosis
The following disorders may also cause absence of stomach visualization:
1. Facial clefts.
2. Central nervous system malformation that results in absent swallowing. Many of these, such as the fetal akinesia sequence, or the lethal pterygium syndrome, are lethal conditions.
3. Diaphragmatic hernia.
4. Situs inversus.

Where Else to Look   Associated malformations are seen in at least 50% of cases of TEF. The following abnormalities should be sought: anorectal atresia, duodenal atresia, malrotation, cardiovascular anomalies, renal obstruction, vertebral problems such as scoliosis, and hydronephrosis. Tracheoesophageal fistula is associated with the VACTERL association as well as chromosomal abnormalities (trisomy 18 and 21).

PREGNANCY MANAGEMENT

Investigations and Consultations Required   Chromosome studies should be done, as well as fetal echocardiography. Consultation with a pediatric surgeon is appropriate. A neonatology consult also should be obtained because of the high risk of preterm delivery.

Fetal Intervention   There is no direct fetal intervention indicated. Serial amniocenteses have no place in management, except for a short-term benefit in cases where steroid therapy has been given to enhance fetal lung maturity. Decreasing amniotic fluid volume, when there is polyhydramnios, may diminish the risk of preterm labor and allow adequate time for the therapeutic effect.

Monitoring Because of the high risk of preterm labor, care should be under the direction of a perinatologist. Tocolytic agents are often necessary. Frequent clinical and sonographic examinations are necessary to monitor the degree of polyhydramnios and for early evidence of preterm labor. Monitoring of the cervix by ultrasound is desirable to detect early funneling of the internal os.

Pregnancy Termination Issues In rare cases with an early diagnosis, the procedure for termination should provide an intact fetus for a complete autopsy.

Delivery Every attempt should be made to reach term. However, significant polyhydramnios often results in preterm delivery. The site for delivery should be a tertiary center with the capabilities of managing very premature infants.

NEONATOLOGY

Resuscitation If the infant is born prematurely or there are associated major organ system anomalies, there may be difficulty with the onset of respiration. When the diagnosis is suspected from prenatal studies and there is delay in onset of respiration, immediate endotracheal intubation is preferable to bag and mask ventilation to avoid overdistension of the stomach. (For technique see Nursery Management below.) Excessive oral secretions may be encountered necessitating placement of an esophageal catheter for continuous drainage.

Transport Transfer to a tertiary perinatal center with a pediatric surgeon is always indicated. The infant should be transported in a semisitting position to minimize the risk of regurgitation of gastric contents into the airway by way of the fistula. An esophageal catheter should be placed to drain the pooled secretions to avoid aspiration from the proximal pouch.

Testing and Confirmation Newborns present with excessive salivation and choking with feedings. Postnatal radiologic studies will define the defect. A radiopaque catheter is carefully passed into the esophagus until resistance is met. Air is injected through the catheter and chest and abdomen radiographs are obtained. Chromosomal analysis, if not obtained prenatally, echocardiography, and careful physical examinations for any associated anomalies are performed.

Nursery Management The priority in the early care is to avoid aspiration of either oral or gastric secretions and thus to decrease the likelihood of pneumonia. Continuous evacuation of esophageal secretions, positioning semisitting, avoiding overdistension of the stomach from crying or positive pressure ventilation, and avoiding compression of the abdomen are useful maneuvers to prevent aspiration.

If endotracheal intubation is required, an attempt should be made to locate the tip of the tube distal to the fistula insertion. This can be accomplished either by placement under endoscopic control or with careful auscultation over the stomach as a positive pressure breath is given, advancing the tube until air is no longer heard entering the stomach.

SURGERY

Preoperative Assessment There are several forms of tracheoesophageal anomalies, but the most common (85%) is a combination of proximal esophageal pouch with a distal TEF.

Preoperative surgical goals consist of identifying the degree of postdelivery aspiration pneumonitis and preventing further airway contamination. This includes assessment of the infant's clinical status as well as the radiographic appearance of the lungs. The latter is a late-occurring sign and more unreliable than clinical and metabolic (blood gas) determinations. A preoperative evaluation for all possible VACTERL anomalies is carried out with particular attention to cardiac lesions.

Operative Indications The decision to perform an urgent gastrostomy to relieve gastric distension and potential aspiration due to reflux or to perform an immediate thoracotomy for division of the TEF and a primary repair of the esophageal atresia is contingent on the preoperative assessment. The former approach is chosen if significant signs of preexisting pulmonary aspiration exist and the latter is used if no significant respiratory distress is evident or if other associated lesions contraindicate primary repair.

Types of Procedures A right thoracotomy by way of a retropleural approach is used to facilitate better control of postoperative drainage in instances of an esophageal leak (5% to 20%). The TEF is divided and the tracheal opening closed carefully to prevent airway stenosis. Care must be exercised so that a double tracheal connection is not missed intraoperatively. A retropleural chest tube is left in position for any potential esophageal leakage. A separate abdominal procedure to place a gastrostomy tube may or may not be used according to surgeon's preference.

Surgical Results/Prognosis As noted, the early complications include respiratory infection, esophageal anastomotic leak, and recurrent TEF as well as potential complications associated with the VACTERL anomalies in those patients. Late complications consist of esophageal strictures, gastroesophageal reflux (GER), dysphagia, and various manifestations of reactive airway disease such as recurrent bronchitis or even asthmatic symptoms. The symptoms of GER can be difficult to treat.

The operative mortality for a full-term infant with uncomplicated esophageal atresia and TEF should approach 0% in tertiary children's centers. Premature infants with associated cardiac anomalies have a survival rate of 50% to 70%. The overall survival rate is approximately 90%.

Surviving children are frequently "slow eaters" who drink increased amounts of fluids with their meals. They also have increased susceptibility to the lodging of esophageal foreign bodies such as meat particles and especially pieces of hot dog. Both of these problems are related to a persistence of esophageal dysmotility due to the atresia.

Long-term survival is good and further morbidity after 2 to 4 years of age is minimal, however, effects of reactive airway disease can be documented in adult post-TEF patients.

BIBLIOGRAPHY

Bovicelli L, Rizzo N, Orsini LF et al: Prenatal diagnosis and management of fetal gastrointestinal abnormalities. *Semin Perinatol* 1983; 7:109–117.

Chittmittrapap S, Spitz L, Kiely EM et al: Oesophageal atresia and associated anomalies. *Arch Dis Child* 1989; 64:364-368.

Dillon PW, Cilley RE: Newborn surgical emergencies, gastrointestinal anomalies, abdominal wall defects. *Pediatr Clin North Am* 1993; 40:1289-1314.

Dudgeon DL, Morrison CW, Woolley MM: Congenital proximal tracheoesophageal fistula. *J Pediatr Surg* 1972; 7:614-619.

Ein SH, Shandling B, Wesson D et al: Esophageal atresia with distal tracheoesophageal fistula: associated anomalies and prognosis in the 1980s. *J Pediatr Surg* 1989; 24:1055-1059.

Evans JA, Reggin J, Greenberg C: Tracheal agenesis and associated malformations: a comparison with tracheoesophageal fistula and the VACTERL association. *Am J Med Genet* 1985; 21:21-38.

Eyheremendy E, Pfister M: Antenatal real-time diagnosis of esophageal atresia. *J Clin Ultrasound* 1983; 11:395-397.

Greenwood RD, Rosenthal A: Cardiovascular malformations associated with tracheoesophageal fistula and esophageal atresia. *Pediatrics* 1976; 57:87-91.

Holder TM, Ashcraft KW: Developments in the care of patients with esophageal atresia and tracheoesophageal fistula. *Surg Clin North Am* 1981; 61:1051-1061.

Jassani MN, Gauderer MW, Faranoff AA et al: A perinatal approach to the diagnosis and management of gastrointestinal malformations. *Obstet Gynecol* 1982; 59:33-39.

Jolley SG, Johnson DG, Roberts CC et al: Patterns of gastroesophageal reflux in children following repair of esophageal atresia and distal tracheoesophageal fistula. *J Pediatr Surg* 1980; 15:857-862.

Louhimo I, Lindahl H: Esophageal atresia: primary results of 500 consecutively treated patients. *J Pediatr Surg* 1983; 18:217-229.

Millener PB, Anderson NG, Chisholm RJ: Prognostic significance of nonvisualization of the fetal stomach by sonography. *Am J Roentgenol* 1993; 160:827-830.

Nyberg DA: Intra-abdominal abnormalities. In: *Diagnostic ultrasound of fetal anomalies: text and atlas*. St. Louis. Mosby–Year Book, 1990. pp. 358-350.

Pretorius DH, Drose JA, Dennis MA et al: Tracheoesophageal fistula in utero: twenty-two cases. *J Ultrasound Med* 1987; 6:509-513.

Pretorius DH, Meier PR, Johnson ML: Diagnosis of esophageal atresia in utero. *J Ultrasound Med* 1983; 2:475-476.

Quan L, Smith DW: The VATER association: vertebral defects, anal atresia, T-E fistula with esophageal atresia, radial and renal dysplasia: a spectrum of associated defects. *J Pediatr* 1973; 82:104-107.

Randolph JG, Newman KD, Anderson KD: Current results in repair of esophageal atresia with tracheoesophageal fistula using physiologic status as a guide to therapy. *Ann Surg* 1989; 209:524-530.

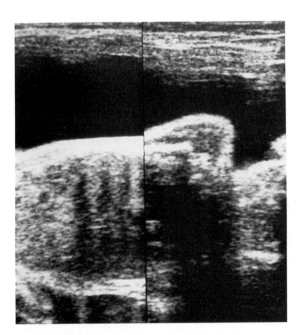

Tracheoesophageal atresia. Longitudinal view of fetus. There is severe polyhydramnios with no visible stomach.

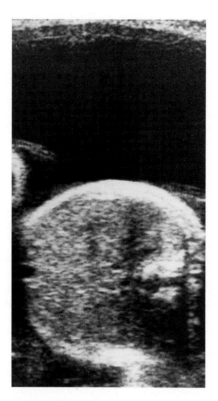

Transverse view of the abdomen. Despite prolonged observation, no stomach could be found.

5.4 Pleural Effusion

EPIDEMIOLOGY/GENETICS

Definition   A pleural effusion is an accumulation of fluid in the pleural space. Effusions can be either chylous or clear (hydrothorax) with most primary congenital effusions being chylous and occurring on the right.

Epidemiology   1 out of 10,000 births (M2:F1).

Embryology   The etiology of pleural effusions is not known, but they may result from either overproduction of lymph or impaired reabsorption. Pleural effusions are divided into primary effusions, which are usually chylous, and secondary effusions that are clear and occur as part of nonimmune hydrops. Over 50 genetic, chromosomal, and sporadic syndromes have been reported, including pleural effusion.

Inheritance Patterns   A number of genetic syndromes including Caffey's cortical hyperostosis (autosomal dominant [AD]) and the Opitz-Frias hypertelorism hypospadias syndrome (AD) have been reported with pleural effusions, hydrops, or chylothorax.

Teratogens   None.

Prognosis   Overall mortality for pleural effusions presenting in the neonatal period is 25%, ranging from 15% for isolated effusions to 95% for those with associated hydrops. Overall mortality for antenatally diagnosed cases is approximately 50%. Mortality is related to hydrops, pulmonary hypoplasia, and prematurity.

SONOGRAPHY

Findings
1. **Fetus**
   Fluid surrounds the lungs on one or both sides. If the effusion is bilateral and everts the diaphragms, secondary hydrops may occur. Assess the size of the lung on the side of the pleural effusion. Lung hypoplasia or agenesis in utero are associated with pleural effusion development. The associated lung will be very small or not seen.
2. **Amniotic Fluid:** If polyhydramnios develops, the prognosis is poor.
3. **Placenta:** Normal.
4. **Measurement Data:** Usually normal.
5. **When Detectable:** About 16 weeks.

Pitfalls   Pericardial and pleural effusions may be confused. With a large pericardial effusion, the lungs are compressed posteriorly.

Differential Diagnosis   Severe primary pleural effusion with secondary hydrops may be confused with primary hydrops. If the pleural effusion is the primary cause the diaphragms are everted. A trial of pleural fluid aspiration may be necessary to make the distinction.

Where Else to Look   Look for stigmata of Down syndrome (neck thickening, femur and humerus shortening, cardiac anomalies, duodenal atresia) and Turner's syndrome (cystic hygroma).

PREGNANCY MANAGEMENT

Investigations and Consultations Required
1. Chromosome studies and viral cultures.
2. Maternal serum studies for toxoplasmosis, other, rubella, cytomegalovirus, and herpes simplex virus (TORCH) and parvovirus.
3. The significant incidence of congenital heart disease requires fetal echocardiographic evaluation of the fetus.
4. Consultation with a neonatologist or pediatric surgeon is helpful.

Fetal Intervention   There is no clear evidence to support active surgical intervention. A management plan that is conservative seems to be the best approach. Following initial evaluation, a follow-up ultrasound scan in 2 to 3 weeks is done. If the effusion is enlarged or has increased, diagnostic/therapeutic thoracentesis should be done. If the lung expands, but the effusion recurs, consideration should be given to placement of a pleuroamniotic shunt. The use of multiple thoracenteses does not appear justified. Thoracentesis, just prior to delivery, may be helpful, if the degree of effusion suggests that respiratory compromise may be an issue at birth.

Monitoring   Persistent effusions require that management is coordinated at a tertiary center. Ultrasound examinations should be performed every 1 to 3 weeks to detect progression and development or hydrops. The frequency will vary with the size of the collections. The pleural effusion may disappear or worsen and require thoracentesis.

Pregnancy Course   When polyhydramnios is present (42%), perinatal mortality is high. Mortality is related to the development of hydrops, prematurity, and pulmonary hypoplasia. Bilateral pleural effusions have a much worse prognosis and may cause in utero death. Small unilateral pleural effusions tend to regress and disappear. Persistent isolated effusions may require prenatal or postnatal drainage.

Pregnancy Termination Issues   In cases in which an accurate diagnosis cannot be made prior to delivery, a nondestructive method of termination should be performed to allow complete fetal evaluation.

Delivery Because immediate resuscitation may be necessary, delivery should occur at a tertiary perinatal center. Early delivery is not indicated except in cases where hydrops occurs after 32 weeks gestation.

NEONATOLOGY

Resuscitation Preparations should be made for intubation, assisted ventilation, and immediate postdelivery thoracentesis. Three factors are important in the decision for immediate intubation and assisted ventilation at birth: 1. gestational age, 2. bilateral collections of fluid, and 3. predelivery drainage either by thoracentesis or pleuroamniotic shunt. Term infants who have had drainage of the fluid collections within 24 hours of delivery may not require assistance with the onset of respirations. In all other cases immediate intubation is usually required.

Transport Delivery at a tertiary perinatal center is preferable. Transfer after delivery is indicated if respiratory support is required, bilateral effusions are present or fluid reaccumulates after initial drainage. The infant should be accompanied by a skilled transport team in transit.

Testing and Confirmation A chest radiograph will show the extent of the pleural effusion.

Nursery Management Facilitation of normal cardiorespiratory adaptation is the primary goal. Respiratory distress syndrome may complicate the course if the infant is delivered prematurely, in which case surfactant replacement therapy is indicated. Continuing pleural drainage for several days may be required.

BIBLIOGRAPHY

Adams H, Jones A, Hayward C: The sonographic features and implications of fetal pleural effusions. *Clin Radiol* 1988; 39:398-401.

Bovicelli L, Rizzo N, Orsini LF et al: Ultrasonic real-time diagnosis of fetal hydrothorax and lung hypoplasia. *J Clin Ultrasound* 1981; 9:253-254.

Estroff JA, Parad RB, Frigoletto FD Jr et al: The natural history of isolated fetal hydrothorax. *Ultrasound Obstet Gynecol* 1992; 2:162-165.

Laberge JM et al: The fetus with pleural effusions. In: Harrison MR et al (eds): *The unborn patient, prenatal diagnosis and treatment.* Philadelphia. WB Saunders, 1991. pp. 314-319.

Longaker MT, Laberge JM, Dansereau J et al: Primary fetal hydrothorax: natural history and management. *J Pediatr Surg* 1989; 24:573-576.

Mandelbrot L, Dommergues M, Aubry MC et al: Reversal of fetal distress by emergency in utero decompression of hydrothorax. *Am J Obstet Gynecol* 1992; 167:1278-1283.

Porembski M, Laughrin TJ, Brown G et al: Ultrasonic antenatal diagnosis of pleural effusion (chylothorax). *J Med Ultrasound* 1981; 5:51-52.

Rodeck CH, Fisk NM, Fraser DI et al: Long-term in utero drainage of fetal hydrothorax. *N Engl J Med* 1988; 319:1135-1138.

Weber AM, Philipson EH: Fetal pleural effusion: a review and meta-analysis for prognostic indicators. *Obstet Gynecol* 1992; 79:281-286.

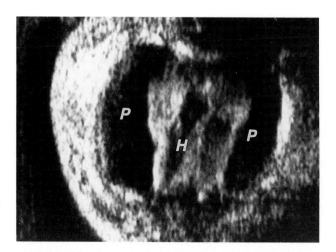

Bilateral pleural effusion (*P*). The heart (*H*) can be seen between the pleural effusions on this transverse view. This fetus was stillborn.

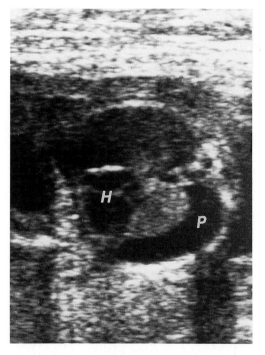

Unilateral pleural effusion (*P*). The heart (*H*) is mildly deviated to the right on this transverse view. Following neonatal aspiration of the effusion the neonate did well.

6 The Gastrointestinal System

6.1 ANAL ATRESIA
IMPERFORATE ANUS

EPIDEMIOLOGY/GENETICS

Definition Anal atresia is the congenital absence of an anal opening.

Epidemiology 1 out of 5,000 births (M3:F2).

Embryology Anal atresia results from an arrest in the division of the cloaca into the urogenital sinus and rectum that occurs during the ninth week of fetal development. Over 80 genetic, chromosomal, and sporadic syndromes have been reported with anal atresia. Associated abnormalities occur in 50% of cases and include spinal/skeletal abnormalities (30%), genitourinary abnormalities (38%), tracheoesophageal fistula (TEF) (10%) and cardiac malformations (5%). The vertebral abnormalities, anal atresia, cardiac abnormalities, tracheoesophageal fistula, esophageal atresia, renal agenesis and dysplasia, and limb defects (VACTERL) association should be considered in these cases.

Inheritance Patterns Sporadic. Rare families show autosomal recessive inheritance.

Teratogens Alcohol, thalidomide, and maternal diabetes.

Prognosis Dependent on associated malformations. Greater than 70% of isolated cases will have successful functional repair.

SONOGRAPHY

Findings
1. **Fetus:** The anus can be visualized as an echogenic dot on transverse view at the level of the genitalia. The echogenic dot will be absent in anal atresia. Although rarely diagnosed prenatally, dilated colon may be noted in the pelvis or periphery of the abdomen. Echogenic foci with acoustic shadowing may be seen within the obstructed colon representing calcified meconium. Associated anomalies are present in 90% of cases diagnosed prenatally including genitourinary (renal agenesis or dysplasia, horseshoe kidney, uterine duplications); cardiovascular, cental nervous system (CNS), gastrointestinal (particularly TEF), and skeletal abnormalities. Anal atresia is associated with the VACTERL syndrome, the syndrome of caudal regression, and trisomies 18 and 21.
2. **Amniotic Fluid:** Usually, the fluid volume is normal in isolated anorectal atresia, but may be decreased if associated with bilateral renal dysplasia or increased if associated with TEF.
3. **Placenta:** Normal.
4. **Measurement Data:** Normal, if isolated.
5. **When Detectable:** The earliest prenatal diagnosis reported was at 29 weeks.

Pitfalls Differentiation of dilated small and large bowel may be very difficult. Location is a help if the descending colon can be traced to the rectum. Apparent haustra can be seen with large and small bowel.

Differential Diagnosis The major differential diagnostic issue is to exclude associated abnormalities that will result in a poor prognosis, and would not benefit from aggressive obstetric management.

Where Else to Look Due to the high association with other anomalies, a careful examination of the fetal genitourinary, skeletal, cardiovascular, CNS, and gastrointestinal structures is recommended.

PREGNANCY MANAGEMENT

Investigations and Consultations Required
1. Fetal echocardiography should be performed to diagnose associated cardiovascular anomalies.
2. Amniocentesis can be performed for chromosome analysis, especially if other anomalies are present.
3. Computed tomography (CT) scan with intraamniotic iodinated contrast injection can resolve diagnostic uncertainty.
4. Consultation with a pediatric surgeon is appropriate.

Monitoring Standard obstetric care is appropriate.

Pregnancy Course No specific obstetric complications are to be expected.

Pregnancy Termination Issues The late clinical presentation of this malformation will preclude the option of pregnancy termination.

Delivery   The high association with other abnormalities makes delivery at a tertiary center the best option. A pediatric dysmorphologist should be available to evaluate the neonate for a possible genetic syndrome.

NEONATOLOGY

Resuscitation   There are no special issues for delivery room management with isolated anal atresia. If other associated anomalies exist then management may need to be directed toward their related issues.

Transport   Transfer to a tertiary center having a pediatric surgeon is always indicated. Beyond orogastric decompression, there are no special precautions during transfer.

Testing and Confirmation   Obvious on newborn examination. Postnatal radiologic studies will define the defect.

Nursery Management   Once the lack of patency of the anus has been established, all enteral intake is contraindicated. Maintenance intravenous fluids should be administered. Nasogastric decompression should be maintained.

SURGERY

Preoperative Assessment   Nasogastric decompression and intravenous (IV) access for fluid resuscitation should be immediately achieved. Evaluation for a high versus low imperforate anus deformity is then carried out. This may be by standard radiographic techniques but is usually by sonography or CT scan.

Operative Indications   The lesion that results in a prenatal sonographic diagnosis is on the severe end of the spectrum of imperforate anus deformities. The anal "fistula" usually ends in the urethra in males and the vagina in females. It is rarely a "blind pouch."

Types of Procedures   The immediate goal is to decompress the blocked colon with a proximal colostomy and prevent further urinary tract contamination. The definitive repair of this condition is delayed until the other associated anomalies have been stabilized and the patient has gained weight. Repair usually takes place at 6 months to 1 year of age or 15 to 20 lbs. body weight.

Surgical Results/Prognosis   The overall survival is excellent unless there is a major associated cardiac defect. Although all patients can be reconnected to achieve stooling by way of the anus, only 70% will achieve socially acceptable anal continence due to insufficient sphincter innervation and poor anorectal sensation. Secondary operations for apparent incontinence should be delayed, because continence tends to improve with age. Although secondary muscle wrapping procedures such as the gracilis sling can be used for secondary incontinence, they are seldom totally successful.

BIBLIOGRAPHY

Grant T, Newman M, Gould R et al: Intraluminal colonic calcifications associated with anorectal atresia: prenatal sonographic detection. *J Ultrasound Med* 1990; 9:411–413.

Harris RD, Nyberg DA, Mack LA et al: Anorectal atresia: prenatal sonographic diagnosis. *Am J Roentgenol* 1987; 149:395-400.

Hertzberg BS, Bowie JD: Fetal gastrointestinal abnormalities. *Radiol Clin North Am* 1990; 28:101-114.

Langemeijer RATM, Molenaar JC: Continence after posterior sagittal anorectoplasty. *J Pediatr Surg* 1991; 26:587-590.

Nyberg DA: Intra-abdominal abnormalities. In: *Diagnostic ultrasound of fetal anomalies: text and atlas.* St Louis. Mosby–Year Book, 1990. pp. 363-368.

Pe A: Imperforate anus and cloacal malformations. In: Ashcraft KW, Holder TM (eds): *Pediatric surgery,* 2nd ed. Philadelphia. WB Saunders, 1993. pp. 372-373.

Pena A: Surgical management of anorectal malformation: a unified concept. *Pediatr Surg Int* 1988; 3:82-93.

Samuel N, Dicker D, Landman J et al: Early diagnosis and intrauterine therapy of meconium plug syndrome in the fetus: Risks and benefits. *J Ultrasound Med* 1986; 5:425-428.

Santulli TV, Schullinger JN, Kiesewetter WB et al: Imperforate anus: a survey from the members of the Surgical Section of the American Academy of Pediatrics. *J Pediatr Surg* 1971; 6:484-487.

Shalev E, Weiner E, Zuckerman H: Prenatal ultrasound diagnosis of intestinal calcifications with imperforate anus. *Acta Obstet Gynecol Scand* 1983; 62:95-96.

Smith ED: The bath water needs changing, but don't throw out the baby: An overview of anorectal anomalies. *J Pediatr Surg* 1987; 22:335-348.

Vermesh M, Mayden KL, Confino E et al: Prenatal sonographic diagnosis of Hirschsprung's disease. *J Ultrasound Med* 1986; 5:37-39.

Vintzileos AM, Campbell WA, Nochimson DJ et al: Antenatal evaluation and management of ultrasonically detected fetal anomalies. *Obstet Gynecol* 1987; 69:640-660.

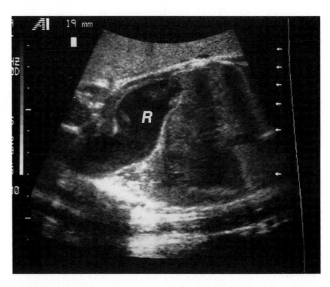

Coronal view of the fetal abdomen. A dilated loop of bowel can be seen (*R*). This represents a dilated rectum and sigmoid colon. Anal atresia was found at delivery.

6.2 Duodenal Atresia

EPIDEMIOLOGY/GENETICS

Definition   Duodenal atresia is characterized by complete obliteration of the lumen of the duodenum, and is the most common type of congenital small bowel atresia.

Epidemiology   1 out of 10,000 births. One third have trisomy 21.

Embryology   At 5 weeks of embryonic life, the lumen of the duodenum is obliterated by proliferating epithelium. Patency is usually restored by the eleventh week. Failure of this recanalization results in duodenal atresia. Associated abnormalities occur in 30% to 50% of patients and include skeletal defects (vertebral, rib, and sacral agenesis; radial anomalies; and club foot), gastrointestinal (GI) abnormalities (annular pancreas, esophageal atresia, TEF, intestinal malrotation, Meckel's diverticulum and anal atresia), cardiac malformations and renal defects. More than 15 genetic, chromosomal, and sporadic syndromes have been reported with duodenal atresia.

Inheritance Patterns   Generally sporadic with rare familial reports.

Teratogens   Maternal diabetes.

Prognosis   Mortality is due to associated abnormalities or preterm labor and can be as high as 36%. Successful surgical repair is possible in essentially all cases of isolated duodenal atresia.

SONOGRAPHY

Findings
1. **Fetus:** The "double bubble" sign, an enlarged fluid-filled stomach and proximal duodenum separated by the pylorus, is seen. The stomach fails to empty. No fluid-filled bowel, distal to the duodenum, is seen.
2. **Amniotic Fluid:** Severe polyhydramnios occurs, although it may not be present until after 24 weeks.
3. **Placenta:** Normal.
4. **Measurement Data:** The abdominal circumference may be increased due to the distended stomach.
5. **When Detectable:** May be detectable as early as 18 to 20 weeks, but appearances may be normal until after 24 weeks.

Pitfalls
1. A prominent normal stomach with a visible incisura angularis may be confused with a double bubble sign. The amniotic fluid will be normal and stomach dilatation will not persist on repeat exams.
2. A bile-filled gallbladder might be misinterpreted as a distended duodenum, as might other right upper quadrant cystic masses such as choledochal cyst or hepatic cyst. Appropriate angulation should show the two cystic structures of the stomach and duodenum connecting.

Differential Diagnosis
1. Annular pancreas—The sonographic appearances are indistinguishable
2. Duodenal stenosis—The obstruction site is usually at a more distal level.
3. Ladd's bands—The typical obstruction site is in the third portion of the duodenum.
4. Proximal jejunal atresia—The entire duodenum and proximal jejunum will be dilated.
5. Midgut volvulus—More dilated small bowel will be visible.
6. Proximal intestinal duplications—A normal-sized stomach should be visible as well.

Where Else To Look
1. Look for the other findings of Down syndrome (there is a 30% association).
2. Skeletal problems are often found—vertebral deformities, radial ray problems, and club feet are seen.
3. Other gastrointestinal malformations such as malrotation, other atresias, and Meckel's diverticulum should be sought.
4. Cardiovascular malformations can occur in the absence of Down syndrome.
5. Genitourinary malformatons such as hydronephrosis and multicystic dysplastic kidney may be seen.
6. Examine the cervix to see if it is still long and closed.

PREGNANCY MANAGEMENT

Investigations and Consultation Required   Consultation with a pediatric surgeon is indicated for the family to discuss neonatal management. Chromosome studies should be done at any gestation by either amniocentesis, percutaneous umbilical blood sampling, or late chorionic villi sampling (CVS). Detailed fetal echocardiography is warranted, even in the absence of trisomy 21, due to the high association of cardiac abnormalities (20%).

Fetal Intervention   No intervention is warranted. Serial amniocentesis has no benefit in prolonging pregnancy.

Monitoring   The diagnosis is usually made because of the onset of polyhydramnios. Therefore, preterm labor will occur in the majority of cases, and care should be under the direction of a perinatologist. Regularly scheduled examinations are necessary to detect evidence of preterm labor and for early institution of tocolysis.

Pregnancy Course The major obstetric complication of this disorder is severe polyhydramnios with a high incidence of preterm labor.

Pregnancy Termination Issues Pregnancy termination would not be indicated in a chromosomally normal fetus because of the excellent prognosis following surgical repair. Even in fetuses with Down syndrome, the options for termination are limited by the late clinical presentation of duodenal atresia.

Delivery The site for delivery should be one capable of managing the preterm infant and one where appropriate personnel are available for surgical repair.

NEONATOLOGY

Resuscitation With high obstruction, amniotic fluid may be green stained from regurgitated bilious secretions, giving the erroneous impression that there has been meconium passage in utero. Aspiration of bilious material into the lungs is equally damaging as with meconium aspiration and every effort should be made to prevent its occurrence. Fetal distress can occur, usually from reasons other than the structural anomaly. If there are other indications of distress, it is safer to assume that aspiration may have occurred and therefore laryngoscopy and tracheal suction are indicated before the onset of respiration. In the absence of other markers of fetal distress and if the fluid is thin and without particulate matter, airway instrumentation is probably not indicated.

If positive pressure ventilation is required because of respiratory depression, bag and mask ventilation should be avoided to reduce the likelihood of gaseous distension of the stomach and duodenum.

If there is known or suspected high obstruction (polyhydramnios or other ultrasound findings), the stomach should be emptied prior to transfer of the infant from the delivery room to reduce the risk of regurgitation and aspiration.

Transport Transfer to a tertiary center where there is a pediatric surgeon is always indicated. Orogastric decompression and maintenance of intravenous fluid infusion in transit is essential.

Testing and Confirmation Confirmation of the diagnosis is best established by abdominal radiographs or ultrasound. Air is an excellent and safe contrast media for suspected upper tract obstruction. The classic radiograph shows the double bubble of an air-filled stomach and proximal duodenum.

Additional diagnostic evaluation for associated anomalies should be obtained as indicated.

Nursery Management If cardiorespiratory resuscitation has been required, the first priority is to facilitate cardiorespiratory adaptation with oxygen, fluids, and ventilatory support as needed.

Intravenous access should be established by the most rapid and reliable route and fluid and electrolyte support instituted. If "third spacing" or dehydration is suspected, the rate of infusion should be increased until there is urine production. Nasogastric decompression should be maintained to minimize the risk of aspiration and respiratory complication. Parenteral nutrition is usually required in the postoperative period as there is usually a significant interval before adequate enteral intake is established.

SURGERY

Preoperative Assessment Acute management includes a radiographic upper gastrointestinal contrast study or radiographic enema examination to attempt to rule out an associated intestinal malrotation and potential volvulus. If this lesion can be excluded then the surgery can be delayed long enough to rule out other significant anomalies included in the VACTERL syndrome.

Operative Indications If an associated intestinal malrotation can be ruled out, preoperatively, then the surgical management of the duodenal atresia is semielective. That is, the operation can be safely delayed while possible associated anomalies are evaluated and the patient is stabilized.

Types of Procedures Nasogastric decompression is immediately instituted as well as intravenous fluid management. The defect usually occurs at the level of the second to third portion of the duodenum and frequently is in close association with the sphincter of Oddi. The operation of choice is a duodenoduodenostomy or duodenojejunostomy. The dilated proximal duodenum can have poor peristalsis with slow emptying across the anastomotic site, making delayed enteral nutrition a possibility. Total parenteral nutrition via a central venous line can be required or a trans-anastomotic feeding jejunostomy can be used for earlier enteral nutrition.

Associated VACTERL gastrointestinal deformities such as esophageal atresia with TEF or imperforate anus must be considered when establishing the order of preference for surgical repair.

Surgical Results/Prognosis A major associated and potentially lethal problem is the presence of a cardiac defect in 20% of patients, which accounts for both a high mortality and chronic complication rate. Uncomplicated duodenal atresia has an excellent prognosis with a greater than 95% survival rate.

BIBLIOGRAPHY

Barss VA, Benecerraf BR, Frigoletto FD Jr: Antenatal sonographic diagnosis of fetal gastrointestinal malformations. *Pediatrics* 1985; 76:445-449.

Cragun JD, Martin ML, Moore CA et al: Descriptive epidemiology of small intestinal atresia. Atlanta, GA. *Teratology* 1993; 48:441-450.

Fonkalsrud EW, DeLorimier AA, Hays DM: Congenital atresia and stenosis of the duodenum: a review compiled from the members of the Surgical Section of the American Academy of Pediatrics. *Pediatrics* 1969; 43:79-83.

Haller JA Jr, Tepas JJ, Pickard LR et al: Intestinal atresia: current concepts of pathogenesis, pathophysiology, and operative management. *Am Surg* 1983; 49:385-391.

Irving IM: Duodenal atresia and stenosis: annular pancreas. In: Lister J, Irving IM (eds): *Neonatal surgery*, 3rd ed. London. Butterworths, 1990.

Kimura K, Tsugawa C, Ogawa K et al: Diamond-shaped anastomosis for congenital duodenal obstruction. *Arch Surg* 1977; 112:1262-1263.

Mooney D, Lewis JE, Connors RH et al: Newborn duodenal atresia: an improving outlook. *Am J Surg* 1987; 153:347-349.

Nelson LH, Clark CE, Fishburne JI et al: Value of serial sonography in the in utero detection of duodenal atresia. *Obstet Gynecol* 1982; 59:657-660.

Nixon HH, Tawes R: Etiology and treatment of small intestinal atresia: analysis of a series of 127 jejunoileal atresias and comparison with 62 doudenal atresias. *Surgery* 1971; 69:41-51.

Nyberg DA: Intra-abdominal abnormalities. In: *Diagnostic ultrasound of fetal anomalies: text and atlas*. St Louis. Mosby–Year Book, 1990. pp. 352-355.

Rescorla FJ, Grosfeld JL: Intestinal atresia and stenosis: analysis of survival in 120 cases. *Surgery* 1985; 98:668-676.

Romero R, Jeanty P, Gianluigi P et al: The prenatal diagnosis of duodenal atresia. Does it make any difference? *Obstet Gynecol* 1988; 71:739.

Touloukian RJ: Intestinal atresia and stenosis. In: Ashcraft KW, Holder TM (eds): *Pediatric surgery*, 2nd ed. Philadelphia. WB Saunders, 1993. pp. 305-319.

Wayne ER, Burrington JD: Management of 97 children with duodenal obstruction. *Arch Surg* 1973; 107:857.

Wesley J, Mahour GH: Congenital intrinsic duodenal obstruction: a 25 year review. *Surgery* 1977; 82:716-720.

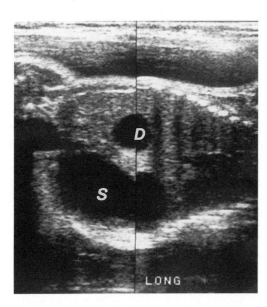

Coronal view of the fetal trunk. Two cystic structures can be seen. These represent the body of the stomach (*S*) and the duodenal bulb (*D*). Polyhydramnios was present.

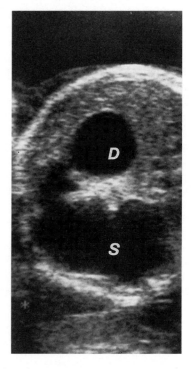

Angled view to show the two cystic structures connecting. The pylorus between the stomach (*S*) and the duodenum (*D*) is visible.

6.3 GASTROINTESTINAL ATRESIA OR STENOSIS

EPIDEMIOLOGY/GENETICS

Definition   Nonduodenal bowel atresias with congenital obliteration of the lumen of segments of the large or small intestine.

Epidemiology   Small intestinal atresias occur in 2 to 3 out of 10,000 births (jejunal—50%, ileal—43%, multiple—7%). Colonic atresia occurs in 1 out of 20,000 births.

Embryology   Most isolated cases of bowel atresias are thought to be due to ischemic injury from hypotension, vascular accidents, volvulus, intussusception, or vascular malformations. Forty-four percent of cases have associated findings including: small for gestational age (30%), meconium peritonitis (12%), meconium ileus (10%), cystic fibrosis (15%), omphalocele (7.5%), gastroschisis (12.5%), malrotation, imperforate anus, cardiovascular defects (7%) and chromosomal abnormalities (7%). More than 15 genetic, chromosomal, and sporadic syndromes have been described with intestinal atresia.

Inheritance Patterns   Rare autosomal recessive (AR) genetic syndromes including multiple intestinal atresias and jejunal atresia have been described. Approximately 25% of cases of jejunal and ileal atresia have cystic fibrosis (AR).

Teratogens   Thalidomide and cocaine.

Prognosis   Outcome is excellent in greater than 95% of patients if the atresia occurs as an isolated abnormality. Otherwise, the prognosis is dependent on the associated abnormalities or syndrome diagnosis.

SONOGRAPHY

Findings
1. **Fetus:** Multiple dilated fluid-filled bowel loops are noted within the abdomen proximal to the stenotic or atretic segment. The exact site of obstruction may be difficult to determine sonographically because large and small bowel are more or less the same size in utero. Small bowel dilatation is much more common.
2. **Amniotic Fluid:** Polyhydramnios is usually present and is more severe in more proximal atresias. Large bowel atresias are often not associated with polyhydramnios.
3. **Placenta:** Normal.
4. **Measurement Data:** The abdominal circumference may be large due to bowel dilatation.
5. **When Detectable:** Usually detected after 24 weeks.

Pitfalls
1. Cystic abdominal masses, such as duplication, mesenteric, and ovarian cysts, may be confused with dilated bowel loops.
2. Hydronephrosis and hydroureter or very large multicystic kidneys may also be confused with fluid-filled, dilated bowel. Renal anomalies, however, are rarely associated with polyhydramnios.
3. In utero, the small and large bowel are approximately equal in size. Significantly dilated loops of bowel are much more likely to be due to small bowel atresia, especially if there is polyhydramnios. The distribution of the bowel is of little value in determining whether it is large or small bowel.

Differential Diagnosis
1. Midgut volvulus.
2. Meconium ileus.
3. Congenital chloridorrhea.

Where Else to Look
1. Meconium peritonitis (ascites, intraperitoneal calcifications or cysts) occurs in 6% of cases due to bowel perforation. Either ascites or a meconium cyst will be visible (see Chapter 6.5).
2. Associated bowel anomalies are common and include malrotation, volvulus, intestinal duplications, gastroschisis, and other bowel atresias (anorectal, esophageal, colonic).
3. Extraintestinal anomalies are seen in less than 5% of small bowel atresias distal to the duodenum.

PREGNANCY MANAGEMENT

Investigations and Consultations Required   Chromosome studies should be performed even for more distal lesions. If sonographic findings are suggestive of meconium ileus, an evaluation for cystic fibrosis should be done. Fetal echocardiography should be done to exclude associated cardiac malformations. A management plan should be devised in consultation with a pediatric surgeon.

Monitoring   The high risk of prematurity makes it mandatory that prenatal care is under the direction of a perinatologist. Ultrasound examinations should be performed every 3 to 4 weeks to detect polyhydramnios and monitor the degree of bowel dilatation. Polyhydramnios is, however, rare in lesions beyond the jejunum. Careful assessment for signs of preterm labor is essential.

Pregnancy Course   The risk of preterm labor is high in lesions from the jejunum proximal.

Pregnancy Termination Issues   Pregnancy termination is rarely entertained because of the late clinical presentation of these malformations and their potential for surgical correction.

Delivery   In general, management should be delivery at term in a facility with appropriate support services. In theory, early delivery might be beneficial in cases with massive bowel dilatation, but no data are available to support this approach.

NEONATOLOGY

Resuscitation   With high obstruction, amniotic fluid may be green stained from regurgitated bilious secretions giving the erroneous impression that there has been meconium passage in utero. Aspiration of bilious material into the lungs is equally damaging as with meconium aspiration and every effort should be made to prevent its occurrence. Fetal distress can occur, usually from reasons other than the structural anomaly. If there are other indications of distress, it is safer to assume that aspiration may have occurred and, therefore, laryngoscopy and tracheal suction are indicated before the onset of respiration. In the absence of other markers of fetal distress and if the fluid is thin and without particulate matter, airway instrumentation is probably not indicated.

If positive pressure ventilation is required because of respiratory depression, bag and mask ventilation should be avoided to reduce the likelihood of gaseous distension of the stomach and proximal small bowel. If there is known or suspected high obstruction (polyhydramnios or other ultrasound findings), the stomach should be emptied prior to transfer of the infant from the delivery room to reduce the risk of regurgitation and aspiration.With known or suspected distal obstruction there are usually no special resuscitation issues.

Transport   Transfer to a tertiary center with a pediatric surgeon is always indicated. Orogastric decompression and maintenance of intravenous fluid infusion in transit is essential.

Testing and Confirmation   Confirmation of the diagnosis is best established by abdominal radiographs and ultrasound. Air is an excellent and safe contrast media for suspected upper tract obstruction. The typical pattern is to see multiple dilated loops and air-fluid levels proximally with no visualization of bowel distally. Additional diagnostic evaluation for associated anomalies should be obtained as indicated.

Nursery Management   If cardiorespiratory resuscitation has been required, the first priority is to facilitate cardiorespiratory adaptation with oxygen, IV fluids, and ventilatory support as needed.

Intravenous access should be established by the most rapid and reliable route and fluid and electrolyte support instituted. If "third spacing" or dehydration is suspected, the rate of infusion should be increased until there is urine production. Orogastric decompression should be maintained to minimize the risk of aspiration and respiratory complication. Parenteral nutrition is usually required in the postoperative period as there is usually a significant interval before adequate enteral intake is established.

SURGERY

Operative Indications   All neonates with obstructed small bowel require surgery.

Types of Procedures   Intestinal decompression and IV access with maintenance fluids are begun immediately. Antibiotics are also started. The infant then has an exploratory laparotomy.

Surgical repair usually consists of the excision of a portion of the dilated proximal intestine and a modified end to end or end to side primary anastomosis. If the atresia involves a large portion of bowel, it can result in potential short-gut syndrome. Under these circumstances, tapering of the dilated proximal bowel with primary anastomosis is utilized. This avoids increased loss of length, facilitates early gut function, and diminishes bacterial overgrowth in the proximal intestine. The use of proximal intestinal stomas is reserved only for those cases complicated by severe meconium peritonitis or perforation with bacterial contamination and secondary peritonitis.

Surgical Results/Prognosis   The long-term prognosis is primarily related to the length and functional capability of the remaining small bowel or associated defects such as cystic fibrosis. Uncomplicated short-segment intestinal atresias have an excellent prognosis. Extensive areas of gut atresia can result in the short-gut syndrome. Infants can be kept alive by intravenous alimentation but undergo progressive worsening of liver function with eventual death from portal hypertension.

BIBLIOGRAPHY

Cragun JD, Martin ML, Moore CA et al: Descriptive epidemiology of small intestinal atresia. Atlanta, GA. *Teratology* 1993; 48:441-450.

DeLorimier AA, Fonkalsrud EW, Hays DM: Congenital atresia and stenosis of the jejunum and ileum. *Surgery* 1969; 65:819-827.

Haller JA Jr, Tepas JJ, Pickard LR et al: Intestinal atresia: current concepts of pathogenesis, pathophysiology, and operative management. *Am Surg* 1983; 49:385-391.

Howard EF, Othersen HB: Proximal jejunoplasty in the treatment of jejunal atresia. *J Pediatr Surg* 1973; 8:685-690.

Kjoller M, Holm-Nielsen G, Meiland H et al: Prenatal obstruction of the ileum diagnosed by ultrasound. *Prenat Diagn* 1984; 5:427.

Lister J: Intestinal atresia and stenosis, excluding the duodenum. In: Lister J, Irving IM (eds): *Neonatal surgery*. London, Butterworths', 1990.

Louw J: Resection and end to end anastomosis in the management of atresia and stenosis of the small bowel. *Surgery* 1967; 62:940-950.

Nixon HH, Tawes R: Etiology and treatment of small intestinal atresia: analysis of a series of 127 jejunoileal atresias and comparison with 62 duodenal atresias. Surgery 1971; 69:41-51.

Nyberg DA: Intra-abdominal abnormalities. In: *Diagnostic ultrasound of fetal anomalies: text and atlas*, St. Louis. Mosby–Year Book, 1990. pp. 355-358.

Rescorla FJ, Grosfeld JL: Intestinal atresia and stenosis: analysis of survival in 120 cases. *Surgery* 1985; 98:668-676.

Rickham PP, Karplus M: Familial and hereditary intestinal atresia. *Helv Paediatr Acta* 1971; 26:561-564.

Samuel N, Dicker D, Feldberg D et al: Ultrasound diagnosis and management of fetal intestinal obstruction and volvulus in utero. *J Perinat Med* 1984; 12:333-337.

Touloukian RJ: Intestinal atresia and stenosis. In: Ashcraft KW, Holder TM (eds): *Pediatric surgery*, 2nd ed. Philadelphia. WB Saunders, 1993. pp. 305-319.

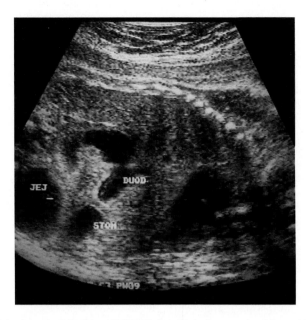

Jejunal atresia. A few loops of distended small bowel greater than 2.5 cm wide are seen, but most of the bowel is not fluid filled. The relatively few distended loops allowed a diagnosis of a high small bowel obstruction. Polyhydramnios was present.

6.4 GASTROSCHISIS

EPIDEMIOLOGY/GENETICS

Definition   Gastroschisis is the intrauterine evisceration of fetal intestine through a paraumbilical wall defect.

Epidemiology   Occurs in 1 out of 4,000 births (M1:F1).

Embryology   The etiology is probably heterogeneous with some cases of gastroschisis resulting from vascular accident or error in development of the right omphalo-mesenteric artery leading to infarction and necrosis at the base of the umbilical cord. The umbilical cord arises intact, medial to the defect. Thickening, edema, and matting together of the intestines occurs in some cases. It used to be thought that these abnormalities were due to the irritating effects of amniotic fluid, but they are more likely the result of vascular compromise from kinking of the blood vessels coming through the small paraumbilical defect. Intestinal atresias and other gastrointestinal disruptions are found in approximately 5% to 15% of cases. Malrotation is almost universal. Extraintestinal abnormalities occur in less than 5% of cases.

Inheritance Patterns   Rare familial recurrences suggest a few families may have an autosomal dominant inheritance of isolated gastroschisis.

Teratogens   None known.

Screening   Maternal serum alpha-fetoprotein (MSAFP) screening can detect approximately three fourths of gastroschisis cases. Values of 4 to 5 MOM are often seen.

Prognosis   Liveborns have a greater than 90% survival rate with modern surgical treatment and neonatal intensive care.

SONOGRAPHY

Findings
1. **Fetus:** Small or large bowel herniates through the anterior abdominal wall. The bowel exits through the right lower quadrant. Cord vessels can be seen to the left of the exiting bowel. If the anterior abdominal wall defect is small, bowel loops within or outside the abdomen are dilated. Small bowel dilatation to a width of greater than 1.8 cm is associated with greater long-term morbidity. Gut malrotation is common, so the stomach may be inverted or malpositioned. The stomach or bladder may be included in the gastroschisis contents.
2. **Amniotic Fluid:** Amniotic fluid volume is usually normal or slightly diminished. Polyhydramnios can occur if the gut is obstructed.
3. **Placenta:** Normal placenta.

4. **Measurement Data:** Intrauterine growth retardation (IUGR) often develops. Abdomen measurements are unreliable because some of the bowel is in the gastroschisis.
5. **When Detectable:** At 13 weeks. Prior to 13 weeks, there is confusion with physiological gut herniation.

Pitfalls
1. The extraabdominal bowel can be overlooked and thought to be umbilical cord coiled alongside the abdomen.
2. In large patients with oligohydramnios and in third trimester prone fetuses, the condition can easily be missed.

Differential Diagnosis
1. Limb body wall complex—Gastroschisis is a component of the syndrome, but in addition, the liver will be outside of the abdomen and there will be spine and limb problems.
2. Ruptured omphalocele—In this extremely rare entity, the liver, as well as bowel, is usually outside of the abdomen.
3. Tangled cord adjacent to the fetal abdomen—Color flow Doppler will show vascular flow.

Where Else to Look
1. Look for bowel dilatation of greater than 18 mm in gastroschisis or in the abdomen—this finding is associated with delay in time to oral feeding.
2. Check stomach position for malrotation.
3. Look elsewhere for anomalies. Ruptured omphalocele containing only gut, indistinguishable by ultrasound, is associated with chromosomal anomalies.

PREGNANCY MANAGEMENT

Investigations and Consultations Required   Although the risk of chromosome abnormalities is low, amniocentesis should be discussed with the patient. Fetal echocardiography should be performed in all cases of gastroschisis. The family should be referred to a pediatric surgeon for a thorough discussion of the neonatal management issues.

Monitoring   Care should be coordinated in a tertiary center because of the potential need for early intervention. Serial ultrasound examinations should be performed every 3 to 4 weeks to detect thickening or dilatation of the fetal bowel and to assess fetal growth. Fetal assessment, such as nonstress testing, should be initiated if there is evidence of a lag in growth.

Pregnancy Course   The increased incidence of IUGR in fetuses with gastroschisis may complicate the obstetric management.

Pregnancy Termination Issues   There are no special concerns regarding the method or location for pregnancy termination.

Delivery   For the fetus with normal-appearing bowel on ultrasound examination, delivery at term is appropriate. The mode of delivery is controversial. Some studies have shown no clear benefit of cesarean section over vaginal delivery, but a recent study by Sakala et al showed an improved perinatal outcome in neonates delivered by elective cesarean section prior to labor. In the fetus where bowel dilatation or thickening develops, the prognosis may be improved by early delivery when fetal lung maturity is achieved. A pediatric surgeon and a tertiary neonatal intensive care unit (NICU) should be available at the delivery site.

NEONATOLOGY

Resuscitation   Assistance with the onset of respiration is usually not required, unless there is concurrent prematurity associated respiratory distress. If assisted ventilation is required, bag and mask ventilation is contraindicated to avoid gaseous distension of the stomach and bowel.

The major concern is the protection of the extruded bowel. Extreme care must be taken to avoid torsion of the bowel loops, which could further compromise perfusion. If there is marked distension of the bowel, perfusion can be compromised by the kinking of the mesenteric vessels as they exit through the abdominal wall defect. Prompt decompression of the stomach is important. The bowel should be covered with warmed saline-soaked gauze and supported to avoid torsion and the trunk should be encased in a sterile plastic bag with a drawstring ("bowel bag"). This not only reduces evaporative heat and water loss, but also reduces the likelihood of surface contamination.

Transport   Transfer to a tertiary center having a pediatric surgeon is always indicated. Care of the bowel, as outlined above, should be provided during the transport. Reliable venous access should be established and a balanced electrolyte solution administered. Gastric decompression is essential.

Testing and Confirmation   Once there is recovery from the initial surgery and the exposed bowel is covered, additional diagnostic evaluation may be instituted if there is concern for associated anomalies.

Nursery Management   Protection of the bowel and intravenous fluid support as described above should be provided in the time prior to surgical repair. In some instances, it may be necessary to provide ventilatory support in the early postoperative period as there may be increased intraabdominal pressure from the reduction of the extruded bowel back into the abdominal cavity. Parenteral nutrition is required during the postoperative recovery period as there is always a significant interval before adequate enteral intake is established.

SURGERY

Preoperative Assessment   The immediate postdelivery goals are to preserve infant temperature, avoid excess fluid loss from the exposed bowel surface, prevent further surface contamination, and maintain circulation to the exposed bowel loops. Nasogastric decompression is essential and intravenous fluids calculated at 1.5 times normal maintenance rates are begun. Broad spectrum antibiotic therapy should be started.

Operative Indications   All neonates with gastroschisis require surgery shortly after birth.

Types of Procedures   The operative repair consists of enlarging the narrowed abdominal wall opening and evaluating the exposed viscera. The abdominal wall is stretched gently and an attempt is made to reduce the extraabdominal contents into the abdomen. If the intraabdominal pressure is less than 20 mm Hg by intragastric or intravesical pressure measurement, a primary fascial closure can be achieved. Excessive intraabdominal pressures necessitate delayed fascial closure using temporary coverage with a silastic/dacron intraabdominal pouch or the use of mobilized lateral skin flaps. The former method requires a secondary closure of fascia after the bowel has been gradually reduced into the abdomen over the ensuing 5 to 7 days. The latter requires a secondary closure of fascia at several months of age. Both techniques can result in infections and chronic incisional herniae.

Complications   The infant may have had intrauterine intestinal ischemia with necrosis of an exposed bowel loop requiring an excision and primary bowel anastomosis or possible temporary intestinal stomas. Intestinal atresias can also be a complication. Their repair as a primary or secondary procedure depends on the degree of chemical peritonitis with "matting" of the bowel that is present. Delayed intestinal function with poor enteral nutrition is expected in most patients. Central venous access and early total parenteral nutrition are therefore required. A "short bowel" syndrome can be a significant functional problem with long-term parenteral nutrition and liver failure as potential complications.

Surgical Results/Prognosis   Ultimate survival approaches 90%. A small abdominal cavity that cannot be closed with the techniques described above has a poor outcome. Postoperative infection and delayed total enteral nutrition are the major acute and chronic complications. Large defects can be associated with lung hypoplasia requiring long-term ventilatory support resulting in chronic respiratory insufficiency.

BIBLIOGRAPHY

Chescheir NC, Azizkhan RG, Seeds JW et al: Counseling and care for the pregnancy complicated by gastroschisis. *Am J Perinatol* 1991; 8:323-329.

Colombani PM, Cunningham MD: Perinatal aspects of omphalocele and gastrochisis. *Am J Dis Child* 1977; 131:1386-1388.

Fries MH, Filly RA, Callen PW et al: Growth retardation in prenatally diagnosed cases of gastroschisis. *J Ultrasound Med* 1993; 12:583-588.

Guzman ER: Early prenatal diagnosis of gastroschisis with transvaginal ultrasonography. *Am J Obstet Gynecol* 1990; 162:1253-1254.

Hoyme HE, Jones MC, Jones KL: Gastroschisis: abdominal wall disruption secondary to early gestational interruption of the omphalomesenteric artery. *Semin Perinatol* 1983; 7:294-298.

Irving IM: Umbilical abnormalities. In: Lister J, Irving IM (eds): *Neonatal surgery*. London, Butterworth, 1990.

Kushnir O, Izquierdo L, Vigil D et al: Early transvaginal sonographic diagnosis of gastroschisis. *J Clin Ultrasound* 1990; 18:194-197.

Langer JC, Khanna J, Caco C et al: Prenatal diagnosis of gastroschisis: development of objective sonographic criteria for predicting outcome. *Obstet Gynecol* 1993; 81:53-56.

Luck SR, Sherman JO, Raffensperger JG et al: Gastroschisis in 106 consecutive newborn infants. *Surgery* 1985; 98:677-683.

Nakayama DK, Harrison MR, Gross BH et al: Management of the fetus with an abdominal wall defect. *J Pediatr Surg* 1984; 19:408-413.

Perrella RR, Ragavendra N, Tessler FN et al: Fetal abdominal wall mass detected on prenatal sonography: gastroschisis vs omphalocele. *Am J Roentgenol* 1991; 157:1065-1068.

Philippart AI, Canty TG, Filler RM: Acute fluid volume requirements in infants with anterior abdominal wall defects. *J Pediatr Surg* 1972; 7:553-558.

Rubin SZ, Martin DJ, Ein SH: A critical look at delayed intestinal motility in gastroschisis. *Can J Surg* 1978; 21:414-416.

Sakala EP, Erhard LN, White JJ: Elective caesarean section improves outcomes of neonates with gastroschisis. *Am J Obstet Gynecol* 1993; 169:1050-1053.

Swartz KR, Harrison MW, Campbell JR et al: Ventral hernia in the treatment of omphalocele and gastroschisis. *Ann Surg* 1985; 201:347-350.

Yang P, Beaty TH, Khoury MJ et al: Genetic-epidemiologic study of omphalocele and gastroschisis: evidence for heterogeneity. *Am J Med Genet* 1992; 44:668-675.

Yaster M, Scherer TL, Stone MM et al: Prediction of successful primary closure of congenital abdominal wall defects using intraoperative measurements. *J Pediatr Surg* 1989; 24:1217-1220.

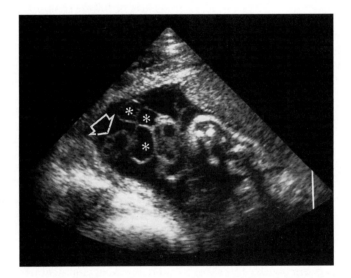

Gastroschisis. Fluid-filled bowel loops (*) are seen adjacent to the fetal abdomen. Note the different appearance of the loop of cord (*arrow*) with the two small umbilical arteries. Gastroschisis loops can be mistaken for cord loops.

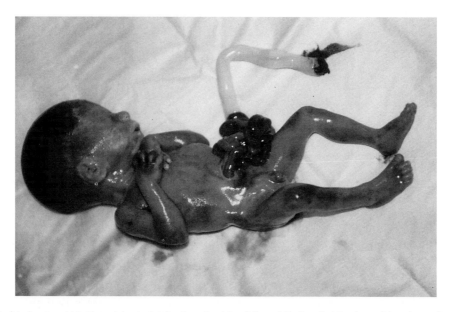

22-week fetus with isolated gastroschisis. Note abdominal defect is to the right of the umbilical cord with only small bowel extruding from the abdomen.

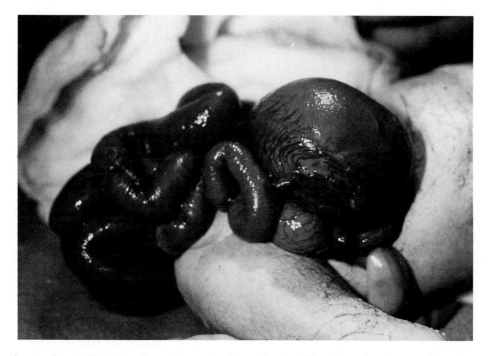

Close-up of gastroschisis in a newborn with extrusion of stomach and small bowel through a right paraumbilical defect.

6.5 Meconium Cyst
Meconium Peritonitis

EPIDEMIOLOGY/GENETICS

Definition   A meconium cyst forms as the result of peritoneal inflammation from recurrent meconium spillage from an intrauterine bowel perforation.

Epidemiology   Unknown, but rare.

Embryology   Meconium peritonitis is a chemical peritonitis resulting from fetal bowel perforation of any cause. Continued leakage of meconium results in cyst formation. Sixty-five percent of cases are due to meconium ileus or small bowel atresia with the majority of cases of meconium ileus associated with a diagnosis of cystic fibrosis. Other commonly associated conditions include volvulus and intussusception.

Inheritance Patterns   Cystic fibrosis is an autosomal recessive single-gene disorder.

Teratogens   None.

Prognosis   Most meconium cysts disappear spontaneously during pregnancy. Surgery for gut torsion or perforation is occasionally required.

SONOGRAPHY

Findings
1. **Fetus**
   a. Echogenic foci, with or without shadowing, are seen anywhere in the peritoneal cavity or scrotum. Calcifications are often linear. A common site is just below the diaphragm on the right.
   b. Meconium pseudocysts—a more or less echofree cyst with irregular echogenic borders. Calcification is often present in the wall. Cysts result from a walled-off bowel perforation. Serial sonograms will show a gradual reduction in size often with increased calcification. They usually resolve before delivery.
   c. Generalized ascites occurs in about 50% of cases of meconium peritonitis. The ascitic fluid may appear echogenic due to leakage of meconium through a recent bowel perforation.
   d. Dilated small bowel is seen in only about 25% of cases of prenatally diagnosed meconium peritonitis and reflects mechanical bowel obstruction leading to perforation. In prenatally diagnosed cystic fibrosis, echogenic foci are intermixed with mildly dilated small bowel loops. Calcification is rarely, if ever, seen with cystic fibrosis.
2. **Amniotic Fluid:** Polyhydramnios is present in the majority of cases (60%).

3. **Placenta:** Normal.
4. **Measurement Data:** The abdominal circumference may be large if the ascites is severe or if the bowel is markedly dilated.
5. **When Detectable:** Usually not detected until after 24 weeks.

Pitfalls
1. Very echogenic meconium may be difficult to distinguish from calcifications.
2. A few meconium cysts have smooth walls and echofree contents.
3. Single, small intraabdominal echogenic foci with shadowing are normal and not associated with cystic fibrosis or postpartum gut perforation.

Differential Diagnosis
1. Of fetal abdominal calcifications:
   a. Intraluminal meconium calcification (seen in small bowel and anorectal atresia).
   b. Parenchymal calcification (hepatic, splenic, adrenal, ovarian)—may be related to toxoplasmosis or cytomegalovirus (CMV).
   c. Cholelithiasis.
   d. Echogenic small bowel—Localized echogenic small bowel is of the same echogenicity as adjacent bone and may be due to:
      i. cystic fibrosis;
      ii. trisomy 21;
      iii. CMV;
      iv. intragut bleed;
      v. normality.
2. Of meconium cyst:
   a. Ovarian cyst—females only; smooth walls often echofree
   b. Duplication cyst—usually tubular shape
   c. Mesenteric cyst—rare, may be septated.
   d. Dilated gallbladder and liver cyst—partially within, or adjacent, to the liver.

Where Else to Look
1. Secondary cystic fibrosis changes in pancreas, gallbladder, and lungs are not seen in utero.
2. Look for changes of CMV and Down syndrome.

PREGNANCY MANAGEMENT

Investigations and Consultations Required   Because the exact etiology often cannot be determined by sonographic findings, amniocentesis should be performed for chromosome studies, viral cultures, and DNA studies for cystic fibrosis. Consultation with a pediatric surgeon should be arranged to plan both fetal and neonatal management.

Fetal Intervention   Early delivery may be appropriate if there is marked bowel dilatation. However, no guidelines exist for judging when intervention might be indicated. For cases with massive fetal ascites, fetal paracentesis just prior to delivery may prevent dystocia.

Monitoring   Careful sonographic monitoring is necessary to assess fluid volume, fetal growth, degree of bowel dilatation, and amount of ascites. Most cysts disappear within a few weeks.

Pregnancy Course   The prognosis for obstetric complications will depend on the etiology of the cyst. Significant fetal ascites may result in dystocia. Concomitant bowel obstruction may lead to polyhydramnios and preterm labor. Most meconium cysts regress and cause no problem postpartum.

Pregnancy Termination Issues   Unless a precise diagnosis has been established, the technique for termination should allow for delivery of an intact fetus for a complete autopsy.

Delivery   Because of the significant risk of premature delivery, and the potential need for immediate surgical intervention for the neonate, the pregnancy should be managed in a tertiary center.

NEONATOLOGY

Resuscitation   Severe abdominal distension may be present at birth, hindering the onset of respiration and necessitating endotracheal intubation. If ascites is known to be present from prenatal ultrasound, then it is probably safe to perform paracentesis to relieve some of the distension.

Transport   Transfer to a tertiary center having a pediatric surgeon is always indicated. Gastric decompression during transport, to avoid aspiration, is essential. Reliable intravenous access and infusion of fluid and electrolyte solution are also indicated.

Testing and Confirmation   The major diagnostic questions are the co-existence of an obstructive lesion and an open perforation allowing continuing meconium spillage. Abdominal radiography without contrast media is usually sufficient to answer both concerns. If meconium ileus is determined to be the cause of the obstruction leading to the perforation, then iontophoresis (sweat testing) for cystic fibrosis is indicated and is known to be reliable after 1 week of age in term infants.

Nursery Management   The primary issues are avoidance of aspiration by gastric decompression, maintenance of hydration and electrolyte balance, and confirmation of the diagnosis. Often, hypotension develops rapidly after birth and large volumes of plasma expanders are required to maintain perfusion.

SURGERY

Preoperative Assessment   Intestinal decompression and IV access with fluid resuscitation and antibiotics are started immediately. An evaluation for an intestinal obstruction is completed. An exploratory laparotomy is performed when and if an intestinal obstruction or peritoneal signs of infection are identified.

Operative Indications   As previously noted, meconium cysts may not produce intestinal obstruction. However, a meconium cyst can maintain a fistulous connection to the bowel lumen and become secondarily infected.

Types of Procedures   Such cysts require antibiotics, drainage, and eventual excision with closure of the fistula. Intestinal obstruction with meconium peritonitis presents a significant surgical challenge. Frequently, temporary enteral stomas are needed with delayed closure after resolution of the extensive peritoneal inflammatory response.

Surgical Results/Prognosis   Depending on etiology, the remaining small intestine or colon may be very short resulting in chronic short-gut syndrome. This may result in long-term parenteral nutrition with secondary liver failure. Long-term surgical survival for non-short–gut infants is good with the ultimate prognosis dependent on associated factors such as cystic fibrosis.

BIBLIOGRAPHY

Andrassy RJ, Nigiotis JG: Meconium disease of infancy: meconium ileus, meconium plug syndrome, and meconium peritonitis. In Ashcraft K, Holder T (eds): *Pediatric surgery*. Philadelphia. WB Saunders, 1993.

Boix-Ochoa J: Meconium peritonitis. *J Pediatr Surg* 1968; 3:715.

Careskey JM, Grosfeld JL, Weber TR et al: Giant cystic meconium peritonitis (GCMP): improved management based on clinical and laboratory observations. *J Pediatr Surg* 1982; 17:482-489.

Forouhar F: Meconium peritonitis: pathology, evolution, and diagnosis. *Am J Clin Pathol* 1982; 78:208-213.

Foster MA, Nyberg DA, Mahony BS et al: Meconium peritonitis: prenatal sonographic findings and their clinical significance. *Radiology* 1987; 165:661-665.

Hertzberg BS, Bowie JD: Fetal gastrointestinal abnormalities. *Radiol Clin North Am* 1990; 28:101-114.

McGahan JP, Hanson F: Meconium peritonitis with accompanying pseudocyst: prenatal sonographic diagnosis. *Radiology* 1983; 148:125-126.

Nicolaides KH, Campbell S: Ultrasound diagnosis of congenital abnormalities. In: Harrison MR, Golbus MS, Filly RA (eds): *The unborn patient, antenatal diagnosis and treatment.* Philadelphia. WB Saunders, 1991; pp 593-648.

Nyberg DA: Intra-abdominal abnormalities. In: *Diagnostic ultrasound of fetal anomalies: text and atlas.* St Louis. Mosby–Year Book, 1990. pp. 378-382.

Yankes JR, Bowie JD, Effman EL: Antenatal diagnosis of meconium peritonitis with inguinal hernias by ultrasonography. *J Ultrasound Med* 1988; 7:221-223.

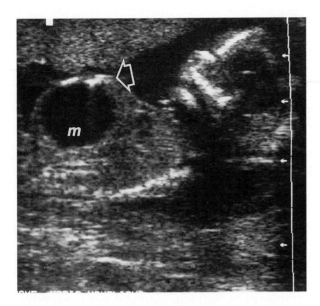

Sagittal longitudinal view. There is a cystic mass in the fetal abdomen (*m*). Note the echogenic areas in the wall that represent areas of calcification (*arrow*). This meconium cyst has a relatively smooth wall. An irregular wall is not uncommon.

6.6 MECONIUM ILEUS

EPIDEMIOLOGY/GENETICS

Definition   Meconium ileus is a cause of congenital intestinal obstruction due to inspissated meconium.

Epidemiology   1 out of 50,000 births (M1:F1).

Embryology   The cause of inspissated meconium is usually unknown, but commonly associated conditions include small bowel atresias, cystic fibrosis, volvulus, and intussusception.

Inheritance Patterns   Cystic fibrosis is an autosomal recessive single-gene disorder, but the other known etiologies are generally sporadic.

Teratogens   None.

Prognosis   In those cases proven to be secondary to cystic fibrosis (CF), the latter diagnosis determines the long-term outcome. In the non-CF related cases, the etiologies are mixed and the prognosis variable, though most resolve and have normal bowel function.

SONOGRAPHY

Findings
1. **Fetus:** Dilated bowel develops due to impacted meconium in the distal ileum. Echogenic meconium may be seen within dilated bowel or within bowel of normal caliber. Echogenic, but nonshadowing masses may be seen within the abdomen and represent impacted meconium. Colonic dilatation may be seen if the meconium plug obstructs the colon.
2. **Amniotic Fluid:** Polyhydramnios may be present if the bowel is dilated.
3. **Placenta:** Normal.
4. **Measurement Data:** Abdominal circumference may be increased if the bowel is significantly dilated.
5. **When Detectable:** Cases have been diagnosed prior to 24 weeks.

Pitfalls
In normal fetuses, echogenic bowel may be seen prior to 20 weeks, but this is usually a transient and nonobstructive phenomenon. No small bowel dilatation will be seen.

Differential Diagnosis
1. Echogenic bowel associated with chromosomal abnormalities particularly trisomy 21 may mimic that seen in meconium ileus.
2. Echogenic bowel may be seen in congenital infections such as CMV.
Cases of meconium ileus with perforation will present with a sonographic picture of meconium peritonitis, and those conditions, such as CMV, that have a poor prognosis must be excluded.

Where Else to Look   Look for stigmata of Down syndrome or CMV.

PREGNANCY MANAGEMENT

Investigations and Consultations Required   Molecular studies for CF should be considered. The best approach is probably amniocentesis, which also can provide information regarding chromosome status. Measurement of amniotic fluid proteins, such as alkaline phosphatase, will not be helpful, as low levels would be expected in any condition that causes intestinal obstruction. If there is a question of peritonitis, amniotic fluid culture for CMV should be performed. Consultation with a pediatric surgeon is appropriate. If a diagnosis of CF is established, referral of the family to a pediatrician with special expertise in the management of CF should be done.

Fetal Intervention   Theoretically early delivery prior to bowel perforation will improve prognosis. However, at present no criteria have been established to indicate when intervention would be appropriate.

Monitoring   Serial ultrasounds and regular clinical assessment is essential to detect increased amniotic fluid volume and evidence of preterm labor. No other special fetal assessment is necessary. Prenatal care should be coordinated in a tertiary center.

Pregnancy Course   Polyhydramnios secondary to intestinal obstructions may result in preterm labor.

Pregnancy Termination Issues   There are no special concerns if a diagnosis has been established. Without a diagnosis a complete autopsy and appropriate molecular studies on fetal tissue are essential.

Delivery   Prenatal care and delivery should be at a tertiary center. The degree of bowel distension will rarely be significant enough to cause abdominal dystocia.

NEONATOLOGY

Resuscitation   No special resuscitation measures required.

Transport   Transfer to a tertiary perinatal center having a pediatric surgeon is always indicated. Gastric decompression during transport is essential.

Testing and Confirmation   Reliable iontophoresis is possible after 1 week in term infants.

Nursery Management   The primary issues are avoidance of aspiration by gastric decompression, maintenance of hydration and electrolyte balance, and confirmation of the diagnosis. Relief of the obstruction by use of water-soluble high osmolality contrast media enemas can be obtained in the majority of cases.

SURGERY

Preoperative Assessment   Initial management includes nasogastric decompression, IV fluid resuscitation, and a water-soluble contrast enema radiographic study. The latter will definitively make a diagnosis and may be therapeutic by dislodging the impacted firm meconium from the distal ileum. The hypertonic intestinal contrast material can acutely dehydrate the infant. Compensation for this fluid shift must be made with increased IV fluids up to 1.5 to 2.0 times normal maintenance levels.

Operative Indications   Failure with two separate radiographic efforts or the presence of peritoneal irritation or free intraperitoneal air warrants subsequent surgical management.

Types of Procedures   Surgical management includes intraoperative irrigation of the meconium-obstructed bowel by way of an enterotomy. Successful evacuation is followed by primary bowel closure. Necrotic intestine, meconium peritonitis, or extensive proximal intestinal meconium blockage can necessitate the use of enteral stomas with a subsequent reanastomosis at a later time.

Surgical Results/Prognosis   The short-term prognosis is excellent (80%) and the long-term outcome is related to the cause of the meconium ileus.

BIBLIOGRAPHY

Benacerraf BR, Chaudhury AK: Echogenic fetal bowel in the third trimester associated with meconium ileus secondary to cystic fibrosis. *J Reprod Med* 1989; 34:299-300.

Caniano DA, Beaver BL: Meconium ileus: a fifteen-year experience with forty-two neonates. *Surgery* 1987; 102:699-703.

Caspi B, Elchalal U, Lancet M et al: Prenatal diagnosis of cystic fibrosis: Ultrasonographic appearance of meconium ileus in the fetus. *Prenat Diagn* 1988; 8:379-382.

Chang PY, Huang FY, Yeh ML et al: Meconium ileus-like condition in Chinese neonates. *J Pediatr Surg* 1992; 27:1217-1219.

Denholm TA, Crow HC, Edwards WH et al: Prenatal sonographic appearance of meconium ileus in twins. *Am J Roentgenol* 1984; 143:371-372.

Estroff JA, Parad RB, Benacerraf BR: Prevalence of cystic fibrosis in fetuses with dilated bowel. *Radiology* 1992; 183:677-680.

Goldstein RB, Filly RA, Callen PW: Sonographic diagnosis of meconium ileus in utero. *J Ultrasound Med* 1987; 6:663-666.

Hertzberg BS, Bowie JD: Fetal gastrointestinal abnormalities. *Radiol Clin North Am* 1990; 28:101-114.

Kalayoglu M, Sieber WK, Rodnan JB et al: Meconium ileus: a critical review of treatment and eventual prognosis. *J Pediatr Surg* 1971; 6:290-300.

Muller F, Aubry MC, Gasser B et al: Prenatal diagnosis of cystic fibrosis. II: meconium ileus in affected fetuses. *Prenat Diagn* 1985; 5:109-117.

Nicolaides KH, Campbell S: Ultrasound diagnosis of congenital abnormalities. In: Harrison MR, Golbus MS, Filly RA (eds): *The unborn patient: antenatal diagnosis and treatment*. Philadelphia. WB Saunders, 1991. pp. 593-648.

Noblett H: Treatment of uncomplicated meconium ileus by gastrografin enema: a preliminary report. *J Pediatr Surg* 1969; 4:190-197.

Shigemoto H, Endo S, Isomoto T et al: Neonatal meconium obstruction in the ileum without mucoviscidosis. *J Pediatr Surg* 1978; 13:475-479.

6.7 OMPHALOCELE

EPIDEMIOLOGY/GENETICS

Definition   An omphalocele is a transparent sac of amnion attached to the umbilical ring that contains herniated abdominal viscera.

Epidemiology   Occurs in 1 out of 4,000 births (M1:F5).

Embryology   Omphaloceles, which contain liver, are thought to result from failure of lateral body-fold migration and body-wall closure. Omphaloceles containing gut only are said to result from the embryonic persistence of the body stalk. Omphaloceles have associated malformations in over half of all cases discovered, including congenital heart defects, bladder exstrophy, imperforate anus, neural tube defects, cleft lip with or without cleft palate, and diaphragmatic hernias. In addition, approximately 25% have associated chromosomal abnormalities, especially trisomies 13 and 18. The Beckwith-Wiedemann syndrome, which includes omphalocele with macrosomia, macroglossia, organomegaly and neonatal hypoglycemia, and a number of rare skeletal dysplasias, should be considered in these patients.

Inheritance Patterns   Rare autosomal dominant and X-linked recessive families have been reported with isolated omphaloceles. Some cases of the Beckwith-Wiedemann syndrome show autosomal dominant inheritance.

Teratogens   None known.

Screening   MSAFP screening detects approximately 40% of omphaloceles.

Prognosis   The prognosis is generally dependent on associated malformations and/or the size of the defect in the anterior abdominal wall for an isolated omphalocele. Giant lesions containing both solid and hollow viscera have limited potential for successful closure.

SONOGRAPHY

Findings
1. **Fetus:** Liver or gut bulge into a circumscribed mass at the cord insertion site. An umbilical hernia represents a very small omphalocele. Eighty percent of omphaloceles contain liver, sometimes with small bowel. A membrane surrounds the mass; and usually, some fluid lies between the omphalocele contents and the membrane. Ascites may be present within the omphalocele or in the abdomen. Twenty percent of omphaloceles contain gut and fluid only. Most chromosomal anomalies are seen in this subgroup. Ruptured omphalocele is a rare complication—there are similar appearances to gastroschisis, except that the liver may be present and the cord runs through the center of the mass.
2. **Amniotic Fluid:** Polyhydramnios is often present.
3. **Placenta:** Normal.
4. **Measurement Data:** The abdominal circumference cannot be accurately measured because of the omphalocele.
5. **When Detectable:** Can be detected at 11 weeks, although confusion with physiological gut herniation at that age is possible.

Pitfalls
1. If the liver lies outside of the abdomen at 10 or 11 weeks, then a true omphalocele is present. In "pseudoomphalocele," only gut will be seen in the hernia.
2. A few omphaloceles are said to be only intermittently visible; presumably, they act like a hernia and return to the abdomen now and then.
3. Confusion with gastroschisis may occur. Typically, a surrounding membrane is seen with omphalocele and not with gastroschisis. It is said that omphaloceles can rupture. Liver within the ventral mass is not seen with gastroschisis, unless another anomaly, such as the limb body-wall complex, is present. The cord may occasionally exit at the site of an omphalocele.
4. Undue transducer pressure on a flaccid fetal abdomen can cause an anterior bulge that can resemble an omphalocele, however there is no waist to the apparent omphalocele and it is dependant on fetal position.

Differential Diagnosis
1. Gastroschisis—A surrounding membrane is present with omphalocele. The cord exits the left side of a gastroschisis.
2. Umbilical hernia—indistinguishable from a small omphalocele.
3. Bladder exstrophy—No bladder is visible. A mass is seen below the cord insertion site.
4. Cloacal exstrophy—Dilated vagina and renal systems are also seen.
5. Body stalk anomaly—There are usually limb problems and the placenta is attached to the fetus.
6. Allantoic cyst—Does not arise from the fetus. The contents are cystic and the cyst is attached to the cord. A urachal cyst may also be present so that the allantoic and urachal cysts lie adjacent.
7. Pentalogy of Cantrell—There is ectopia cordis present in addition to a large omphalocele.

Where Else to Look   At least 50% of fetuses with omphalocele have defects elsewhere.
1. Look for findings of trisomy 13 and 18, which are seen in about one third of omphalocele patients, including heart defects, and facial and limb problems.

2. Look for stigmata of the Beckwith-Wiedeman syndrome, including macrosomia; renal, liver, and spleen enlargement; macroglossia; and polyhydramnios. Tumors may be seen.

3. Look for findings of body stalk anomaly and limb body-wall complex. Spinal distortion, limb absence, and ectopia cordis may be seen.

4. Omphalocele is a component of Pentalogy of Cantrell (ectopia cordis and diaphragmatic and sternal defects are seen as well as omphalocele).

5. In the absence of other syndromes, cardiac defects, such as ventricular septal defect (VSD) and other gastrointestinal problems, such as bowel malrotation, atresias, and stenoses, occur.

6. Look for cord cysts—The chances of a chromosomal anomaly increase if one or more cord cysts are present in addition to the omphalocele.

PREGNANCY MANAGEMENT

Investigations and Consultations Required   Chromosome studies are an essential component of the initial evaluation. The high incidence of associated congenital heart defects requires that fetal echocardiography be performed in all cases. Consultation with a pediatric surgeon will prepare the family for the issues regarding neonatal management, such as primary versus secondary closure, and allow a coordinated management plan to be developed.

Monitoring   No special modifications are needed. Serial ultrasound examinations should be done every 4 weeks to monitor growth. Fetal evaluations, such as nonstress testing, are not necessary unless there is evidence of alteration in normal growth parameters.

Pregnancy Course   There are no specific obstetric complications to be expected.

Pregnancy Termination Issues   In cases with multiple abnormalities and in which a precise etiology has not been determined, consideration should be given to using a nondestructive method of termination, for example, prostoglandin, followed by a careful autopsy.

Delivery   There appears to be no advantage to cesarean section except in those cases where a large lesion might result in obstructed labor. Delivery should be performed at term, in a center with appropriate perinatal facilities for surgical management of the neonate.

NEONATOLOGY

Resuscitation   Assistance with the onset of respiration is usually not required unless there is concurrent prematurity, associated respiratory distress, or an associated anomaly that interferes with the onset of cardiorespiratory adaptation. If assisted ventilation is required, bag and mask ventilation is contraindicated to avoid gaseous distension of the stomach and bowel.

The major concern is to avoid trauma to and contamination of the omphalocele sac. Once respiration and circulation are established, the sac should be covered with warmed saline moistened gauze, covered by additional wrapping, to avoid evaporative heat and water loss. It is always safe to enclose the trunk and legs in a sterile plastic drawstring bag (bowel bag). Prompt decompression of the stomach is important initially, followed by intermittent gastric suction.

Transport   Transfer to a tertiary center with a pediatric surgeon is always indicated. Protection of the sac, as described above, as well as gastric decompression, should be maintained during transport. Reliable IV access should be established and infusion of a balanced electrolyte solution should be instituted.

Testing and Confirmation   Because of the very high incidence of associated anomalies, appropriate diagnostic testing including chromosomal analysis, echocardiography, and renal sonography should be obtained expeditiously before surgical intervention.

Nursery Management   Care of the omphalocele sac, gastric decompression, and intravenous fluids, as noted above, should be maintained. In some instances, it may be necessary to provide ventilatory support in the early postoperative period as there may be increased intraabdominal pressure from the reduction of the extruded viscera back into the abdominal cavity. Parenteral nutrition is required during the postoperative recovery period as there is always a significant interval before adequate enteral intake can be established.

SURGERY

Preoperative Assessment   Preoperative and postdelivery goals include a thorough evaluation for associated anomalies, particularly of the cardiac system, including echocardiography. Preoperative broad-coverage antibiotics are administered.

Operative Indications   Surgical repair is required on a semiurgent schedule, after resuscitation and the evaluation for associated anomalies, to prevent further contamination of the permeable membrane covering the defect. Some surgeons prefer nonoperative management of the intact omphalocele using frequent applications of a desiccating antiseptic solution and undertaking a delayed closure of the secondarily produced skin-covered hernia. This process is associated with acute complications of toxicity due to absorption of the antiseptic solutions and delayed complications secondary to attempted repair of the resultant hernia in the face of significant associated intraperitoneal adhesions. For these reasons most surgeons prefer the acute reduction and total surgical repair of omphaloceles. However, in the case of the "giant" omphalocele, which is frequently associated with severe pulmonary insufficiency, the topical form of therapy may be the preferred procedure.

Types of Procedures Intraoperative management consists of removal of the amniotic sac, evaluation for associated intestinal malrotation with lysis of bands obstructing the duodenum, and evaluation of the intestine for possible associated atresias. Primary fascial and abdominal-wall closure can be accomplished if intraabdominal pressure, measured by either the intragastric route using a nasogastric tube or the intravesical method using a bladder catheter, does not exceed 20 mm Hg after return of the viscera to the abdominal cavity. A temporary silastic/dacron extraabdominal pouch is used if the intraabdominal pressure is too high for primary closure. Gradual reduction of the viscera can usually be accomplished over 5 to 7 days with subsequent surgical removal of the pouch and secondary abdominal wall closure.

Giant omphaloceles usually are associated with primary respiratory distress, due to lung hypoplasia, and make primary abdominal-wall repair less likely. Even with the use of an initial silastic pouch, they eventually may require mobilized lateral skin flaps with prosthetic material to achieve coverage of the exposed viscera. The alternative method is the previously described acute nonoperative therapy. Secondary closure of the remaining ventral wall defect after either nonoperative or incomplete surgical closure of the fascia can be achieved following further body growth and development.

Surgical Results/Prognosis If there are no associated anomalies such as an intestinal atresia, resumption of postoperative intestinal function is prompt. Overall survival depends on the severity of the associated anomalies, most commonly cardiac defects, and can vary from 30% to 70%. Long-term morbidity is also related to the associated anomalies, most notably cardiac.

BIBLIOGRAPHY

Bowerman RA: Sonography of fetal midgut herniation: normal size criteria and correlation with crown-rump length. *J Ultrasound Med* 1993; 5:251-254.

Colombani PM, Cunningham MD: Perinatal aspects of omphalocele and gastrochisis. *Am J Dis Child* 1977; 131:1386-1388.

Fink IJ, Filly RA: Omphalocele associated with umbilical cord allantoic cyst: sonographic evaluation in utero. *Radiology* 1983; 149:473-476.

Getachew MM, Goldstein RB, Edge V et al: Correlation between omphalocele contents and abnormalities: sonographic study in 37 cases. *Am J Roentgenol* 1992; 158:133-6.

Irving IM: Umbilical abnormalities. In: Lister J, Irving IM: *Neonatal surgery*. London. Butterworth, 1990; 376-402.

Lodeiro JG, Byers JW III, Chuipek S et al: Prenatal diagnosis and perinatal management of the Beckwith-Wiedeman syndrome: a case and review. *Am J Perinatol* 1989; 6:446-449.

Luck SR, Sherman JO, Raffensperger JG et al: Gastroschisis in 106 consecutive newborn infants. *Surgery* 1985; 98:677-683.

Nakayama DK, Harrison MR, Gross BH et al: Management of the fetus with an abdominal wall defect. *J Pediatr Surg* 1984; 19:408-413.

Nicolaides KH, Snijders RJM, Cheng HH et al: Fetal gastro-intestinal and abdominal wall defects: associated malformations and chromosomal abnormalities. *Fetal Diagn Ther* 1992; 7:102-115.

Nyberg DA, Fitzsimmons J, Mack LA et al: Chromosomal abnormalities in fetuses with omphalocele. *J Ultrasound Med* 1989; 8:299-308.

Philippart AI, Canty TG, Filler RM: Acute fluid volume requirements in infants with anterior abdominal wall defects. *J Pediatr Surg* 1972; 7:553-558.

Salzman L, Kuligowska E, Semine A: Pseudoomphalocele: pitfalls in fetal sonography. *AJR* 1986; 146:1283-1285.

Schmidt W, Yarkoni S, Crelin ES et al: Sonographic visualization of physiologic anterior abdominal wall hernia in the first trimester. *Obstet Gynecol* 1987; 69:911-915.

Swartz KR, Harrison MW, Campbell JR et al: Ventral hernia in the treatment of omphalocele and gastroschisis. *Ann Surg* 1985; 201:347-350.

Van de Gijn EJ, Van Vugt JMG, Sollie JE et al: Ultrasonographic diagnosis and perinatal management of fetal abdominal wall defects. *Fetal Diagn Ther* 1991; 6:2-10.

Yang P, Beaty TH, Khoury MJ et al: Genetic-epidemiologic study of omphalocele and gastroschisis: evidence for heterogeneity. *Am J Med Genet* 1992; 44:668-675.

Yaster M, Scherer TL, Stone MM et al: Prediction of successful primary closure of congenital abdominal wall defects using intraoperative measurements. *J Pediatr Surg* 1989; 24:1217-1220.

Yazbeck S, Ndoye M, Khan AD: Omphalocele: a 25 year experience. *J Pediatr Surg* 1986; 21:761-763.

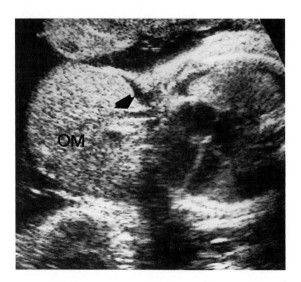

Large liver filled omphalocele (*OM*). Note the cord entering the abdomen at the center of the point where the liver exits the abdomen (*arrow*). A small rim of fluid can be seen at the edge of the liver.

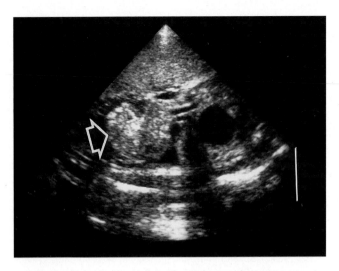

Gut-filled omphalocele. The omphalocele again exits at the cord insertion site (*arrow*) but the entire contents of the omphalocele are gut. This form of omphalocele is much more likely to be karyotypically abnormal.

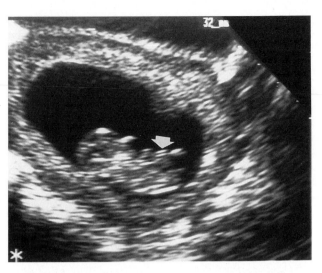

Pseudoomphalocele. Eleven-week fetus with a bulge on the anterior aspect of the abdomen (*arrow*), which represents physiological gut herniation. A repeat sonogram a month later showed a normal anterior abdominal appearance.

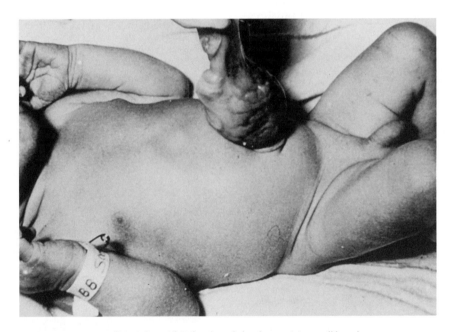

Newborn infant with isolated omphalocele containing small bowel.

7 The Neck and Face

7.1 CLEFT LIP AND PALATE

EPIDEMIOLOGY/GENETICS

Definition   A facial cleft involving the upper lip and/or palate, usually occurring to the left or right of midline. Cleft lip and/or cleft palate may occur as an isolated malformation or as part of a multiple malformation syndrome. Midline facial clefts may be associated with underlying brain malformations, especially holoprosencephaly.

Epidemiology   1 out of 1000 births (M>F) for cleft lip and/or cleft palate; five out of 1000 births for isolated cleft palate (M1:F2). There is marked ethnic and racial variation in incidence. Medial facial clefts account for less than 1% of all facial clefts.

Embryology   Cleft lip and cleft palate are due to a failure of union of the frontonasal process of the face with the lateral maxillary prominences at about 3 to 4 weeks of gestation. Almost 300 multiple malformation syndromes have been described with cleft lip or cleft palate. Midline facial clefts are the result of a deficient frontonasal development process that is normally induced by the underlying brain. Midline facial clefts with underlying brain abnormalities are seen in trisomy 13.

Inheritance Patterns   Most isolated cleft lips or cleft palates show multifactorial inheritance, but dominant, recessive and X-linked syndromes have been described. The pattern of inheritance depends upon an accurate diagnosis.

Teratogens   Alcohol, maternal PKU, hyperthermia, hydantoin, trimethadione, aminopterin and methotrexate.

Prognosis   The prognosis for a good cosmetic and functional repair with isolated cleft lip and/or cleft palate is excellent. Otherwise, the prognosis is dependent upon any associated malformations or a syndrome diagnosis. Midline clefts, if they are associated with underlying brain malformations, usually carry a poor prognosis.

SONOGRAPHY

Findings
1. **Fetus**
   a. Unilateral cleft lip with or without palate—obliquely aligned gap in the lip that extends up to the nose. The profile view shows a nose with a hooked appearance. A gap in the maxilla and palate is sometimes present.
   b. Bilateral cleft lip with or without palatal defect—A central mass protrudes below the nose so there is an abnormal profile view with an infranasal premaxillary mass. Standard views of the lips are not obtainable. A bony gap in the maxilla is present.
   c. Central cleft lip and palate—There is an absence of the central maxilla and upper lip with a deformed nose that may be absent and replaced by a proboscis. There may be only one nostril in a small nose. This type of cleft lip and palate is always associated with other facial findings such as hypotelorism or cyclops and there is usually holoprosencephaly, often with trisomy 13.
2. **Amniotic Fluid:** Amniotic fluid is generally normal, but may be increased due to defective swallowing.
3. **Placenta:** Normal.
4. **Measurement Data:** Assuming this is an isolated process, growth should be normal.
5. **When Detectable:** Cleft lip is detectable by about 13 weeks, but the palatal defect may not be detectable until approximately 18 weeks. Prior to this, the maxilla is still in the process of fusion.

Pitfalls
1. Bilateral cleft lip and palate is often mistaken for a facial mass such as a teratoma or proboscis.
2. The detection of cleft lip and palate is difficult and depends on a cooperative fetus that is not always face down.
3. Isolated cleft palate is usually missed because the maxilla may be spared.
4. A central echo-free area may be seen prior to 18 weeks in the maxilla as development is completed.

Differential Diagnosis
1. Epignathus (facial teratoma). The mass is asymmetrical and enters the mouth. Confusable with bilateral cleft lip and palate
2. Normal variant delayed maxillary fusion.

Where Else to Look
1. All types of cleft lip and palate may well be associated with anomalies elsewhere, particularly congenital heart disease and intracranial malformations. Amniotic bands may be seen with unilateral clefts.
2. The central defect form is associated with midbrain fusion problems such as the various types of holoprosencephaly, septooptic dysplasia, trisomy 13, and other facial problems such as hypotelorism and proboscis.

PREGNANCY MANAGEMENT

Investigations and Consultations Required   Chromosome studies should be done in all cases, including apparently isolated cleft lip/palate. Fetal echocardiography is an essential component of the evaluation. The parents should be examined by a pediatric dysmorphologist for possible genetic disorders that are inherited in an autosomal dominant fashion. The necessity for other consultants will depend on what other structural abnormalities are present.

Monitoring   Because of the significant risk of other abnormalities that may be missed by sonographic evaluations, prenatal care should be under the direction of a perinatologist. No special precautions or fetal assessment is necessary. Once a month sonography is worthwhile because additional defects may have been missed and because of the risk of polyhydramnios.

Pregnancy Course   No specific obstetric complications should be expected in the fetus with cleft lip/palate. Mild polyhydramnios may be associated occasionally.

Pregnancy Termination Issues   Pregnancy termination should be by a nondestructive procedure that will allow full evaluation by a fetal pathologist.

Delivery   The site for delivery should be where there are appropriate facilities and support staff for the care and management of an infant with a cleft. In addition, a pediatric dysmorphologist should be available to assess the infant for possible genetic syndromes.

NEONATOLOGY

Resuscitation   Fetal distress is not expected with isolated facial clefting. However, infants with multiple anomalies including clefts frequently develop fetal distress and require resuscitative assistance. The decision to

intervene is based on the prognosis for the specific syndrome or anomaly complex.

Transport   Referral to a tertiary center following birth is not indicated for isolated facial clefts unless a satisfactory feeding technique cannot be established. With multiple anomalies, referral for more extensive diagnostic evaluation is appropriate.

Testing and Confirmation   Usually detected at birth during the newborn physical examination. A careful search for associated malformations is indicated.

Nursery Management   Establishing a successful oral feeding technique and facilitation of parental adaptation are the initial objectives in management. There are multiple special devices available for use and some infants are helped to feed orally by placement of a customized prosthetic device for an extensive palatal defect.

Referral to a multidisciplinary orofacial team for long-term management, including surgical repair and rehabilitation, is essential.

SURGERY

Preoperative Assessment   Visual inspection is made to determine the type of cleft lip and palate that can range from incomplete to complete, unilateral or bilateral, median to craniofacial. With incomplete cleft lip deformity, the orbicularis muscle has an aberrant attachment to the alar wing and the columella. The premaxilla projects beyond the noncleft side and rotates outward. The nasal structures also are involved to a variable degree. The lateral alar base is invariably rotated outward and flares laterally. The orbital involvement may result in a dystopia, microophthalmia, or anophthalmia.

Presurgical splinting or obturation of the cleft to help with feeding or nursing may be necessary. Presurgical orthopedic manipulation may be necessary to reduce the size of the deformity.

Operative Indications   All patients with these types of anomalies will require surgery. The external lip and facial soft tissues are closed first within 10 weeks or 3 months of life. Closure of more extensive facial clefts involving the orbital globes with exposure of the cornea is carried out as soon as possible. The deeper structures such as the palatal or alveolar defects are closed at age 6 months up to a year to allow good speech and language development. The alveolar bony defects or facial clefting defects are corrected at age 6 to 10 years.

Types of Procedures   The most widely used technique for closure of the cleft lip deformities is the rotation-advancement technique for both the unilateral and bilateral deformities. The medial portion of the cleft deformity including the skin, mucosa, and orbicularis oris muscle are rotated from the columella into a more inferior position. Lateral lip advancement carries the flaring alar base into a better alignment with the contralateral nasal alar base and reorients the lateral component of the orbicularis muscle. In the bilateral lip deformities, the reapproximation of the orbicularis muscle will tend to realign the projection premaxilla and approximate the midfacial structures. The more extensive facial clefts are handled with layered Z-plasties that allow closure of the muscles and skin tissues of the face.

The cleft palate is closed with mucoperiosteal flaps from the hard palate to close the midline structures. The soft palate is repaired by closing the nasal lining and realigning the levator palatini muscles 90° from their attachment to the hard palate. During this procedure care is taken to elongate the palatal tissues in the midline again for purposes of improving later speech.

Bone grafting can be carried out after the age of 5 years, but preferably 8 to 10 years to add further support or replacement to the facial skeletal foundation or contouring. This also prevents peridontal disease and allows better dental eruption and support.

Surgical Results/Prognosis   Surgical results in experienced hands are good and usually restore facial aesthetics and functional speech. Complications from cleft palate closure requiring late palatal lengthening or fistula closure ranges from 8% to 20%. The more extensive the deformities the increased number of procedures that will be required to achieve the desired results.

BIBLIOGRAPHY

Bardach J, Salyer K: *Surgical techniques in cleft lip and palate.* Chicago. Mosby–Year Book, 1987.

Bardach J, Morris HL: *Multidisciplinary management of cleft lip and palate.* Philadelphia. WB Saunders, 1990.

Benacerraf BR, Frigoletto FD Jr, Bieber FR: The fetal face: ultrasound examination. *Radiology* 1984; 153:495-497.

Benacerraf BR, Mulliken JB: Fetal cleft lip and palate: sonographic diagnosis and postnatal outcome. *Plast Reconstr Surg* 1993; 92:1045-1051.

Bronshtein M, Mashiah N, Blumenfeld I et al: Pseudoprognathism—an auxiliary ultrasonographic sign for transvaginal ultrasonographic diagnosis of cleft lip and palate in the early second trimester. *Am J Obstet Gynecol* 1991; 165:1314-1316.

Chervenak FA, Tortora M, Mayden K et al: Antenatal diagnosis of median cleft face syndrome: sonographic demonstration of cleft lip and hypertelorism. *Am J Obstet Gynecol* 1984; 149:94-97.

Dufresne C, Jelks G: Classification of craniofacial anomalies. In: Smith B (ed): Ophthalmic plastic and reconstructive surgery. Philadelphia. Mosby–Year Book, 1987. p 1185.

Dufresne C, So I: Facial clefting malformations. In: Dufresne C, Carson B, Zinreich SJ (eds): *Complex craniofacial problems.* New York. Churchill Livingstone, 1992. p 195.

Jones MC: Etiology of cacial clefts: prospective evaluation of 428 patients. *Cleft Palate J* 1988; 25:16-20.

Kaufman FL: Managing the cleft lip and palate patient. *Pediatr Clin North Am* 1991; 38:1127-1147.

Nyberg DA, Hegge FN, Kramer D et al: Premaxillary protrusion: a sonographic clue to bilateral cleft lip and palate. *J Ultrasound Med* 1993; 12:331-335.

Pilu G, Reece A, Romero R et al: Prenatal diagnosis of craniofacial malformations with ultrasonography. *Am J Obstet Gynecol* 1986; 155:45-50.

Saltzman DH, Benacerraf BR, Frigoletto FD Jr: Diagnosis and management of fetal facial clefts. *Am J Obstet Gynecol* 1986; 155:377-379.

Shields ED: Cleft palate: a genetic and epidemiologic investigation. *Clin Genet* 1981; 20:13-24.

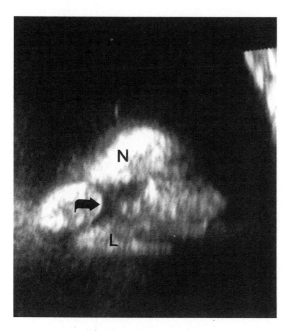

Unilateral cleft palate (*arrow*). *N*, nose; *L*, lip.

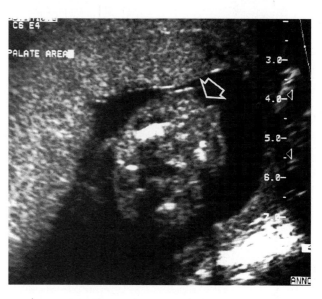

Coronal view showing unilateral cleft lip (*arrow*).

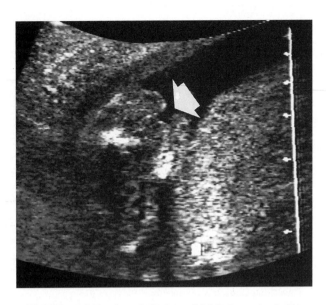

Central cleft lip and palate (*arrow*). This form of cleft lip is associated with gross facial malformations, such as cyclops and absent nose, and intracranial malformations such as holoprosencephaly.

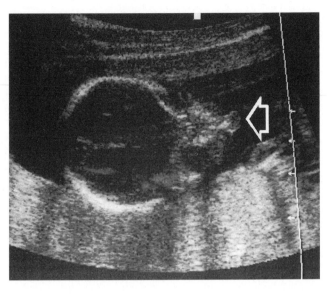

This coronal view of the face shows the apparent central mass that develops when the cleft is bilateral (*arrow*).

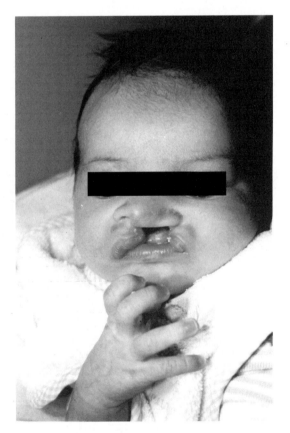

A 2-week-old infant with a unilateral cleft lip and palate deformity with the typical flaring of the nasal alar cartilage and aberrant muscular insertions of the orbicularis oris onto the base of the columella and lateral nasal alar base. Bunching of the orbicularis muscular is noted both medially and laterally to the cleft. Greater segment of the cleft alveolus and palate is rotated outward accentuating the size of the cleft.

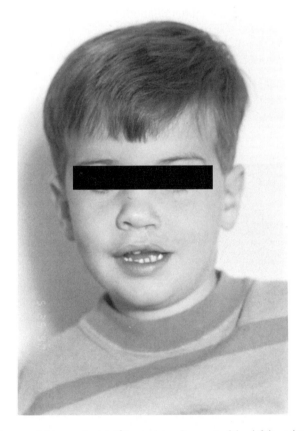

The same child approximately 2¹/₂ years later after repair of the cleft lip, palate, and nasal components. Facial aesthetics and palatal function are also restored.

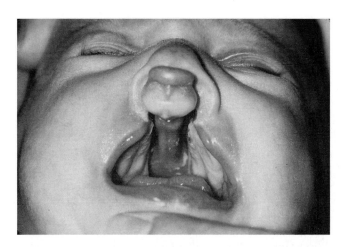

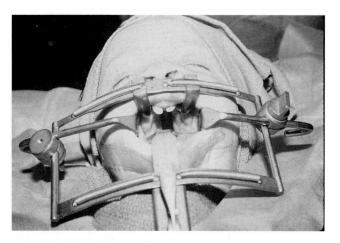

A 3-week-old female infant with a typical bilateral cleft lip and palate deformity. The premaxilla is projecting far forward from the lateral palatal segments, exaggerating the deformity. The lateral palatal shelves are more upright than normal and the vomer is readily noted. The lower lip has two paramedian lip pits, thereby establishing the diagnosis of Van der Woude's syndrome. The lip pits will be removed at the time of the bilateral lip repair at 10 weeks of age.

At 6 months of age the palate will be repaired as shown intraoperatively. Following the lip repair the premaxilla and palatal shelves are in better approximation.

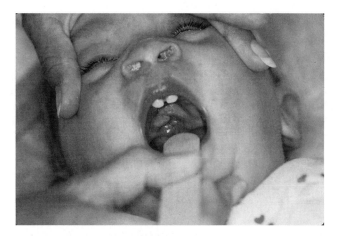

The final appearance at 8 months of age with the cleft lip and nose having been repaired and the palate also repaired.

7.2 CYSTIC HYGROMA

EPIDEMIOLOGY/GENETICS

Definition   Cystic hygromas are characterized by single or multiple congenital cysts of the lymphatic system most commonly found within the soft tissues of the neck.

Epidemiology   1 out of 875 spontaneous abortions (M<1:F1).

Embryology   Nuchal cystic hygromas are the clinical consequence of a delay or absence of the communications that normally develop between the jugular lymph sacs and the internal jugular veins at approximately 40 days gestation. The obstructed jugular lymph sacs dilate along the paths of least resistance into the posterior and lateral cervical areas. Late communication of the sacs with the internal jugular vein may be manifest by redundancy of the posterior nuchal skin, neck webbing, and elevation and anterior rotation of the ears. Complete lymphatic obstruction may be associated with nonimmune fetal hydrops, which is frequently fatal.

Inheritance Patterns   Multiple malformation syndromes with cystic hygromas include the Turner's syndrome, multiple pterygium syndrome (autosomal recessive [AR], X-linked), Noonan syndrome (autosomal dominant [AD]) and the Roberts' syndrome (AR).

Teratogens   Alcohol.

Prognosis   Most severe cases with hydrops die antenatally. Survivors with lymphatic recanalization may present with a webbed neck or redundant nuchal skin.

SONOGRAPHY

Findings
1. **Fetus**
    a. Large bilateral cystic areas termed cystic hygroma develop within the skin in the posterolateral aspect of the neck. They may grow so large that they lie adjacent to each other. It then appears that there is a cystic mass arising from the back of the neck with one to three septa in the center.
    b. Skin thickening—Skin thickening, most pronounced in the upper torso and cranium, soon develops. Septa can be seen within the thickened skin and, as the thickening becomes more severe, lakes of fluid can be seen within the skin.
    c. Hydrops—In more severe examples, hydrops develops with large pleural effusions, pericardial effusions, and ascites. The fetus adopts a Buddha-like position.

2. **Amniotic Fluid:** The amniotic fluid is often reduced.
3. **Placenta:** Normal or thickened with hydrops.
4. **Measurement Data:** Normal, if hydrops does not develop.
5. **When Detectable:** This entity can be first detected at 10 weeks, preferably using the vaginal probe.

Pitfalls
1. Because small cystic hygromata can spontaneously disappear, patients who had cystic hygromata early on may later appear normal and yet have syndromes such as Turner's at birth.
2. A separate entity, also called cystic hygroma, is a unilateral mass in the lateral aspect of the neck or upper torso seen close to term or in neonates. This mass is not associated with karyotypic abnormalities. There is a complex internal structure with multiple septa—surgical removal is required.
3. If the cystic hygroma is incompletely seen, the amniotic band syndrome may be suggested. Skin thickening will not be seen with the amniotic band syndrome.

Differential Diagnosis
1. Nuchal translucency is a similar, although not identical, process in which there is fluid within the skin along the fetal back without the bilateral cystic areas in the neck (see Down syndrome, Chapter 1.4).
2. Encephalocele or meningocele—The mass is posterior and is a single mass. Septum and solid contents may be seen within.
3. Unfused amniotic membrane—Before 13 weeks, an unfused amniotic membrane may lie adjacent to the fetus and be confused with a cystic hygroma.

Where Else to Look
Several syndromes are associated with cystic hygroma:
1. Multiple pterygium syndrome. Pterygia—bands of tough skin—prevent the arms from extending. The fetal limbs are acutely flexed and do not move.
2. Turner's syndrome—(see Chapter 1.5). Look for other stigma of Turner's syndrome—congenital heart disease and renal anomalies.
3. Noonan syndrome—fetuses with a syndrome similar to Turner's, but with normal chromosomes. Cardiac disease with pulmonary stenosis is typical.
4. Pena-Shokeir syndrome—a chromosomally normal syndrome with features similar to trisomy 18.
5. Roberts' syndrome (see Appendix II).

PREGNANCY MANAGEMENT

Investigations and Consultations Required   About 60% of cystic hygromas are chromosomally abnormal, most having Turner's syndrome, a minority having Down syndrome, and a few having trisomy 18. Chromosome analysis and fetal echocardiography are essential components of the evaluation of isolated cystic hygromas. The consultants used will depend very much on the etiology that is established for the cystic hygroma.

Fetal Intervention   In utero drainage procedures have no role in management. Spontaneous resolution is common. Progression to fetal hydrops suggests a generalized severe condition that will not respond to drainage of one body cavity

Monitoring   Serial ultrasound examinations every 3 to 4 weeks should be performed for those conditions likely to progress to fetal hydrops. Assessment for signs of polyhydramnios and preeclampsia should be done in cases with hydrops.

Pregnancy Course   Conditions that are associated with fetal hydrops may be complicated by both polyhydramnios and preeclampsia. Cystic hygroma with hydrops is almost always a lethal combination with death within a short time period. Cystic hygromas without hydrops usually regress completely.

Pregnancy Termination Issues   Unless a precise diagnosis has been established prenatally, the method of termination should be nondestructive and examinations by both a fetal pathologist and a dysmorphologist should be performed.

Delivery   Unless it is of markedly excessive size, the presence of a cystic hygroma should not necessitate a cesarean section. Delivery should occur in a tertiary center with capabilities for managing any complications that may arise.

NEONATOLOGY

Resuscitation   Airway compromise at birth occurs infrequently as the form of cystic hygroma that presents as a mass, cervical cystic hygroma, is not usually midline. However, extensive invasion of the tongue and pharyngeal structures can occur and airway compromise may then be seen. If a large mass is suspected from prenatal sonography, delivery should be planned at a tertiary center with an appropriate team available to establish a reliable airway.

Transport   Time of transfer is dictated by the presence of airway compromise. If the airway is functional then transfer to a tertiary center having a pediatric surgeon can be delayed until cardiorespiratory adaptation is established.

Testing and Confirmation   Cystic hygromas are usually obvious on physical examination in the newborn unless they are small. A webbed neck and excessive nuchal skin, suggesting a resolved antenatal cystic hygroma, are also noted on the newborn examination. Diagnostic evaluation should be directed toward excluding other co-existing abnormalities as indicated by prenatal findings and physical examination. Computed tomography (CT) scan or magnetic resonance imaging (MRI) of the neck and upper thorax are the better imaging studies to delineate the extent and anatomic location of neck masses.

BIBLIOGRAPHY

Azar GB, Snijders RJM, Gosden C: Fetal nuchal cystic hygromata: associated malformations and chromosomal defects. *Fetal Diagn Ther* 1991; 6:46-57.

Bronshtein M, Bar-Hava I, Blumenfeld I et al: The difference between septated and nonseptated nuchal cystic hygroma in the early second trimester. *Obstet Gynecol* 1993; 81:683-687.

Byrne J: The significance of cystic hygroma in fetuses. *Hum Pathol* 1984; 15:61-67.

Chervenak FA, Isaacson G, Blakemore KJ et al: Fetal cystic hygroma. Cause and natural history. *N Engl J Med* 1983; 309:822-825.

Johnson MP, Johnson A, Holzgreve W et al: First-trimester simple hygroma: cause and outcome. *Am J Obstet Gynecol* 1993; 168:156-161.

Langer JC, Fitzgerald PG, Desa D et al: Cervical cystic hygroma in the fetus: clinical spectrum and outcome. *J Pediatr Surg* 1990; 25:58-61.

Ninh TN, Ninh TX: Cystic hygroma in children: a report of 126 cases. *J Pediatr Surg* 1974; 9:191.

Van Zalen-Sprock MM, Van Vugt JMG, Van der Harten HJ et al: Cephalocele and cystic hygroma: diagnosis and differentiation in the first trimester of pregnancy with transvaginal sonography: report of two cases. *Ultrasound Obstet Gynecol* 1992; 2:289-292.

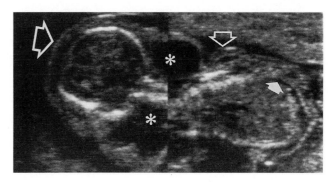

Bilateral cystic hygromata with hydrops. The bilateral cystic masses (*asterisks*) by the neck are the cystic hygroma. There is skin thickening around the body (*open arrows*). A small amount of ascites is present (*closed arrow*).

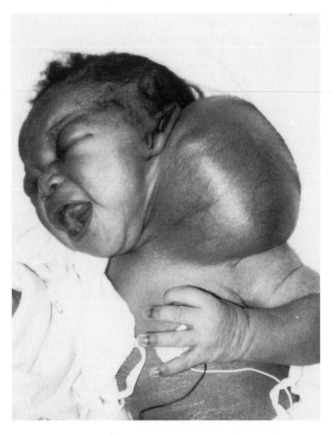

Newborn with large lateral neck lymphangioma. Surgical removal resulted in normal function with an excellent cosmetic repair. For the typical appearance with the usual in utero cystic hygromas see Turner's syndrome (Chapter 1.5)

7.3 THYROID ENLARGEMENT/GOITER

EPIDEMIOLOGY/GENETICS

Definition   A goiter is an enlarged thyroid gland.

Epidemiology   Rare.

Embryology   Goiters can be associated with hypothyroidism (most common), hyperthyroidism, or a euthyroid state. Goiters associated with hypothyroidism are due to iodine deficiency, iodine intoxication, maternal antithyroid medications, or inborn errors in thyroid hormone synthesis. Goiters associated with hyperthyroidism are the result of transplacental passage of maternal thyroid-stimulating antibodies whether or not the mother has active Graves' disease. One in seventy women with Graves' disease will have a fetus with a goiter.

Inheritance Patterns   Generally sporadic. Pendred's syndrome, however, is an autosomal recessive disorder with sensorineural deafness and goiter due to an inborn error in thyroid hormone synthesis.

Teratogens   Propylthiouracil, iodine preparations, lithium.

Prognosis   The prognosis depends on the etiology of the goiter. Polyhydramnios may induce prematurity.

SONOGRAPHY

Findings
1.   **Fetus:** The fetal thyroid is visibly enlarged. There will be a symmetrical anterior echogenic mass in the neck. This goiter may result in posterior extension of the neck. Normal thyroid size measurements exist.
2.   **Amniotic Fluid:** Severe polyhydramnios may occur if the esophagus is compressed.
3.   **Placenta:** Normal.
4.   **Measurement Data:** Intrauterine growth retardation (IUGR) is common.
5.   **When Detectable:** This entity has not been reported as detected before 26 weeks.

Pitfalls   The extended head position may make it difficult to examine the anterior aspect of the neck if the fetus is prone.

Differential Diagnosis   Cervical teratoma—the mass will have a much more coarse and varied internal texture and will extend above or below the thyroid region. The mass may well be asymmetric.

Where Else to Look   Look for cardiomegaly and cardiac rhythm problems—tachycardia and heart block.

PREGNANCY MANAGEMENT

Investigations and Consultations Required   Amniocentesis should be performed for chromosome studies, measurement of alpha-fetoprotein (AFP), and for determination of thyroid-stimulating hormone (TSH) concentration.

Fetal Intervention   Cases of fetal goiter secondary to hypothyroidism may be successfully treated by intraamniotic injection of thyroid hormone.

Monitoring   No specific changes in obstetric management are indicated. Serial sonograms about every 3 weeks, to check for polyhydramnios, are helpful.

Pregnancy Course   Goiter may cause dystocia by preventing the normal flexion of the fetal head during labor.

Pregnancy Termination Issues   In the absence of a precise diagnosis, termination should be done by a nondestructive approach.

Delivery   Because of the high potential for respiratory complications, delivery should be in a tertiary center. Cesarean section may be required as a result of the excessive extension of the fetal head.

NEONATOLOGY

Resuscitation   In the delivery room, the establishment of an adequate airway is the major concern. Rarely does this require emergency tracheostomy, but if the mass is very large, endotracheal intubation can be difficult. Once an airway is secured, other specific resuscitative measures are not required.

Transport   Referral to a tertiary perinatal center is always indicated for diagnostic evaluation and treatment. If airway compromise is present, emergency transfer is important.

Testing and Confirmation   Thyroid enlargement will be visible on clinical examination. Radionuclide scanning, thyroid function studies, and cervical sonography are useful to define both the anatomy and functional status of the gland.

Nursery Management   Once adequate ventilation is assured, the focus of care is the diagnosis of the functional abnormality in thyroid production causing the goiter. Prompt relief of a congenital hypothyroid state or control of neonatal thyrotoxicosis is necessary to suppress the stimulus for hyperplasia and facilitate resolution of the goiter.

BIBLIOGRAPHY

Avni EF, Rodesch F, Vandemerckt C et al: Detection and evaluation of fetal goiter by ultrasound. *Br J Radiol* 1992; 65:302-305.

Belfar HL, Foley TP Jr, Hill LM et al: Sonographic findings in maternal hyperthyroidism. *J Ultrasound Med* 1991; 10:281-284.

Bromley B, Frigoletto FD Jr, Cramer D: The fetal thyroid: normal and abnormal sonographic measurements. *J Ultrasound Med* 1992; 11:25-28.

Fraser GR: Association of congenital deafness with goiter (Pendred's syndrome): a study of 207 families. *Ann Hum Genet* 1965; 28:201-249.

Muir A, Daneman D, Daneman A et al: Thyroid scanning, ultrasound, and serum thyroglobulin in determining the origin of congenital hypothyroidism. *Am J Dis Child* 1988; 142:214-216.

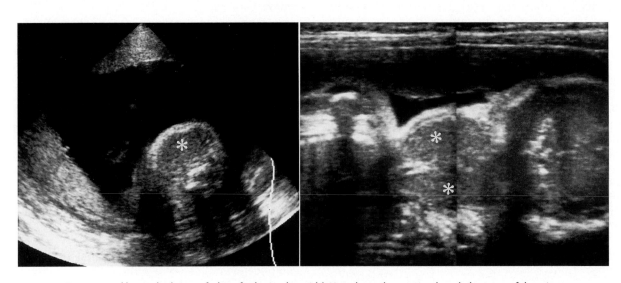

Transverse and longitudinal views of a large fetal goiter (*asterisks*). Note the trachea running through the center of the goiter

8 The Limbs

8.1 Achondrogenesis

EPIDEMIOLOGY/GENETICS

Definition Achondrogenesis is a group of lethal skeletal dysplasias, characterized by severe limb and trunk shortening with a disproportionately large head.

Epidemiology Rare. Presumably, M1:F1, but reported cases show an excess of males.

Embryology These fetuses have severe micromelia, trunk shortening, edema of the soft tissues, and a disproportionately large head. Ossification of the lumbar vertebrae is minimal (type I) or absent (type II), and the sacral, pubic, and ischial bones show little ossification. The ribs are thin and often fracture. Characteristic craniofacial features include micrognathia, flat face, and frontal bossing. Molecular defects, in type II collagen, have been found in a few cases.

Inheritance Patterns Most families show autosomal recessive inheritance.

Teratogens None.

Screening DNA analysis for recurrence in a family with a previously identified type II collagen defect is possible. Genetic heterogeneity is a major concern, so linkage studies are not useful for prenatal diagnosis.

Prognosis Lethal antenatally or in the newborn period.

SONOGRAPHY

Findings
1. **Fetus:** There are several subtypes, some indistinguishable from thanatophoric dwarfism. Most typical is the form with very short limbs, small chest, poorly ossified spine and skull. Nuchal thickening with a cystic area within is sometimes seen. Thick soft tissue on the arms is typical. Ascites may develop.
2. **Amniotic Fluid:** Severe polyhydramnios is invariable.
3. **Placenta:** Normal.
4. **Measurement Data:** The abdomen and head size are large. The limbs and chest size are extremely small.
5. **When Detectable:** 13 or 14 weeks.

Pitfalls Easily confused with osteogenesis imperfecta because both have deossified spine and skulls, but in achondrogenesis, the cranium is not compressible and limb fractures are not seen.

Differential Diagnosis Thanatophoric dwarfism—the bones are more ossified.

Where Else to Look An entire fetal survey is required.

PREGNANCY MANAGEMENT

Investigations and Consultations Required
1. Fetal echocardiography should be performed looking for congenital heart disease, a feature of a number of skeletal dysplasias, but not achondrogenesis.
2. Fetal radiographs should be reviewed by an individual experienced in the diagnosis of skeletal dysplasias.
3. Once a diagnosis of a lethal condition is established, and if the pregnancy is beyond the legal limits for termination, the family should meet with a neonatologist to discuss neonatal management.

Monitoring Once a diagnosis of a lethal condition has been established, routine maternal care and supportive psychological service should be provided. No attempts to treat preterm labor or to monitor fetal status are appropriate.

Pregnancy Course Polyhydramnios is a common complicating factor and may result in preterm labor.

Pregnancy Termination Issues An intact fetus must be delivered and the postmortem examination, including radiologic, morphologic, biochemical, and molecular studies, must be performed by individuals with extensive experience in skeletal dysplasias. Cultured cell lines and frozen chondroosseous tissue should be obtained.

Delivery Vaginal delivery without electronic monitoring is appropriate. Delivery should occur in a center with expertise in the diagnostic evaluation of skeletal dysplasias, or one with an interest and expertise in fetal pathology.

NEONATOLOGY

Neonatal Resuscitation   When the diagnosis is known prior to delivery, a prenatal decision for nonintervention, made after discussion with the family, is appropriate. If the diagnosis is uncertain, resuscitation and ventilatory support are appropriate to allow time for diagnostic evaluation and parental adaptation.

Neonatal Transport   Referral to a tertiary perinatal center is appropriate for confirmation of a diagnosis. Mechanical ventilatory support is often required during the transport.

Testing and Confirmation   Postnatal radiographs can help determine the specific type of achondrogenesis.

Nursery Management   Confirmation of the diagnosis, comfort care for the infant, and counselling and support of the family are the primary goals. Provision of mechani-

cal life support in the interim is appropriate. Liveborn infants who were not given life support survived less than 24 hours.

BIBLIOGRAPHY

Borochowitz Z, Ornoy A, Lachman R et al: Achondrogenesis II—hypochondrogenesis: variability versus heterogeneity. *Am J Med Genet* 1986; 24:273-288.

Borochowitz Z, Lachman R, Adomian GE et al: Achondrogenesis type I: delineation of further heterogeneity and identification of two distinct subgroups. *J Pediatr* 1988; 112:23-31.

Godfrey M, Hollister DW: Type II achondrogenesis-hypochondrogenesis: identification of abnormal type I collagen. *Am J Hum Genet* 1988; 43:904-913.

Graham D, Tracey J, Winn K et al: Early second trimester sonographic diagnosis of achondrogenesis. *J Clin Ultrasound* 1983; 11:336-338.

Mahony BS, Filly RA, Cooperberg PL: Antenatal sonographic diagnosis of achondrogenesis. *J Ultrasound Med* 1984; 3:333-335.

Whitley CB, Gorlin RJ: Achondrogenesis: nosology with evidence of genetic heterogeneity. *Radiology* 1983; 148:693-698.

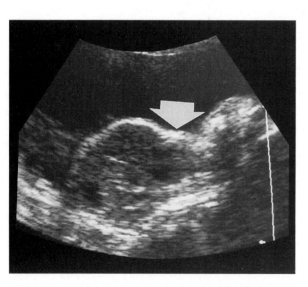

Achondrogenesis. Sagittal view of the chest and abdomen. Note the poorly ossified spine and tiny chest (*arrow*) with a bell shaped relatively large abdomen. There is polyhydramnios.

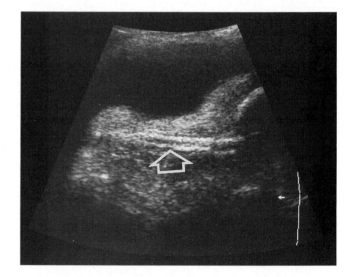

Coronal view of the spine showing the poor quality ossification (*arrow*).

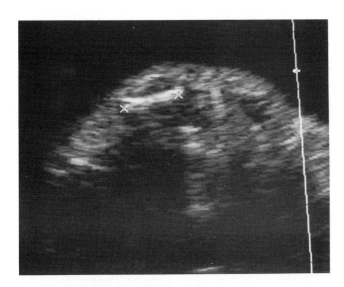

View of the femur (*between the X's*). It is much shorter than normal and fairly well ossified. There is redundant soft tissue present.

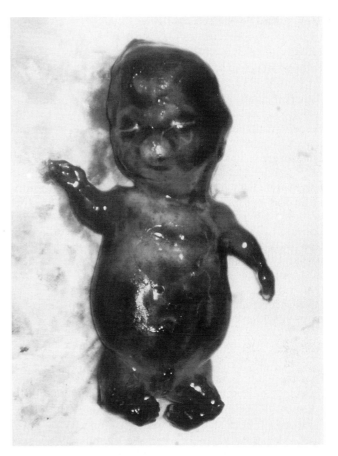

19-week fetus with achondrogenesis. Note very short limbs and normal proportion of head in relation to trunk.

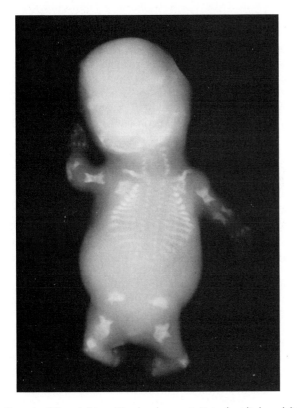

Radiograph of 19-week fetus with achondrogenesis. Note short limbs and deficient ossification of spine.

8.2 ACHONDROPLASIA

EPIDEMIOLOGY/GENETICS

Definition   Achondroplasia is the most common non-lethal skeletal dysplasia and is characterized by rhizomelic limb-shortening with macrocephaly.

Epidemiology   5 to 15 out of 10,000 live births (M1:F1).

Embryology   The phenotype is due to decreased endochondral ossification and is characterized by rhizomelic micromelia, megalencephaly with frontal bossing, and midface hypoplasia. Achondroplasia is due to a mutation in the fibroblast growth factor receptor -3 gene that maps to the distal end of chromosome 4p.

Inheritance Patterns   Autosomal dominant with 80% of cases representing new gene mutations.

Teratogens   None.

Prognosis   Intelligence and life span are usually normal. Affected individuals are at risk for neurologic complications, including spinal cord compression at the foramen magnum and the thoracolumbar region. Other complications include obstructive sleep apnea and obesity. Homozygosity for achondroplasia, which occurs when both parents are affected, is lethal, with either stillbirth or early neonatal death from respiratory failure.

SONOGRAPHY

Findings
1. **Fetus:** Very short limbs (below the fifth percentile) developing in third trimester. There is a similar limb configuration to thanatophoric dwarfism with a relatively small chest, a large head, and a bell-shaped abdomen. A small spine width is seen.
2. **Amniotic Fluid:** Polyhydramnios, developing in third trimester.
3. **Placenta:** Normal.
4. **Measurement Data:** Large abdomen and head. Short limbs.
5. **When Detectable:** After 24 weeks.

Pitfalls   Cannot be diagnosed before 24 weeks in most instances.

Differential Diagnosis
1. Severe intrauterine growth retardation (IUGR)—the limbs will not be as short and there will be markedly decreased fluid.
2. Thanatophoric dwarfism—similar appearances, but it develops earlier and is much more severe.

PREGNANCY MANAGEMENT

Investigations and Consultations Required
1. Fetal echocardiography and chromosome studies should be performed to exclude other conditions with mild shortening of the long bones.
2. Consultation with a pediatric geneticist should be done to assist the family with an understanding of the disorder and the implications for further care.

Monitoring   No change in standard obstetric practice is necessary.

Pregnancy Course   Mild polyhydramnios may develop, but preterm labor or other obstetric complications are unusual.

Pregnancy Termination Issues   The shortening of long bones is not evident until after 24 weeks, the legal limit for termination in most states. A diagnosis of achondroplasia prior to 24 weeks should raise suspicion of other diagnoses (usually thanatophoric dwarfism).

Delivery   Delivery should occur in a tertiary center with full capabilities for neonatal resuscitation, in the event of an incorrect diagnosis. Because of the narrow foramen magnum and upper cervical spine, spinal cord compression is a significant risk with neck manipulation. Therefore, consideration should be given to delivery by elective cesarean section.

NEONATOLOGY

Resuscitation   In the absence of known homozygosity, there are no contraindications for full resuscitative efforts following delivery if there is delay in spontaneous onset of respiration.

Transport: The primary indication for referral in the immediate neonatal period is for confirmation of diagnosis.

Testing and Confirmation   Postnatal skeletal radiographs are pathognomonic and can confirm the clinical phenotype.

Nursery Management   Hydrocephalus may develop though not usually in the neonatal period except in infants with the homozygous form.

SURGERY

Preoperative Assessment   During the first 3 years of life, attention is directed toward spinal development, to detect thoracolumbar kyphosis and foramen magnum stenosis. After walking age, more attention is placed on the problems of angular deformities (usually varus knees). By ages 8 to 10, discussions about lengthening begin to determine the child's and family interest. Plain radiographs help to plan lengthening and angular corrections. During the adult years, spinal stenosis is the major problem to be addressed.

Operative Indications   Thoracolumbar kyphosis in the infant to toddler age usually responds well to nonoperative treatment (bracing). Genu varum (bow legs) requires surgery in the form of either osteotomy or occasionally fibulectomy. If desired, the short stature and disproportion can be treated surgically by limb lengthening of the femurs, tibias, and humeri. Spinal stenosis in adults can be treated with surgical decompression to relieve pain and neurologic deficits.

Types of Procedures   Genu varum with fibular overgrowth leads to lateral collateral ligament laxity. Treatment consists of proximal tibial osteotomy with distraction to pull down the fibular head and tighten the lateral collateral ligament with the Ilizarov technique. This can be coordinated with lengthening.

Lengthening for stature is a complex program to reach minimum normal height for sex at skeletal maturity. This requires 10 to 12 inches (25 to 30 cm) of lengthening in most patients with achondroplasia and 6 to 8 inches (15 to 20 cm) in most patients with hypochondroplasia. The first lengthening can be done between ages 6 and 8 for up to 10 cm in both tibias. The tibia is then repeated with a similar size lengthening at age 10. At age 12, a 10 to 12 cm bilateral humeral lengthening is done. Near skeletal maturity, bilateral femoral lengthenings are done The newest method of femoral lengthening combines it with intramedullary nails in the femurs. This shortens the treatment time.

If patients develop neurologic compromise, which can range from apnea-related to foramen magnum stenosis to more common lumbar spinal stenosis and kyphosis with bladder symptomatology, then decompression of the spinal cord and frequently stabilization of the spine are required.

Surgical Results/Prognosis   Realignment of the tibia by the Ilizarov method has a very low complication rate with the exception of pin-tract infection, which is managed by oral antibiotics. The main risk is that of recurrence because the growth rate of the fibula continues to be faster than the tibia. Care must be taken to avoid injury to the peroneal nerve. An alternative procedure is resection of the fibula, which leaves a nonunion of the fibular bone. However, this does not tighten the lateral collateral ligament.

There are many potential risks of lengthening for stature, including neurovascular injury, stiffness of the ankle or knee joint with a femoral lengthening, joint contractures, premature consolidation requiring reosteotomy, and delayed consolidation. The most common complication is pin-tract infection, which can be treated with oral antibiotics, usually without any sequelae. The risk of late arthritis is a possibility. Extended limb lengthening should only be performed in centers that have significant experience with limb lengthening. The goals of 10 to 12 inches of lengthening over 3 or 4 lengthenings is achievable in most cases. Deformity correction can be combined with the lengthening.

Spinal surgery for achondroplasia is fraught with complications and should only be carried out by experienced individuals. There is a risk of paraplegia in lumbar spinal level surgery and quadriplegia in cervical level surgery. These procedures should only be done when the risk of not proceeding that way outweighs the risk of surgery.

BIBLIOGRAPHY

Andersen PE Jr, Hauge M: Congenital generalized bone dysplasias: a clinical, radiological, and epidemiological survey. *J Med Genet* 1989; 26:37-44.

Clark RN: Congenital dysplasias and dwarfism. *Pediatr Rev* 1990; 12:149-159.

Elejalde BR, de Elejalde MM, Hamilton PR et al: Prenatal diagnosis in two pregnancies of an achondroplastic woman. *Am J Med Genet* 1983; 15:437-439.

Kurtz AB, Filly RA, Wapner RJ et al: In utero analysis of heterozygous achondroplasia: variable time of onset as detected by femur length measurements. *J Ultrasound Med* 1986; 5:137-140.

Leonard CO, Sanders RC, Lau HL: Prenatal diagnosis of the Turner syndrome, a familial chromosomal rearrangement and achondroplasia by amniocentesis and ultrasonography. *Johns Hopkins Med J* 1979; 145:25-30.

Nelson FW, Hecht JT, Horton WA et al: Neurological basis of respiratory complications in achondroplasia. *Ann Neurol* 1988; 24:89-93.

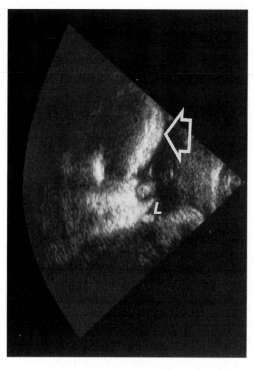

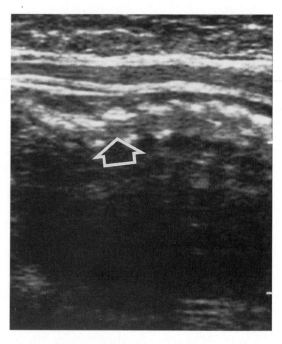

Fetal spine in achondroplasia. The intervertebral distance is decreased and spinal canal is narrowed (*arrow*).

Achondroplasia. Face and forehead view. There is frontal bossing (*arrow*). *L*, lips.

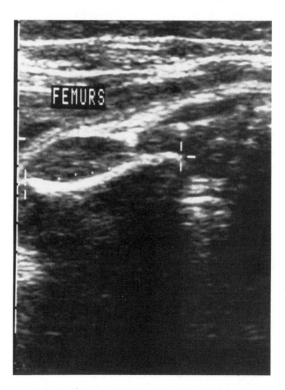

Femur view. The femur (*between X's*) is short and bowed, so there is a resemblance to a telephone receiver.

8.3 Amniotic Band Syndrome

EPIDEMIOLOGY/GENETICS

Definition   Amniotic band syndrome refers to a spectrum of asymmetric disruptive abnormalities and limb amputations thought to result from antenatal rupture of the amnion.

Epidemiology   1 out of 1300 live births (M1:F1).

Embryology   The disruptions and deformities seen in the amniotic band syndrome are asymmetric and highly variable, depending on the gestational timing of amnion rupture and the regions of the fetus involved. Early amnion rupture severely disrupts intrauterine development and may lead to anencephaly, encephaloceles, facial clefting, abdominal wall defects, and ectopia cordis. Later amnion rupture is characteristically associated with ring constrictions, limb amputations, and distal digital fusion, simulating syndactyly.

Inheritance Patterns   Most often sporadic. Very rare cases may be associated with heritable disorders of connective tissue, including Ehlers-Danlos syndromes and epidermolysis bullosa.

Teratogens   None.

Prognosis   In the absence of central nervous system (CNS) involvement, intelligence should be normal. The degree of developmental disruption by the bands will determine the clinical outcome. Digital function is often excellent, despite major amputations.

SONOGRAPHY

Findings
1. **Fetus:** There are numerous forms of amniotic band syndrome, which may occur as isolated problems or as combinations.
    a. Absent digits or portions of limbs (e.g., absent hand or end of digit).
    b. Swollen distal arm—A constriction ring related to an amniotic band causes the hand or foot and adjacent area to swell.
    c. Facial problems—cleft lip and occasionally palate, asymmetrical microphthalmia, and severe nasal deformity.
    d. Cranial problems—Encephalocele and anencephaly may be due to bands (the encephalocele, unlike the type associated with neural crest anomalies, is usually eccentrically placed in, for example, a parietal location).
    e. Club feet or clubbed hands.
    f. Gastroschisis may be due to amniotic bands, especially when both gut and liver lie outside the body. Omphalocele is also occasionally due to amniotic bands.
    g. Amniotic bands are also seen in the limb body wall complex syndrome, which is considered separately (see limb body wall complex, Chapter 8.10).
2. **Amniotic Fluid:** Amniotic bands are occasionally seen in the amniotic fluid, although they are subtle and difficult to see (indeed, they are easy to miss at pathology).
3. **Placenta:** Normal.
4. **Measurement Data:** Providing a structure is not affected by amniotic bands, measurements should be normal.
5. **When Detectable:** 12 to 13 weeks with the vaginal probe.

Pitfalls   The combination of findings with amniotic band syndrome may suggest a neural crest problem, for example, club feet and encephalocele.

Differential Diagnosis
1. Neural crest problems.
2. Radial ray problems such as Fanconi's syndrome or vertebral abnormalities, anal atresia, cardiac abnormalities, tracheoesophageal fistula and esophageal atresia, renal agenesis and dysplasia, and limb defects association (VACTERL), if the arms are affected.
3. Limb swelling may suggest Klippel-Trenaunay-Weber syndrome, but there is no increased vascularity.
4. Membranes within the amniotic fluid, unless associated with the sonographic findings described above, are probably due to: amniotic sheets—infolding of the amnion related to prior synechiae; remnant of blighted twin sac; displaced amnion from chorion due to previous amniocentesis, chorionic villi sampling (CVS) or prior subamniotic bleed; or marginal bleed in subamniotic location with echopenic blood.

Where Else to Look   Look everywhere—virtually any anatomical structure can be affected.

PREGNANCY MANAGEMENT

Investigations and Consultations Required
1. Depending on the pattern of malformations, chromosome evaluation should be performed. Major limb malformations and large nonmembrane covered ventral wall malformations are not likely to be on the basis of aneuploidy.
2. Fetal echocardiography, however, should be performed in all cases, both for diagnostic and prognostic purposes.

Monitoring   Because oligohydramnios may be associated with amniotic band syndrome, a decision must be made regarding the overall prognosis for the fetus before an obstetric management plan can be formulated. Fetal assessment, such as nonstress testing, is inappropriate in cases with major structural malformations or early onset of oligohydramnios where survival is unlikely, even in a full-term infant. Encephaloceles need monitoring for developing hydrocephalus.

Pregnancy Course   No obstetric complications should be expected as a result of the amniotic band sequence, except in those cases complicated by oligohydramnios.

Pregnancy Termination Issues   A precise diagnosis is dependent on the demonstration of amniotic bands. Therefore, the method of termination must ensure an intact fetus and placenta.

Delivery   In cases with uncorrectable structural malformations or prolonged oligohydramnios, strong consideration should be given to labor without fetal monitoring and vaginal delivery.

NEONATOLOGY

Resuscitation   The decision to begin resuscitative measures is contingent upon the extent of the body structure disruption known to be present prior to the onset of labor. With only extremity involvement, full resuscitation is always indicated.

Transport   Referral to a tertiary perinatal center after birth is indicated only if the degree of body structure disruption does not appear to be lethal and to be amenable to reconstructive surgery. Exposed viscera and denuded surfaces should be covered with sterile, moist dressings to prevent excess heat and water loss and to protect from contamination.

Nursery Management   With severe disruption of an uncorrectible nature, comfort care for the infant and counselling and supportive care for the family are the most appropriate measures. Provision of mechanical life support is appropriate when the prognosis is uncertain to allow time for delineation of the defects and for parental adaptation. With extremity involvement only, referral to

a multidisciplinary clinic or team for children with limb deficiencies should be made prior to hospital discharge.

SURGERY

Preoperative Assessment   Classification is according to degree of involvement:
1. simple ring constriction
2. ring constriction with distal bone fusions
3. ring constriction with distal soft tissue fusions
4. intrauterine amputation

A search for associated problems such as syndactyly, clubfoot, and cleft lip/palate should be made. Mild leg length discrepancy can develop during childhood in certain cases.

Operative Indications   In most cases, surgery is largely cosmetic, to eliminate the deep grooves caused by the constriction bands. Urgent surgery is occasionally indicated for unusual cases of impending lymphatic or venous gangrene.

Types of Procedures   Z-plasty skin releases eliminate the cosmetic groove deformity. Although successful single stage releases (360°) have been reported, many surgeons prefer to stage the release, correcting onehalf at a time to prevent the possibility of vascular compromise.

Surgical Results/Prognosis   Recurrence is unlikely after releasing the bands. Parents should be warned, however, that they are trading a groove for a scar.

BIBLIOGRAPHY

Higginbottom MC, Jones KL, Hall BD et al: The amniotic band disruption complex: timing of amniotic rupture and variable spectra of consequent defects. *J Pediatr* 1979; 95:544-549.

Hill LM, Kislak S, Jones N: Prenatal ultrasound diagnosis of a forearm constriction band. *J Ultrasound Med* 1988; 7:293-295.

Jones MC: The spectrum of structural defects produced as a result of amnion rupture. *Semin Perinatol* 1983; 7:281-284.

Lockwood C, Ghidini A, Romero R: Amniotic band syndrome in monozygotic twins: prenatal diagnosis and pathogenesis. *Obstet Gynecol* 1988; 71:1012-1016.

Lubinsky M, Sujansky E, Sanger W et al: Familial amniotic bands. *Am J Med Genet* 1983; 14:81-87.

Mahony BS, Filly RA, Callen PW et al: The amniotic band syndrome: antenatal sonographic diagnosis and potential pitfalls. *Am J Obstet Gynecol* 1985; 152:63-68.

Seeds JW, Cefalo RC, Herbert WNP: Clinical opinion: amniotic band syndrome. *Am J Obstet Gynecol* 1982; 144:243-248.

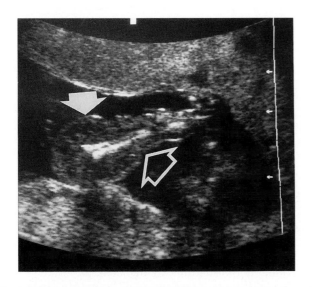

Amniotic band syndrome. Localized swelling of the proximal arm (*closed arrow*) due to a constriction band above the wrist (*open arrow*).

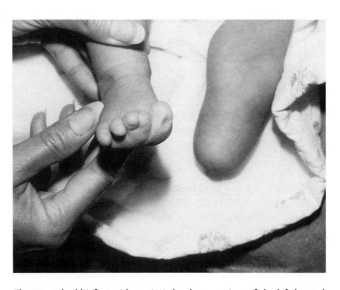

Three-month-old infant with amniotic band amputations of the left leg and toes of the right foot.

8.4 ARTHROGRYPOSIS

EPIDEMIOLOGY/GENETICS

Definition   Arthrogryposis is a term for a group of disorders characterized by congenital, usually nonprogressive, joint contractures at multiple sites.

Epidemiology   1 to 3 out of 10,000 births (M1:F1).

Embryology   Arthrogryposis is a physical finding that results from a heterogeneous group of disorders. These include over 120 genetic, chromosomal, and sporadic multiple malformation syndromes. The arthrogryposes are divided into three groups including: 1. those with only limb involvement; 2. those with generalized neuromuscular involvement; and 3. those with CNS, as well as neuromuscular involvement. Only one half of children with arthrogryposis receive a specific diagnosis. Trisomy 18 is the most common chromosomal diagnosis.

Inheritance Patterns   Autosomal dominant, recessive, and X-linked syndromes have been described.

Teratogens   Maternal hyperthermia and congenital infections.

Prognosis   Prognosis is dependent on an accurate diagnosis and may range from perinatal lethal disorders to those with only mild to moderate orthopedic limitations.

SONOGRAPHY

Findings
1. **Fetus:** The legs are held in one position, either in extension and crossed or persistently flexed. The arms are flexed. The fetus, in the most severe form, is immobile. If the condition only affects the feet, the remainder of the body may have normal movement. The hands are clenched with overlapping of the fingers. The feet are extended, so they are almost in the same axis as the legs, although talipes is also present. Muscle tissue, particularly in the lower limbs, is markedly diminished, however limb edema is sometimes seen.
2. **Amniotic Fluid:** Some examples of arthrogryposis are due to constriction of the cavity by fibroids, uterine anomalies, membranes or oligohydramnios. In others, there is polyhydramnios.
3. **Placenta:** Normal.
4. **Measurement Data:** Normal measurement data.
5. **When Detectable:** There is a variable time of onset with some cases presenting in late second trimester and some developing after 24 weeks.

Differential Diagnosis
1. Multiple pterygium syndrome—Cystic hygroma is present and feet are flexed, rather than extended as in arthrogryposis. All limbs are involved.
2. Pena Shokeir syndrome—Contractures are less exteme. There are rocker-bottom feet with severe growth deficiency.

Where Else to Look   The entire fetus should be surveyed to ensure that the limb abnormalities are not part of a generalized syndrome, such as one of the trisomies.

PREGNANCY MANAGEMENT

Investigations and Consultations Required
1. Fetal karyotype and studies to rule out congenital infections should be considered, especially if additional malformations are detected.
2. Fetal echocardiography may be helpful in establishing a diagnosis and determining prognosis.

Monitoring   Standard obstetric care is appropriate. Serial ultrasounds to assess fluid volume are helpful for prognostic purposes.

Pregnancy Course   Breech presentation is common in fetuses with arthrogryposis syndromes. Polyhydramnios is rare except in lethal disorders.

Pregnancy Termination Issues   The heterogeneous group of disorders that have arthrogryposis as a feature require that a complete autopsy on an intact fetus be performed. Accurate recurrence risk counseling requires a precise diagnosis.

Delivery   The mode of delivery should be based on obstetric indications only. Because an exact diagnosis will rarely be established prenatally, delivery at a tertiary center is appropriate.

NEONATOLOGY

Resuscitation   The decision not to offer resuscitation is easiest when there is a definite diagnosis of a concomitant lethal condition. In all other circumstances, resuscitation should be initiated and support continued, if needed, while a diagnostic evaluation is completed.

Transport   Referral to a tertiary perinatal center for diagnostic evaluation is appropriate. With an otherwise asymptomatic infant, referral for outpatient evaluation and treatment planning is also acceptable.

Testing and Confirmation   As long-term prognosis is heavily influenced by associated or co-existing disorders, complete diagnostic evaluation and etiologic determination are the top priorities. Muscle biopsy and nerve conduction studies are important in determining the potential for rehabilitation.

Nursery Management Treatment is directed toward achieving stable functional weight bearing and manual dexterity. Initially, positioning, physical therapy, and bracing are used, followed by surgery in later infancy and childhood.

SURGERY

Preoperative Assessment The diagnosis is made by physical examination alone. The affected joints are stiff, contracted, and have diminished or absent joint skin creases. Involvement usually includes both hands, both feet, and often both hips, elbows, shoulders, and knees. The joints are typically flexed, with webbing seen on the flexion side in severe cases. Some children have isolated single-limb involvement. Scoliosis develops in about 10% of cases.

Operative Indications The need for surgery depends on the location and extent of involvement. The most common surgery required for arthrogrypotic children in the first year of life is for correction of club foot and reduction of dislocated hips. As these children grow, they often require release of knee flexion contractures in order to stand upright. Upper extremity surgery is occasionally indicated to treat elbow flexion contractures.

Types of Procedures Soft tissue releases (cutting tight muscles and ligaments) are the mainstay of treatment. Instead of lengthening tight tendons, they are simply cut, in order to diminish the chance of recurrence. In nearly every case, the joint capsular ligaments must also be sectioned. For dislocated hips, the tight structures are cut and the hip is placed into the acetabulum. Scoliosis is treated by distraction instrumentation and fusion in older children.

Recurrence of foot deformities often requires talectomy or triple arthrodesis. In older children and teenagers with recurrent contractures, external fixators have been used to gradually correct contracted knees and elbows. Gradual correction with distraction devices (Ilizarov apparatus) is safer for the contracted neurovascular structures than acute correction.

Surgical Results/Prognosis Prognosis is largely dependent on the initial degree of involvement and etiology. Total body involvement may make a child wheel-chair bound. More commonly, involvement of all four extremities responds to surgery, but the child often requires braces and crutches to walk. Isolated single-limb involvement has the best prognosis. Hand deformities preclude many activities, but most children do remarkably well. Mentation is normal in most cases.

BIBLIOGRAPHY

Bui TH, Lindholm H, Demir N et al: Prenatal diagnosis of distal arthrogryposis type I by ultrasonography. *Prenat Diagn* 1992; 12:1047-1053.

Degani S, Shapiro I, Lewinsky R et al: Prenatal ultrasound diagnosis of isolated arthrogryposis. *Acta Obstet Gynecol Scand* 1989; 68:461-462.

Fahy MJ, Hall JG: A retrospective study of pregnancy complications among 828 cases of arthrogryposis. *Genet Couns* 1990; 1:3-11.

Goldberg JD, Chervenak FA, Lipman RA et al: Antenatal sonographic diagnosis of arthrogryposis multiplex congenita. *Prenat Diagn* 1986; 6:45-49.

Gorczyca DP, McGahan JP, Lindfors KK et al: Arthrogryposis multiplex congenita: prenatal ultrasonographic diagnosis. *J Clin Ultrasound* 1989; 17:40-44.

Hageman G, Willemse J: Arthrogryposis multiplex congenita: review with comment. *Neuropediatrics* 1983; 14:6-11.

Hall JG: Arthrogryposis (congenital contractures). In: Emery AA, Rimoin DL (eds): *Principles and practice of medical genetics*, Edinburgh. Churchill Livingstone, 1983. pp. 781-811.

Miskin M, Rothberg R, Rudd NL et al: Arthrogryposis multiplex congenita-prenatal assessment with diagnostic ultrasound and fetoscopy. *J Pediatr* 1979; 463-464

Robinson YJ, Rouse GA, De Lange M: Sonographic evaluation of arthrogryotic conditions. *JDMS* 1994; 10:18-22.

Wynne-Davies R, Lloyd-Roberts GC: Arthrogryposis multiplex congenita: search for prenatal factors in 66 sporadic cases. *Arch Dis Child* 1976; 51:618-623.

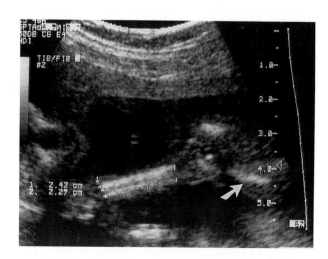

View of the tibia and fibula in a patient with Arthrogryposis. Note the almost complete absence of soft tissue due to severe muscle wasting. The femur can be seen to the right (*arrow*). No change in the straight alignment of the upper and lower leg were seen over a prolonged period.

8.5 CAMPTOMELIC DYSPLASIA

EPIDEMIOLOGY/GENETICS

Definition   Camptomelic dysplasia is a heterogeneous group of lethal skeletal dysplasias with characteristic bowing deformities of the femur and tibia.

Epidemiology   Rare. Phenotypic sex ratio (M1:F2.3), karyotypic sex ratio (M2:F1).

Embryology   The camptomelic dysplasias are comprised of both short-boned and long-boned types and have a flat facial profile, cleft palate, and tracheal abnormalities. An apparent preponderance of females is due to 46 XY males with ambiguous genitalia. Camptomelia or bending of the long bones can also be produced by other genetic disorders including osteogenesis imperfecta.

Inheritance Patterns   Frequently autosomal recessive.

Teratogens   None.

Prognosis   Usually lethal in the neonatal period. Survival duration is related to the degree of respiratory compromise at birth. Infants with less severe manifestations may occasionally survive into early infancy but with significant respiratory and feeding difficulties. All have delayed development and are mentally retarded.

SONOGRAPHY

Findings
1. **Fetus**
   a. Bowed and shortened lower limbs, particularly the tibia and femur. There may be acute angulation of the femur suggesting fracture. The fibulae are hypoplastic.
   b. A bell shaped chest and abdomen is seen due to the narrow chest.
   c. Severe micrognathia with elongated philtrum and flattened nose. Hypotelorism may occur.
   d. Club feet.
   e. Lateral ventriculomegaly may develop.
   f. So far, the tomahawk scapulae have not been diagnosed in utero.
   g. Poorly formed or ambiguous genitalia may be seen.
   h. Renal pelvic dilatation is sometimes seen.
2. **Amniotic Fluid:** Increased fluid is usual because the thorax is small.
3. **Placenta:** Normal.
4. **Measurement Data:** Small chest circumference and markedly shortened lower limbs.
5. **When Detectable:** At about 17 weeks.

Differential Diagnosis   Osteogenesis imperfecta—The lower limbs are also most affected by osteogenesis imperfecta and bowing is often seen. The facial and cranial findings and club feet seen with camptomelic dwarfism do not occur with osteogenesis imperfecta.

Where Else to Look   This is a syndrome that involves all parts of the body, so look everywhere.

PREGNANCY MANAGEMENT

Investigations and Consultations Required
1. Fetal echocardiography should be performed to exclude congenital heart defects that are not usually a feature of camptomelic dysplasia.
2. Neonatology should be consulted to plan the perinatal management approach that will be taken.

Monitoring   Tocolytic agents are contraindicated. There are no benefits to prolonging pregnancy.

Pregnancy Course   Polyhydramnios and preterm labor frequently complicate the fetal malformation.

Pregnancy Termination Issues   An intact fetus must be delivered and the postmortem examination, including radiologic, morphologic, biochemical, and molecular studies, must be performed by individuals with extensive experience in skeletal dysplasias. Culture cell lines and frozen chondroosseous tissue should be obtained.

Delivery   The site for delivery should be one where all personnel are comfortable with a nonaggressive approach to labor, delivery, and neonatal care.

NEONATOLOGY

Resuscitation   When the diagnosis is known prior to delivery, a prenatal decision for non–intervention, made after discussion with the family, is appropriate. If the diagnosis is uncertain, resuscitation and ventilatory support are instituted to allow time for diagnostic evaluation and parental adaptation.

Transport   Referral to a tertiary perinatal center is appropriate for confirmation of a diagnosis. Mechanical ventilatory support is often required during the transport.

Testing and Confirmation   Skeletal radiographs postnatally will establish the diagnosis.

Nursery Management   Confirmation of the diagnosis and counselling and support of the family are the primary goals. Provision of mechanical life support initially is appropriate with concurrence of the family. Withdrawal of support may become a problem subsequently if respiratory insufficiency persists.

BIBLIOGRAPHY

Balcar I, Bieber FR: Sonographic and radiologic findings in camptomelic dysplasia. *Am J Roentgenol* 1983; 141:481-482.

Carlan SJ, Parsons MT, Flasher J: Camptomelic skeletal dysplasia with a narrow thorax. *JDMS* 1990; 1:40-42.

Cordone M, Lituania M, Zampatti C et al: In utero ultrasonographic features of camptomelic dysplasia. *Prenat Diagn* 1989; 9:745-750.

Gillerot Y, Vanheck CA, Foulon M et al: Camptomelic syndrome: manifestations in a 20 week fetus and case history of a 5-year-old child. *Am J Med Genet* 1989; 34:589-592.

Hall BD, Spranger JW: Camptomelic dysplasia: further elucidation of a distinct entity. *Am J Dis Child* 1980; 134:285-289.

Houston CS, Opitz JM, Spranger JW et al: The camptomelic syndrome: review, report of 17 cases, and follow-up on the currently 17-year-old boy first reported by Maroteaux et al in 1971. *Am J Med Genet* 1983; 15:3-28.

Kozlowski K, Butzler HO, Galatius-Jensen F et al: Syndromes of congenital bowing of the long bones. *Pediatr Radiol* 1978; 7:40-48.

Winter R, Rosenkranz W, Hofmann H et al: Prenatal diagnosis of camptomelic dysplasia by ultrasonography. *Prenat Diagn* 1985; 5:1-8.

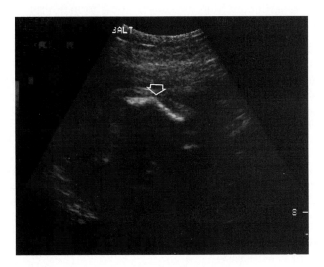

Camptomelic dwarfism. Shortened angulated femur initially thought to be due to osteogenesis imperfecta. Note the apparent fracture (*arrow*).

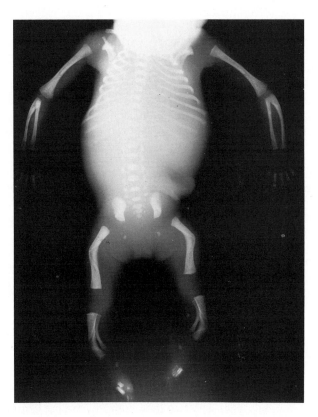

Radiograph showing angulated shortened femurs and shortened bowed tibia and fibula. *From Sanders RC, Greyson-Flag RT, Hogge WA et al: Osteogenesis imperfecta and camptomelic dysplasia: difficulties in prenatal diagnosis.* J Ultrasound Med *1994; 13:691-700; used with permission.*

8.6 CLUB AND ROCKER-BOTTOM FEET
VERTICAL TALUS

EPIDEMIOLOGY/GENETICS

Definition A club foot is a foot malformation characterized by dorsiflexion and eversion of the foot with associated abnormalities in the musculature of the lower leg. A rocker-bottom foot is the phenotypic description of a foot characterized by a prominent heel with a convex sole.

Epidemiology Club foot occurs with a frequency of 1 out of 1000 live births. The frequency of rocker-bottom feet is unknown, but is much less common.

Embryology Club foot can occur as an isolated abnormality or as part of over 200 chromosomal, genetic, or sporadic multiple malformation syndromes. It is frequently secondary to lower extremity paralysis from a neural tube defect. Rocker-bottom feet have been described in association with over 30 chromosomal, genetic, or sporadic multiple malformation syndromes, especially trisomy 18.

Inheritance Patterns Dependent upon the etiology of the foot abnormalities.

Teratogens None specific.

Prognosis Dependent upon the etiology of the foot abnormalities.

SONOGRAPHY

Findings
1. **Fetus**
   a. Club feet—The two long bones of the leg can be seen at the same time as the lateral aspect of the foot because the foot is inverted or, more likely, extraverted. The foot is either flexed or extended (see diagram p. 178 for the various different types). It is fixed in position.
   b. Rocker-bottom foot—The heel of the foot extends posterior to the leg. The midportion of the foot may be inferior to the proximal and distal portions of the foot.
2. **Amniotic Fluid:** If the condition is isolated, the amniotic fluid is normal.
3. **Placenta:** If the condition is isolated, the placenta is normal.
4. **Measurement Data:** Normal, if the condition is isolated.
5. **When Detectable:** At about 13 weeks using the vaginal probe.

Pitfalls The foot may be held in a slightly deviated flexed position, as a normal variant, if there is little fluid and the foot is pushing against the uterine wall.

Differential Diagnosis Arthrogryposis—The foot is very extended, but not necessarily deviated to right or left and there is soft-tissue loss.

Where Else to Look Club and rocker-bottom feet are associated with syndromes that involve every structure. Look particularly for chromosomal malformations.

PREGNANCY MANAGEMENT

Investigations and Consultations Required Chromosome studies and fetal echocardiography are essential components of the work-up, except for an isolated clubfoot. Consultation with a pediatric geneticist/dysmorphologist with evaluation of the parents may be helpful in establishing a diagnosis. Because club feet may be a manifestation of primary CNS disorders, myelomeningocele, fetal akinesia syndromes, and a host of genetic syndromes, the diagnosis of isolated club foot must be made with caution.

Monitoring No change in standard obstetric management is necessary.

Pregnancy Course No obstetric complications should be expected, if these conditions are isolated.

Pregnancy Termination Issues Should termination be chosen, the method used should provide an intact fetus for complete morphologic and pathologic examination.

Delivery The high likelihood that these conditions are not isolated makes delivery in a tertiary center, with full diagnostic and treatment capabilities, the preferable approach.

SURGERY

Preoperative Assessment The diagnosis of neonatal clubfoot is made on clinical examination, with uncorrectable hindfoot equinus and rigid forefoot adductus. The entire foot is internally rotated, relative to the tibia. Radiographs of clubfeet in the neonatal period are less helpful, because the bones are largely nonossified.

The physical findings in rocker-bottom feet are more subtle. The arch of the foot is "flat." In a true vertical talus, the foot is rigid, not flexible. Radiographic confirmation of the vertical talus is required to confirm the diagnosis. In a true vertical talus, stress plantarflexion lateral views of the foot show that the first metatarsal never lies in line with the long axis of the talus. Other causes of flatfoot should be considered in the preoperative assessment, including tarsal coalition, flexible flatfoot, and benign calcaneovalgus flatfoot (from intrauterine molding).

Operative Indications   Nearly every true clubfoot or vertical talus will require surgery in order to obtain a plantigrade, shoeable foot. Serial casting alone will occasionally correct a mild unilateral club foot. However, 90% of cases will require surgery for optimal results.

Types of Procedures   The initial treatment for clubfoot or vertical talus is serial casting. This helps to stretch the contracted soft tissues in preparation for surgery. The optimal age for surgery is 6 to 12 months. For both disorders, surgery consists of tendon lengthenings combined with ligament releases. This allows the bones to be repositioned into normal alignment. Usually, small temporary steel pins are inserted to hold the alignment for the first 6 weeks after surgery. Casts are worn for 6 to 12 weeks after surgery. In more severe cases, follow-up bracing is used to prevent recurrence, particularly in neurogenic and severe cases associated with syndromes.

Surgical Results/Prognosis   For most idiopathic cases, the results of surgery are a nearly normal foot. Most children can walk without a limp. It is always stiffer than a normal foot, and therefore may be prone to develop arthritis in middle age. The calf is noticeably thinner in diameter on the affected side, which may be of cosmetic concern in girls who wear skirts or dresses. Recurrence after surgery is rare, except in teratologic and neurogenic cases. Recurrence requires further surgery, such as triple arthrodesis (fusion of the hindfoot joints). More recently, external fixators (Ilizarov) have been used to stretch out recurrent contracted foot deformities.

BIBLIOGRAPHY
Bronshtein M, Zimmer EZ: Transvaginal ultrasound diagnosis of fetal club feet at 13 weeks, menstrual age. *J Clin Ultrasound* 1989; 17:518-520.

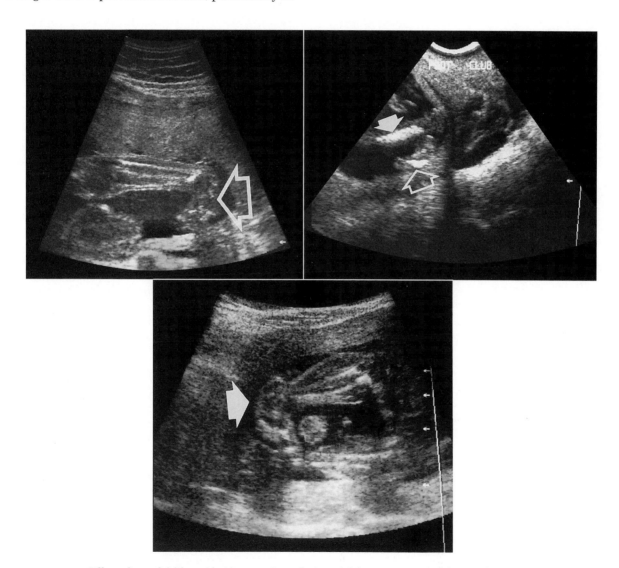

Different forms of clubfoot with either extension or flexion and abduction or inversion deformities (*arrows*).

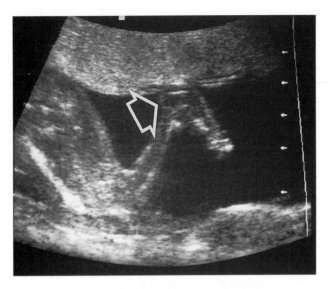

Rocker-bottom foot. Note the prominent heel.

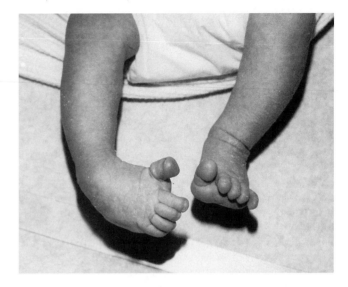

Term newborn with isolated right clubbed foot.

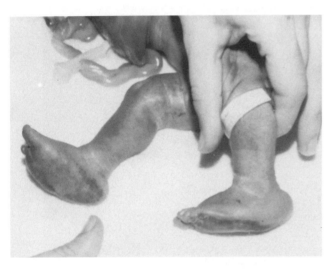

28-week stillborn with trisomy 13. Note typical rocker-bottom feet with prominent calcaneous.

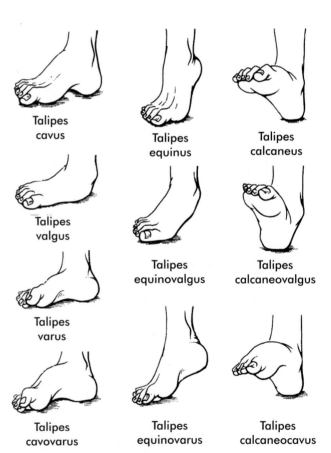

Diagram showing the different types of club feet. *Reprinted with permission from* Dorland's illustrated medical dictionary, *28th ed. Philadelphia. WB Saunders, 1994.*

8.7 Diastrophic Dysplasia

EPIDEMIOLOGY/GENETICS

Definition   Diastrophic dysplasia is a short-limb skeletal dysplasia characterized by club feet, ear swelling, and progressive joint and spine deformity.

Epidemiology   Very rare (M1:F1).

Embryology   Diastrophic dysplasia is characterized by club feet, abducted "hitchhiker" thumbs, inflammatory cystic swelling of the ear pinnae, and cleft palate. The gene for diastrophic dysplasia has been cloned and is called the diastrophic dysplasia suffate transporter (DTDST) and is located on chromosome 5q31-34.

Inheritance Patterns   Autosomal recessive.

Teratogens   None.

Prognosis   Rare neonatal death has been described, but most patients have a normal life span and intellectual development. Adult height is generally under four feet with severe orthopedic abnormalities. A lethal variant has been reported with associated cardiac defects and a high incidence of intrauterine growth retardation. All succumbed shortly after birth or in early infancy.

SONOGRAPHY

Findings
1. **Fetus:** The sonographic features involve much of the body.
   a. Micromelia—All limbs are very short throughout their extent.
   b. Ulna deviation of the hands with short phalanges—The thumbs are abducted and proximally inserted (hitchhiker's thumbs). The big toes have a similar deformity. The feet are severely extended and clubbed.
   c. Micrognathia.
   d. Cleft palate.
   e. Cervical kyphoscoliosis, a major finding later in life, is subtle in utero.
   f. Flexion deformity of the elbows and knees.
   g. The chest is relatively normal sized, considering the small limb size.
2. **Amniotic Fluid:** Normal.
3. **Placenta:** Normal.
4. **Measurement Data:** All limb measurements are well below the fifth percentile.
5. **When Detectable:** At about 13 weeks.

Differential Diagnosis   Other lethal dwarfisms. Long bones are not bowed. The hitchhiker thumb and kyphoscoliosis make for a relatively distinct picture.

Where Else to Look   The entire body needs to be surveyed in detail.

PREGNANCY MANAGEMENT

Investigations and Consultations Required
1. Fetal echocardiography should be performed; the presence of a congenital heart defect would suggest another type of skeletal dysplasia other than diastrophic dysplasia.
2. A neonatology consult should be obtained to assist in planning perinatal management.
3. The gene for diastrophic dysplasia has been mapped to the long arm of chromosome 5q31-34 and prenatal diagnosis is available in at risk families.

Monitoring   Preterm labor secondary to polyhydramnios is frequent. Therefore, obstetric care should be coordinated by a perinatologist. Despite the severity of the disorder, it is not lethal and severe prematurity will only further complicate management.

Pregnancy Course   Polyhydramnios is frequently a complication of this skeletal dysplasia and may result in preterm labor. As is the case for all skeletal dysplasias, the lethal forms should be excluded before establishing an obstetric management plan.

Pregnancy Termination Issues   An intact fetus must be delivered and the postmortem examination, including radiologic, morphologic, biochemical, and molecular studies, must be performed by individuals with extensive experience in skeletal dysplasias. Cultured cell lines and frozen chondroosseous tissue should be obtained.

Delivery   Respiratory complications are common, and intubation may be complicated because of micrognathia. Delivery should occur in a tertiary center with the capabilities to manage these complications.

NEONATOLOGY

Resuscitation   Initiation of resuscitation in liveborn infants is appropriate when the prognosis is in doubt.

Testing and Confirmation   Confirmation of the diagnosis and prognosis are the first priorities. Careful physical examination, skeletal radiographs, echocardiography, and genetic testing are useful in the evaluation.

Nursery Management   Respiratory insufficiency secondary to laryngeal obstruction appears to be the mode of death in the lethal variant. Response to ventilatory support and a mechanical airway is unknown. The long-term treatment plan is directed toward orthopedic correction of the club feet and kyphoscoliosis, should the latter develop.

SURGERY

Preoperative Assessment   Initial problems may include severe clubfoot and dislocated hips. Flexion contractures develop in upper and lower extremities. Scoliosis (or kyphoscoliosis) occurs in early childhood. Growth is retarded, with a mean adult height less than four feet tall. In addition to the orthopedic problems, assess for cleft palate, which is seen in two thirds of cases.

Operative Indications   Orthopedic surgical efforts are directed primarily toward the club feet and hip dysplasia problems. Knee flexion deformity and patellar subluxation can also benefit from surgery. Scoliosis is initially treated with bracing, but ultimately may require surgery to stabilize deformities.

Types of Procedures   These club feet are some of the most difficult club feet to treat. They are very stiff and frequently recur after surgical treatment. Conventional releases frequently cannot achieve full correction, and recurrence of deformity is common. Newer alternatives for treatment include application of a distraction apparatus such as the Joshi or the Ilizarov device.

Conventional treatment resorts to talectomy in the most severe cases. Talectomy, unfortunately, has not had good long-term results and frequently presents with recurrent deformities that are almost impossible to treat.

Surgical Results/Prognosis   Cervical spinal kyphosis in diastrophic dysplasia can lead to neurologic complications if untreated. Flexion contractures frequently lead to severe joint deformities that can preclude walking ability. This is one of the more difficult orthopedic conditions to treat.

BIBLIOGRAPHY

Clark RN: Congenital dysplasias and dwarfism. *Pediatr Rev* 1990; 12:149-159.

Gembruch U, Niesen M, Kehrberg H et al: Diastrophic dysplasia: a specific prenatal diagnosis by ultrasound. *Prenat Diagn* 1988; 8:539-545.

Gollop TR, Eigier A: Prenatal ultrasound diagnosis of diastrophic dysplasia at sixteen weeks. *Am J Med Genet* 1987; 27:321-324.

Gustavson KH, Holmgren G, Jagell S et al: Lethal and non-lethal diastrophic dysplasia: a study of 14 Swedish cases. *Clin Genet* 1985; 28:321-334.

Hastbacka J, Salonen R, Laurilap et al: Prenatal diagnosis of diastrophic dysplasia with polymorphic DNA markers. *J Med Genet* 1993; 30:265-268.

Kaitila I, Ammala P, Karjalainen O et al: Early prenatal detection of diastrophic dysplasia. *Prenat Diagn* 1983; 3:237-244.

Mantagos S, Weiss RR, Mahoney M et al: Prenatal diagnosis of diastrophic dwarfism. *Am J Obstet Gynecol* 1981; 139:111-113.

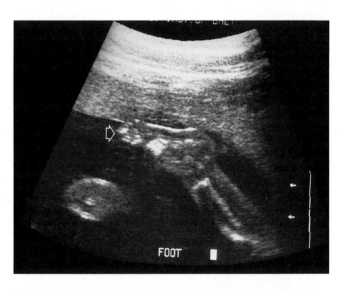

Diastrophic dwarfism—hitchhiker thumb. The thumb (*arrow*) is at right angles to the remaining digits. All are short and stubby.

Severely extended foot (*arrow*) in diastrophic dysplasia. Note the short tibia.

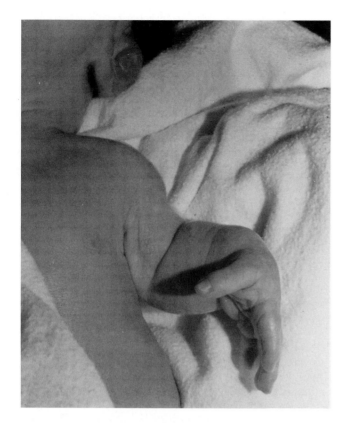

Two month old infant with diastrophic dysplasia. Note angulated (hitchhiker) thumb and ear cartilage hematomas (cauliflower ear).

8.8 FOCAL FEMORAL HYPOPLASIA

EPIDEMIOLOGY/GENETICS

Definition Focal femoral hypoplasia (FFH) is characterized by shortening and/or deformity of the femur.

Epidemiology Rare (M2:F3).

Embryology Focal femoral hypoplasia is a physical finding that may be seen in over 25 genetic and sporadic multiple malformation syndromes, including a number of skeletal dysplasias.

Inheritance Patterns Dependent on diagnosis, but includes dominant and recessive genetic syndromes.

Teratogens Maternal diabetes and fetal vitamin A exposure.

Prognosis Prognosis depends on etiology and can range from lethal skeletal dysplasias to disorders with only mild orthopedic abnormalities.

SONOGRAPHY

Findings
1. **Fetus**
   a. The proximal portion of one femur, including the femoral head, is usually absent. The femur is often angulated or bowed.
   b. There may be absence of the fibula and a bowed tibia on the affected side.
   c. Absence, or partial absence, of other long bones or digits may occur.
2. **Amniotic Fluid:** Normal.
3. **Placenta:** Normal.
4. **Measurement Data:** Normal, except in the affected limb or limbs.
5. **When Detectable:** At about 18 weeks. The abnormality becomes progressively more obvious.

Pitfalls The deformity with angulation of the femur can create an impression of osteogenesis imperfecta with a fracture. However, no additional fractures are seen.

Differential Diagnosis Osteogeneis imperfecta—see Pitfalls in this section. The severe forms of this disorder must be differentiated from sirenomelia, which is generally associated with lethal renal abnormalities.

Where Else to Look
1. Look elsewhere for findings associated with osteogenesis imperfecta.
2. Cleft palate and micrognathia have a rare association.
3. Shortening of other limbs may occasionally occur.

PREGNANCY MANAGEMENT

Investigations and Consultations Required
1. To exclude other syndromes fetal echocardiography should be performed. The presence of a congenital heart defect should prompt a reassessment of the diagnosis of FFH, unless occurring with maternal diabetes.
2. An orthopedic surgeon should meet with the family to discuss the prognosis for the child.

Monitoring The severity of the degree of shortening can be predicted by the rate of growth of the femur, so serial ultrasound studies are worthwhile for surgical preparation.

Pregnancy Course No specific obstetric complications are associated with FFH.

Pregnancy Termination Issues An intact fetus should be delivered in order that the diagnosis can be confirmed. There would be no increased risk for recurrence, if FFH is the only finding.

Delivery There should be no perinatal complications associated with FFH that would require delivery in a tertiary center.

NEONATOLOGY

Resuscitation There are no specific resuscitation measures required.

Transport Referral in the immediate neonatal period is not necessary unless there are associated malformations requiring evaluation and management.

Testing and Confirmation The diagnostic evaluation should include careful physical examination, skeletal radiographs, and pediatric orthopedic consultation. These may be obtained through an outpatient referral.

SURGERY

Preoperative Assessment Determine what the predicted leg length discrepancy will be. This is estimated by measuring the length of the long and short legs at birth. The percent shortening tends to remain constant, while the absolute discrepancy increases with age. Radiographs define both length and angular deformities. Next determine the stability of the hip and knee, and look for contractures.

Operative Indications All children with this diagnosis will require some form of surgery. Problems to be addressed may include the following: femoral shortening, tibial shortening, unstable knee, varus hip, acetabular insufficiency, and external rotation deformity. Usually the necessary corrective surgeries are staged over a series of years. The most important decision to make is whether to lengthen or amputate. More traditional thinking recommends amputation and prosthetic rehabilitation. The indications for leg lengthening are evolving, but the tendency is to recommend lengthening for predicted discrepancies of up to 15 cm and even more. For mild cases, epiphyseodesis (growth arrest) of the normal side can easily equalize length.

Types of Procedures The management controversy for this diagnosis has been reconstruction with lengthening and deformity correction versus Symes amputation with above-knee prosthetic fitting. A modification of amputation has been described in which the joint is removed, and the foot and ankle, are rotated 180°, thereby becoming a "knee" and allowing below-knee prosthetic fitting. Amputations reduce the number of surgeries required. Lengthening requires greater commitment of time and effort.

Surgical lengthening involves application of an external fixator, cutting the short bone, and then gradually distracting the gap, which fills in with regenerated bone. Simultaneous correction of angular and rotational deformities is possible. Because the knee cruciate ligaments are deficient, the external fixator must cross the knee with hinges to prevent joint subluxation. If the hip joint is shallow, a prelengthening pelvic osteotomy is done to stabilize the hip joint. Usually no more than 8 cm of lengthening should be carried out in the femur at any one time. This can be combined with 4 to 6 cm of tibial lengthening. Recently, it has been demonstrated that femoral lengthening can be carried out as early as the toddler-age group.

Surgical Results/Prognosis The main risk of lengthening is loss of knee motion. An intensive rehabilitation program is necessary. Knee and hip subluxation are additional risks, and may be prevented by adhering to certain technical points.

When there is a hip and knee present, the results of lengthening are potentially excellent. It is possible to equalize the leg length and maintain the function of the knee and hip and restore the patient to a normal gait pattern in most children. Many children receive amputation instead of reconstruction because of the surgeon's lack of experience in lengthening. Both options (amputation and lengthening) should be offered, as well as referral to major centers if needed. The cost of lengthenings is initially higher than amputation, but when considering lifetime costs for changing prostheses, lengthening is cost effective. Amputation surgery is quite reliable and has withstood the test of time. Long-term outcome studies are needed to determine the relative place of amputation versus lengthening.

BIBLIOGRAPHY

Burn J, Winter RM, Baraitser M et al: The femoral hypoplasia—unusual facies syndrome. *J Med Genet* 1984; 21:331-340.

Camera G, Dodero D, Parodi M et al: Antenatal ultrasonographic diagnosis of a proximal femoral focal deficiency. *J Clin Ultrasound* 1993; 21:475-479.

Jeanty P, Kleinman G: Proximal femoral focal deficiency. *J Ultrasound Med* 1989; 8:639-642.

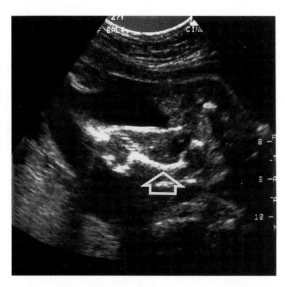

Proximal focal femoral hypoplasia. The left femur is markedly shortened and bowed. In this example the femoral head (*arrow*) is present. All other bones were of normal length and appearance.

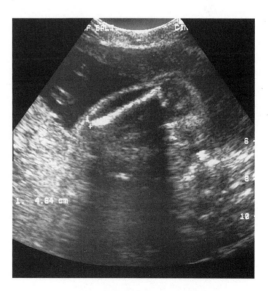

Normal right femur in the same patient.

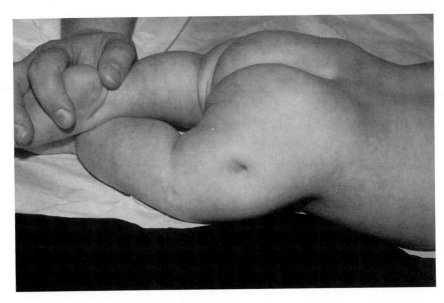

Six-month-old infant with focal femoral deficiency. Dimple marks site of outwardly curved shortened femur.

8.9 Klippel-Trenaunay-Weber Syndrome

EPIDEMIOLOGY/GENETICS

Definition Klippel-Trenaunay-Weber syndrome (KTWS) is the association of various cutaneous hemangiomas, vascular abnormalities, and hemihypertrophy or segmental overgrowth.

Epidemiology Rare (M1:F1).

Embryology The pathogenesis of this disorder is unknown, but may be due to abnormalities in the regulation of local growth factors. The location of the cutaneous hemangiomas, vascular abnormalities, and overgrowth may not correspond and makes simple vascular explanations for the overgrowth unlikely.

Inheritance Patterns Sporadic.

Teratogens None known.

Prognosis Prognosis depends on the type and extent of involvement.

SONOGRAPHY

Findings
1. **Fetus:** One or more areas of localized enlargement of one or more limbs. There may be focal enlargement of a portion of the torso. Color flow Doppler will demonstrate greatly increased arterial flow in the involved area. It is important to determine whether the vascular malformation extends from a limb to the trunk. This makes the prognosis much worse, because the limb cannot be resected. When there is a large arteriovenous shunt, there may be cardiomegaly and other findings of hydrops.
2. **Amniotic Fluid:** Normal.
3. **Placenta:** Normal.
4. **Measurement Data:** Measurement data will be enlarged locally by the abnormal trunk and limb masses.
5. **When Detectable:** At about 18 weeks.

Pitfalls
A high-quality ultrasound system is required to see the abnormal blood flow.

Differential Diagnosis
1. Amniotic band syndrome—Although there may be a localized limb enlargement, no increased blood flow will be seen.
2. Proteus syndrome—hemihypertrophy with subcutaneous hemangioma.

Where Else to Look
Look for evidence of hydrops.

PREGNANCY MANAGEMENT

Investigations and Consultations Required
1. Although the yield will be low, chromosome analysis should be performed.
2. Fetal echocardiography should be done to establish baseline parameters.
3. Magnetic resonance imaging (MRI) may be considered if it is uncertain if there is increased vascularity.
4. Consultations should be obtained with neonatology and pediatric surgery to discuss neonatal management with the family.

Fetal Intervention Theoretically, the administration of digoxin or similar medication to the mother and subsequent placental transfer may have some benefit in cases with high-output cardiac failure. At 32 weeks gestation or greater, early delivery and ex utero management is preferable.

Monitoring The pregnancy should be monitored by serial ultrasound examinations to detect signs of fetal hydrops. Fetal echocardiography may be helpful in the early detection of cardiac decompensation. The high risk of pregnancy complications requires that prenatal care be under the direction of a perinatologist.

Pregnancy Course Nonimmune fetal hydrops or polyhydramnios may complicate pregnancy management.

Pregnancy Termination Issues Pregnancy termination should be done by a nondestructive procedure and an autopsy performed in a center with expertise in fetal pathology.

Delivery Delivery should be in a tertiary center because of the significant risk of pregnancy and neonatal complications. The size and location of the mass may require cesarean section.

NEONATOLOGY

Resuscitation There are no specific resuscitation measures required, unless there is evidence of fetal cardiac decompensation or hydrops fetalis. See Chapter 12.2 for details of management.

Transport Referral, in the immediate neonatal period for diagnostic evaluation, to exclude other etiologies, is indicated only for marked asymmetry of the extremities or for complications of hydrops.

Testing and Confirmation Findings on physical examination after birth easily confirms the diagnosis.

Nursery Management   In the absence of congestive heart failure or hydrops fetalis, routine newborn care is appropriate. Lymphatic obstruction has also been described. Surgical intervention has been delayed usually to early childhood or later in adulthood.

SURGERY

Preoperative Assessment   Diagnostic evaluation of the vascularity of the involved extremity with non-invasive imaging techniques such as ultrasound and MRI may demonstrate either venous obstruction or an arteriovenous malformation. Extremity bone radiographs of the involved and contralateral limbs are important for future consideration in therapy for bony hypertrophy.

Operative Indications   Therapy depends on the degree of vascular involvement and bony hypertrophy. The vascular component is frequently associated with lymphatic obstruction and edema. Angiomatosis with rapidly proliferating skin and subcutaneous lesions may also be present.

Types of Procedures   Compression treatment is effective if started early and strict patient compliance is achieved. Intermittent pneumatic compression can be applied, particularly at night. The technique is improved with associated use of static compression (Jobst) garments. This therapy is particularly difficult in infants and growing children because the garments are warm, they require frequent changes in size and, if not used properly, they can produce local irritation over the damaged skin. Local vascular procedures to correct atrioventricular (A-V) fistulae and varicose veins result in marginal success. Intermittent bouts of cellulitis require antibiotic therapy, but prophylactic antibiotics

are not routinely used. Severe limb hypertrophy can require epiphysiodesis and functional impairment may require major limb procedures and/or amputations.

Surgical Results/Prognosis   These children may be severely handicapped both functionally and cosmetically. This lesion is not usually associated with malignant degeneration or secondary tumors.

BIBLIOGRAPHY

Baskerville PA, Ackroyd JS, Lea Thomas M et al: The Klippel-Trenaunay syndrome: clinical, radiological and haemodynamic features and management. *Br J Surg* 1985; 72:232-236.

Drose JA, Thickman D, Wiggins J et al: Fetal echocardiographic findings in the Klippel-Trenaunay-Weber syndrome. *J Ultrasound Med* 1991; 10:525-527.

Edgerton MT: The treatment of hemangiomas with special reference to the role of steroid therapy. *Ann Surg* 1976; 183:517-532.

McCullough CJ, Kenwright S: The prognosis in congenital lower limb hypertrophy. *Acta Ortho Scand* 1979; 50:307-313.

Meholic AJ, Freimanis AK, Stucka J et al: Sonographic in utero diagnosis of Klippel-Trenaunay-Weber syndrome. *J Ultrasound Med* 1991; 10:111-114.

Mor Z, Schreyer P, Wainraub Z et al: Nonimmune hydrops fetalis associated with angiosteohypertrophy (Klippel-Trenaunay) syndrome. *Am J Obstet Gynecol* 1988; 159:1185-1186.

Servelle M: Klippel and Trenaunay's syndrome: 768 operated cases. *Ann Surg* 1985; 201:365-373.

Stringel G, Dastous J: Klippel-Trenaunay syndrome and other cases of lower limb hypertrophy: pediatric surgical implications. *J Pediatr Surg* 1987; 22:645-650.

Viljoen D, Saxe N, Pearn J et al: The cutaneous manifestations of the Klippel-Trenaunay-Weber syndrome. *Clin Exp Dermatol* 1987; 12:12-17.

Warhit JM, Goldman MA, Sachs L et al: Klippel-Trenaunay-Weber syndrome: appearance in utero. *J Ultrasound Med* 1983; 2:515-518.

Klippel-Trenaunay-Weber syndrome. A large mass (*arrow*) arises from the chest wall. The mass was pulsatile and involved the shoulder joint.

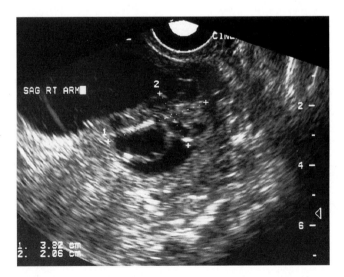

There was a second mass involving the right hand (*between x's*). The arm and hand were swollen and a large soft tissue mass was present.

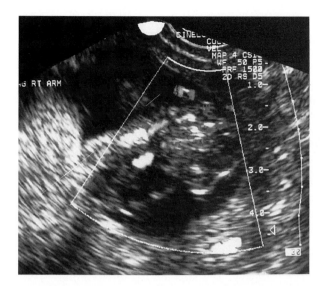

Color flow Doppler image of the same hand. The highly echogenic areas (within box) represent blood flow related to the enlarged, abnormal vasculature of this atrioventricular malformation.

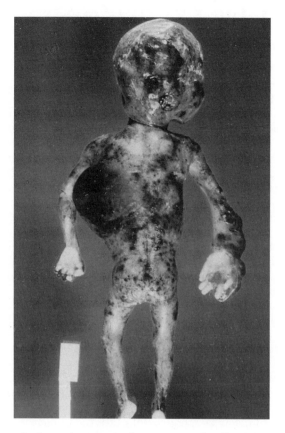

Posttermination specimen showing the masses arising from the trunk and right hand.

8.10 LIMB-BODY WALL COMPLEX
BODY STALK COMPLEX, CYLLOSOMAS

EPIDEMIOLOGY/GENETICS

Definition Limb body wall complex (LBWC) is generally defined as consisting of two out of the three following abnormalities: 1. myelomeningocele or caudal regression; 2. thoracoabdominoschisis or abdominoschisis; and 3. limb defects.

Epidemiology Rare.

Embryology Limb-body wall complex is most frequently thought to arise as a result of early amnion disruptions. Some cases, however, may be due to an early error in embryonic development.

Inheritance Patterns Sporadic.

Teratogens None known.

Prognosis If all components of the syndrome are present, the condition is lethal. Milder forms of amniotic band syndrome, with gastroschisis and absent limb, for example, may be grouped with LBWC, but have a better prognosis.

SONOGRAPHY

Findings
1. **Fetus:** A complex array of sonographic findings is seen.
   a. One or more limbs, or segments of limbs, are missing. Club feet may be present.
   b. Intestines, liver, and even the bladder extend outside of the abdominal wall and may be attached to the placenta. Diaphragmatic absence and bowel atresia occur.
   c. A short, curved spine with sacral regression is common.
   d. Myelomeningocele is frequent, with secondary Arnold-Chiari malformation and hydrocephalus.
   e. Ectopia cordis or other cardiac anomalies may be present.
   f. Facial clefts may be present.
2. **Amniotic Fluid:** There is often oligohydramnios.
3. **Placenta:** The placenta may be attached to the fetus. The umbilical cord is short or absent and is adherent to placental membranes. Occasionally, amniotic membrane remnants are visible.
4. **Measurement Data:** Normal where measurable, but most structures are affected by the process.
5. **When Detectable:** 13 to 14 weeks.

Pitfalls Limited fluid may make limb visualization difficult.

Differential Diagnosis The body stalk anomaly, in which the placenta is attached to the trunk of the fetus and similar deformities occur, is a variant of the same condition.

Where Else to Look The entire fetus needs to be scanned in detail because anomalies can affect any organ.

PREGNANCY MANAGEMENT

Investigations and Consultations Required The pattern and severity of the malformations are inconsistent with the usual chromosomal abnormalities, but chromosome studies should be performed to exclude unbalanced chromosome rearrangements that may have implications for subsequent pregnancies. If the condition does not appear lethal, consultation with a pediatric surgeon may be helpful for discussion with the parents regarding the complications of the malformations.

Monitoring The classic form of limb body wall complex is lethal and prenatal care should focus on maternal issues. Fetal assessment is not appropriate.

Pregnancy Course No specific obstetric complications should be expected.

Pregnancy Termination Issues To establish a precise diagnosis, a termination technique should be used that allows an intact fetus be delivered.

Delivery A diagnosis of LBWC should be an indication for vaginal delivery only, without fetal monitoring.

NEONATOLOGY

Resuscitation Resuscitation is not indicated as this anomaly, reportedly, is lethal.

Transport Not indicated unless the fetus survives delivery and the diagnosis is uncertain.

Testing and Confirmation Careful physical examination and sonography are usually all that are required to determine the extent of organ involvement.

Nursery Management Supportive care is appropriate until the diagnosis is confirmed and time has been allowed for parental adaptation to the prognosis.

BIBLIOGRAPHY

Lockwood CJ, Scioscia AL, Hobbins JC: Congenital absence of the umbilical cord resulting from maldevelopment of embryonic body folding. *Am J Obstet Gynecol* 1986; 155:1049-1051.

Moerman P, Fryns J-P, Vanderberghe K et al: Constrictive amniotic bands, amniotic adhesions, and limb-body wall complex: discrete disruption sequences with pathogenetic overlap. *Am J Med Genet* 1992; 42:470-479.

Patten RM, Van Allen M, Mack LA et al: Limb-body wall complex: in utero sonographic diagnosis of a complicated fetal malformation. *Am J Roentgenol* 1986; 146:1019-1024.

Russo R, D'Armiento M, Angrisani P et al: Limb body wall complex: a critical review and a nosological proposal. *Am J Med Genet* 1993; 47:893-900.

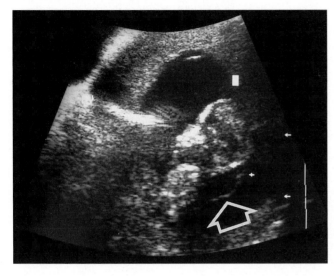

Limb body wall defect. View of the head and upper body. An amniotic band is visible attached to the head (*arrow*).

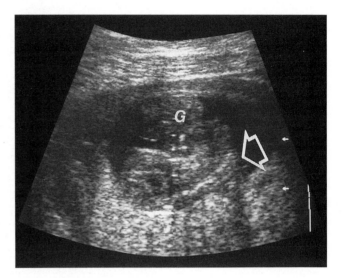

A large mass with liver and gut lies outside the fetal abdomen (*G*). The spine (*arrow*) is short due to caudal regression.

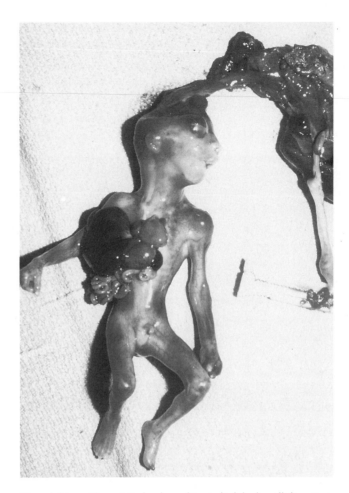

18-week fetus with amniotic bands resulting in limb-body wall disruption. Extruded visceral contents included heart, liver, and gastrointestinal tract components.

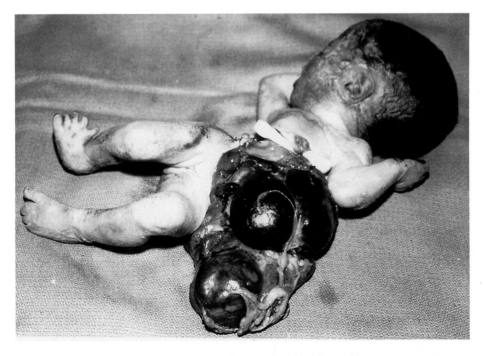

24-week fetus with limb-body wall disruption showing right clubbed foot and massive evisceration.

8.11 MULTIPLE PTERYGIUM SYNDROME

EPIDEMIOLOGY/GENETICS

Definition   The multiple pterygium syndromes are a heterogeneous group of disorders characterized by pterygia or webbing across the neck and other joints.

Epidemiology   Rare (M1:F1).

Embryology   Pterygia, or webs that occur across joint spaces, are thought to be the result of limited in utero movement. Over 25 multiple malformation syndromes have been described with pterygia and have been divided into lethal and nonlethal forms. The lethal forms generally have growth retardation, cystic hygroma, and/or fetal hydrops.

Inheritance Patterns   Most nonlethal cases are sporadic whereas lethal cases usually show autosomal recessive inheritance. Rare X-linked recessive families have been reported.

Teratogens   None.

Prognosis   Life span and intellectual development in nonlethal cases is generally normal. Ambulation and function are dependent upon the severity of the pterygia and success of orthopedic correction.

SONOGRAPHY

Findings
1. **Fetus**
   a. Persistently severely flexed arms and flexed hips with extended, crossed legs. Fetal movement is almost absent.
   b. Cystic hygroma may be present in the second trimester. Hydrops may occur.
   c. There are club feet and the hands are also in a clubbed position. Syndactyly of the second to fourth fingers gives the hands an odd shape.
   d. Micrognathia and cleft palate may be present.
   e. Hypertelorism with corneal opacities may be seen.
   f. Omphalocele and cardiac defects such as ventricular septal defect have been reported.
2. **Amniotic Fluid:** Polyhydramnios is often present.
3. **Placenta:** Normal.
4. **Measurement Data:** Normal.
5. **When Detectable:** About 16 weeks.

Pitfalls   So far, the pterygia have not been detected, so the conditon can be confused with a normal fetus that holds its limbs in a flexed position due to a confined space as with oligohydramnios.

Differential Diagnosis
1. Arthrogryposis—A similar limb position is assumed along with absent fetal movement. However, hydrops and cystic hygroma are not seen.
2. Other syndromes with cystic hygroma. Unusual limb position is not a feature of Turner's or Noonan syndromes.

Where Else to Look   This is a generalized syndrome, so look throughout the body.

PREGNANCY MANAGEMENT

Investigations and Consultations Required   Chromosome studies should be done, as trisomy 18 may present with a similar clinical picture on rare occasions. Fetal echocardiography should be performed as cardiac hypoplasia (generalized) is a frequent feature.

Monitoring   Standard obstetric care without fetal assessment is appropriate. No attempt to stop preterm labor should be made.

Pregnancy Course   Polyhydramnios is a common complication and may be severe, resulting in preterm labor.

Pregnancy Termination Issues   Delivery of an intact fetus for careful assessment of external features and neuropathologic evaluation is essential to establish a precise diagnosis.

Delivery   The site of delivery should be one where the staff is comfortable with a noninterventional approach to labor management and newborn resuscitation. Fetal monitoring during labor is not appropriate.

NEONATOLOGY

Resuscitation   If a lethal variant is suspected from prenatal diagnosis, a decision for nonintervention at delivery is appropriate with concurrence of the family. There may be difficulty in establishing a reliable airway if jaw mobility is affected.

Transport   Referral to a tertiary perinatal center in the immediate neonatal period is appropriate for diagnostic evaluation and confirmation of the prognosis. Mechanical respiratory support during transport may be needed for infants with the lethal variant.

Testing and Confirmation   The diagnostic evaluation should include careful physical examination, genetic consultation, and skeletal radiographs.

Nursery Management   Mechanical life support, to allow time for diagnostic evaluation and parental adaptation, is appropriate. Deaths in the lethal variant are from respiratory failure secondary to pulmonary hypoplasia, which implies that long-term mechanical ventilation is unlikely to be beneficial.

The long-term treatment goal is to establish joint mobility with physical therapy and soft-tissue release surgery.

BIBLIOGRAPHY

Anthony J, Mascarenhas L, O'Brien J et al: Lethal multiple pterygium syndrome. The importance of fetal posture in midtrimester diagnosis by ultrasound: discussion and case report. *Ultrasound Obstet Gynecol* 1993; 3:212-216.

Baty B, Cubberley D, Morris C et al: Prenatal diagnosis of distal arthrogryposis. *Am J Med Genet* 1988; 29:501-510.

De Die-Smulders CEM, Vonsee HJ, Zandvoort JA et al: The lethal multiple pterygium syndrome: prenatal ultrasonographic and postmortem findings: a case report. *Eur J Obstet Gynecol Reprod Biol* 1990; 35:283-289.

Hall JG, Reed SD, Rosenbaum KN et al: Limb pterygium syndromes: a review and report of eleven patients. *Am J Med Genet* 1982; 12:377-409.

Lockwood CL, Irons M, Troiani J et al: The prenatal sonographic diagnosis of lethal multiple pterygium syndrome: a heritable cause of recurrent abortions. *Am J Obstet Gynecol* 1988; 159:474-476.

Meizner I, Hershkovit R, Carmi R et al: Prenatal ultrasound diagnosis of a rare occurrence of lethal multiple pterygium syndrome in two siblings. *Ultrasound Obstet Gynecol* 1993; 3:432-436.

Moerman P, Fryns JP, Cornelis A et al: Pathogenesis of the lethal multiple pterygium syndrome. *Am J Med Genet* 1990; 35: 415-421.

Shenker L, Reed K, Anderson C et al: Syndrome of camptodactyly, ankyloses, facial anomalies, and pulmonary hypoplasia (Pena-Shokeir syndrome): obstetric and ultrasound aspects. *Am J Obstet Gynecol* 1985; 152:303-307.

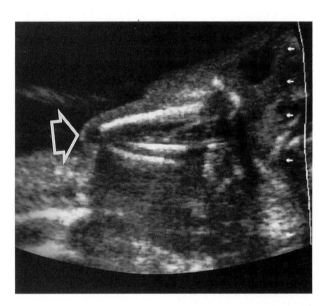

View of the arm. The arrow shows the elbow. The proximal and distal portions of the arm are close together because the arm was in a constantly severely flexed position.

8.12 OSTEOGENESIS IMPERFECTA

EPIDEMIOLOGY/GENETICS

Definition Osteogenesis imperfecta (OI) is a heterogeneous group of brittle-bone diseases characterized by an excessive tendency to antenatal or postnatal fractures.

Epidemiology An Australian study found the incidence of 1.6 to 3.5 out of 100,000 live births (M1:F1).

Embryology Most types of OI are due to type I collagen abnormalities and exhibit a highly variable phenotype. The Sillence classification is frequently used to divide these disorders into phenotypic groups. Type I is the classic form of OI characterized by moderate fractures, blue sclera, variable degrees of hearing loss, and dentinogenesis imperfecta; type II is a severe lethal neonatal form with multiple antenatal fractures; type III is a progressively deforming disorder with severe disability by middle age; and type IV is a mild phenotype with normal sclerae.

Inheritance Patterns Most families demonstrate autosomal dominant inheritance, but some autosomal recessive families have been described, especially for type II.

Teratogens None.

Screening If the precise abnormality in a particular family is known, biochemical analysis of type I collagen or another biochemical or DNA marker may be studied on chorionic villus samples or amniocytes. Because some families do not have type I collagen defects, linkage studies cannot be routinely done. Gonadal mosaicism for type I collagen mutations has been found in phenotypically normal parents, thereby complicating genetic counselling.

Prognosis Highly variable, depending on clinical type. Infants with type II disease are born with multiple fractures and often die in the neonatal period from respiratory compromise. In the milder types I and IV, fractures may not occur until later in life.

SONOGRAPHY

Findings
1. **Fetus**
   a. Types I and IV—There are one or two fractures with normal or mildly shortened bones. Bone length of limbs, on each side, is not equal. Callus formation is visible, the bone is angulated, there is bowing, or the bone has an irregular contour.
   b. Type II—Most in utero cases fall in this group. There is generalized bony deossification with many rib deformities. The head is compressible with too easily seen intracranial structures and absence of skull reverberations. The bones are variably shortened with callus and bone angulation.
   c. Lethal form of type II—Intracranial structures are too well seen with little or no skull ossification. All bones are extremely short with marked fragmentation. There is a very small chest.
2. **Amniotic Fluid:** Normal or increased fluid.
3. **Placenta:** Normal placenta.
4. **Measurement Data:** Variably shortened long bones. Normal head and abdomen size.
5. **When Detectable:** Can be detected at 13 or 14 weeks.

Pitfalls Variable short limb length may be the only clue to the more mild form.

Differential Diagnosis
1. Achondrogenesis—Leg shortening and a small chest may be the predominant findings. Osteogenesis imperfecta may be mistaken for achondrogenesis because bones are echopenic in achondrogenesis also.
2. Camptomelic dwarfism—Tibial and femoral bowing may be the predominant features (the legs are usually more affected than the arms in OI), so camptomelic dwarfism may be diagnosed.
3. Hypophosphatasia—generalized hypoechoic bones, but usually no fractures are seen.

Where Else To Look Look at the eyes for cataract. The lens has a very thick border.

PREGNANCY MANAGEMENT

Investigations and Consultations Required
1. Many of the skeletal dysplasias, but not OI, are associated with congenital heart disease. Therefore, a fetal echocardiogram should be done.
2. Fetal radiographs may be helpful in establishing a more precise diagnosis.
3. A neonatologist should be consulted to plan perinatal management, if a lethal dwarfism is expected.

Monitoring No obstetric intervention should be performed for the fetus with OI, type II. Other types are not lethal; they are associated with a less severe deformity and standard obstetric management should be used.

Pregnancy Course Polyhydramnios may occur, but, if present, is usually mild.

Pregnancy Termination Issues An intact fetus must be delivered for a complete postmortem evaluation, including radiologic, morphologic, biochemical, and molecular studies. There is a special need for establishing cultured cell lines to determine the exact molecular or biochemical defect in order that early diagnosis will be possible in future pregnancies.

Delivery   For the nonlethal forms of OI, cesarean delivery is theoretically of benefit to decrease the risk of fractures and intracranial hemorrhage. Delivery should occur in a tertiary center.

NEONATOLOGY

Resuscitation   Given that the prenatal differentiation between the various types may be difficult, it is appropriate to initiate resuscitative efforts. However, if the prenatal diagnosis of OI II is definite, a prenatal decision for nonintervention, after discussion with the parents, is appropriate.

Transport   Referral to a tertiary perinatal center for confirmation of the diagnosis is always indicated for a liveborn infant with OI. Mechanical ventilatory support may be required during transport. Caution in handling is required to reduce the risk of inadvertent fractures.

Testing and Confirmation   Careful physical examination and skeletal radiographs are helpful in determining classification. Multiple prenatal fractures and blue sclerae at birth strongly suggest OI II, the ultimately lethal form.

Nursery Management   Assistive devices (plastic shells) may be needed to facilitate handling while protecting the infant from additional fractures.

Long-term ventilatory support is possible, but controversial for some infants with OI II. Survival beyond early childhood has not been reported.

SURGERY

Preoperative Assessment   Type II OI patients die in early infancy, although we are aware of one child who survived and is ventilator-dependent and wheelchair-bound at age 9 years. In general, the severity of the phenotype will determine the level of treatment needed. Radiographs show osteoporosis and healed or healing fractures. Mild cases may be confused with child abuse. One should not forget that a child may be both abused and suffer from OI. Therefore, having the diagnosis of OI does not rule out abuse.

Operative Indications   When children with OI fracture, they generally heal at a normal rate. The important issue is to prevent progressive bowing deformities from developing in the long bones. The usual treatment for childhood fractures is cast immobilization. More aggressive treatment with internal or external fixation is occasionally indicated to prevent deformity. In severe cases, such as type III, this is often a losing battle, with the patient eventually becoming wheelchair bound. For more functional patients, bowing deformities represent a mechanical and cosmetic problem.

Corrective osteotomies can help, although the technical nature of these procedures can be difficult in thin, gracile, bowed bones. Scoliosis frequently develops in severe cases, and requires operative stabilization with special techniques to accommodate the frail bone. Bracing is not helpful in controlling spinal deformities in OI. However, leg braces can help improve walking ability in selected cases.

Types of Procedures   Acute fractures are treated usually with casts or splints, occasionally with surgery and internal fixation. Established bowing and angular deformities may be treated by corrective osteotomies and internal fixation. Severely bowed bones require the so-called "shish kabob" procedure, in which the bowed bone is cut at multiple levels into small sections and then "skewered" onto a straight intramedullary rod to heal in the corrected alignment. Special telescopic intramedullary nails that elongate during growth are used in young children.

Surgical Results/Prognosis   Ultimate prognosis depends on the severity of the specific phenotype. In general, if fractures appear before walking age, there is a 30% chance that the child will eventually be wheelchair bound. Nonunion of fractures, although rare in normal children, can be seen in up to 20% of children with OI.

BIBLIOGRAPHY

Andersen PE Jr, Hauge M: Osteogenesis imperfecta: a genetic, radiological, and epidemiological study. *Clin Genet* 1989; 36:250-255.

Chervenak FA, Romero R, Berkowitz RL et al: Antenatal sonographic findings of osteogenesis imperfecta. *Am J Obstet Gynecol* 1982; 143:228-230.

Sillence DO, Barlow KK, Garber AP et al: Osteogenesis imperfecta type II: delineation of the phenotype with reference to genetic heterogeneity. *Am J Med Genet* 1984; 17:407-423.

Sillence DO: Osteogenesis imperfecta nosology and genetics. *Ann NY Acad Sci* 1988; 543:1-15.

Willing MC, Pruchno CJ, Byers PH: Molecular heterogeneity in osteogenesis imperfecta. *Am J Med Genet* 1993; 45:223-227.

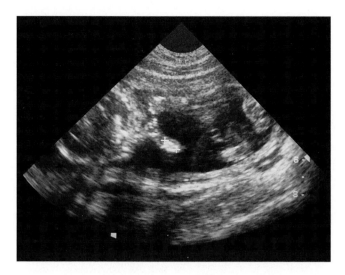

Lethal form of osteogenesis imperfecta. The humerus (*between x's*) is extremely short and fractured into several fragments.

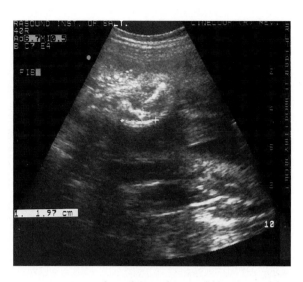

Type III osteogenesis imperfecta. There is a fracture of the midpoint of the tibia (*X*).

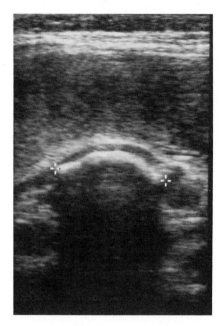

Type II osteogenesis imperfecta. The femur is mildly shortened and bowed. Note the irregular texture indicating previous fractures.

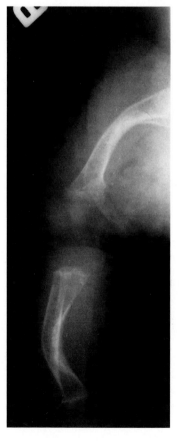

Radiograph of the same bone after birth. There has been remodeling with repair of the fracture . The bones are deossified.

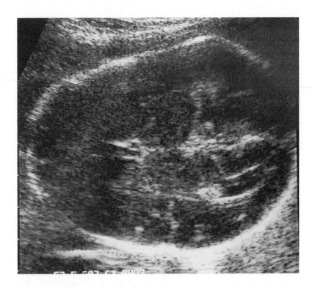

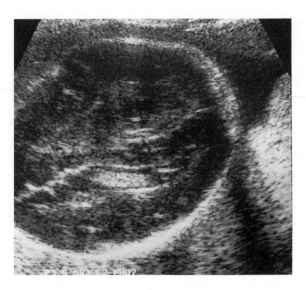

View of the head. Note the unduly well seen intracranial structures and the poorly ossified cranium. The area closest to the transducer is flattened due to the transducer pressure because the skull is so weak.

The same skull reexamined with a light touch. The skull deformity is no longer present.

8.13 POLYDACTYLY

EPIDEMIOLOGY/GENETICS

Definition   Polydactyly is a phenotypic abnormality of the limbs characterized by excessive partitioning of the digital rays of the hands and feet. This is clinically manifested as extra digits, broad digits, or bifid digits.

Epidemiology   Postaxial (ulnar or fibular side of the limb) polydactyly occurs in 1 out of 3000 Caucasian live births, but it is 10 times more common in blacks than Caucasians (M1.5:F1). Preaxial (radial or tibial side of limb) polydactyly is much less common with a frequency in Caucasians of 0.15 out of 1000.

Embryology   Over 100 multiple malformation syndromes have been described with polydactyly, including many short-limb skeletal dysplasias and chromosome abnormalities including trisomies 13, 18, and 21.

Inheritance Patterns   Isolated postaxial polydactyly is most often inherited as an autosomal dominant trait. Isolated preaxial polydactyly is most often unilateral and not familial.

Teratogens   Alcohol, valproate, maternal diabetes.

Prognosis   Excellent for isolated polydactylies, otherwise, it is dependent upon the associated abnormalities and syndrome diagnosis.

SONOGRAPHY

Findings
1. **Fetus:** Hands and/or feet have one or more extra digits that may be normally sited and sized as a sixth finger or they may small, abnormally located, and angled.
2. **Amniotic Fluid:** Normal, if the only finding is polydactyly.
3. **Placenta:** Normal, if the only finding is polydactyly.
4. **Measurement Data:** Normal, if isolated.
5. **When Detectable:** About 18 weeks.

Pitfalls   Inappropriate oblique angulation can create an appearance of polydactyly when none exists.

Differential Diagnosis   Abnormally located fifth digit.

Where Else to Look
1. Limb lengths—Meckel-Gruber syndrome, Ellis-van Creveld syndrome, short-rib polydactyly, and chondroectodermal dysplasia all commonly have extra digits.
2. Trisomy 13—look for stigmata; commonly has polydactyly.

PREGNANCY MANAGEMENT

Investigations and Consultations Required
1. Chromosome analysis to exclude trisomy 13 is essential.
2. Fetal echocardiography is necessary because a number of the syndromes with polydactyly also have congenital heart defects.
3. Additional consultations will depend upon the presumptive diagnosis and the types of malformations seen in association with the polydactyly.

Monitoring   Unless the condition can clearly be established as lethal (e.g., Meckel-Gruber syndrome, short-rib polydactyly syndrome), obstetric management should not be modified.

Pregnancy Course   Obstetric complications will vary, depending on the associated abnormalities. Those conditions with skeletal dysplasias may be associated with polyhydramnios.

Pregnancy Termination Issues   Except for cases with chromosomal abnormalities, all other situations require a nondestructive termination procedure and a complete postmortem evaluation by a fetal pathologist and a dysmorphologist.

Delivery   Because an exact diagnosis may be difficult to establish prenatally, delivery should occur in a tertiary center where a full array of diagnostic and management options exist.

BIBLIOGRAPHY
Temtany SA, McKusick VA: The genetics of hand malformations. New York. Alan R. Liss, for the National Foundation-March of Dimes, 1987.

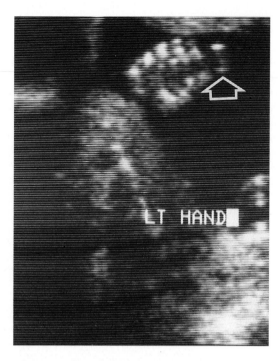

Polydactyly. An extra digit (*arrow*) is present and appears to be about the same size and location as the others.

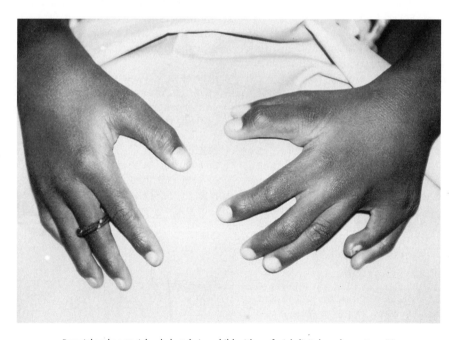

Preaxial and postaxial polydactyly in a child with orofacial-digital syndrome type IV.

8.14 RADIAL RAY PROBLEMS
RADIAL RAY APLASIA/HYPOPLASIA

EPIDEMIOLOGY/GENETICS

Definition   Radial aplasia/hypoplasia is a physical and radiographic abnormality characterized by partial or complete absence of the radius or radial-ray structures (thumb and radial carpal bones). The etiology is heterogeneous with most defects being unilateral and sporadic.

Epidemiology   0.3 to 0.8 out of 10,000 births.

Embryology   The distal upper limbs are composed of two major developmental fields: a radial (preaxial) field and an ulnar (postaxial) field. Most major limb defects result from abnormalities in one of these fields, causing preaxial or postaxial limb defects. Defects occurring at the junction of these fields result in split-hand (ectrodactyly) malformations.

Inheritance Patterns   Most radial defects are unilateral and sporadic with bilateral defects being much more likely to be part of a multiple malformation syndrome. Syndromes with radial aplasia/hypoplasia (see index) include hematologic syndromes like Fanconi's anemia, Aase syndrome, and thrombocytopenia-absent radius (TAR) syndrome; sporadic associations like the VACTERL association and the Goldenhar's syndrome; chromosome syndromes including trisomy 13, 18, and triploidy; and some miscellaneous syndromes like the acrofacial dysostoses, Baller-Gerold syndrome, Cornelia de Lange syndrome, Townes-Brock syndrome, and the Holt-Oram syndrome.

Teratogens   Thalidomide, cocaine, valproate, and vitamin A.

Prognosis   Dependent upon associated abnormalities and syndrome diagnosis. Good function possible in most cases with aggressive orthopedic treatment.

SONOGRAPHY

Findings
1.   **Fetus:** Arm bones—The radius can be short or absent. The ulna can be short, bowed, or sometimes also absent. The hand is usually clubbed and the thumb may be absent along with some of the carpal bones.
    a.   In TAR syndrome, the lower limbs may also be short or absent. The condition is symmetrical.
    b.   In Holt-Oram, the bony deformity may be asymmetrical and lower limb involvement does not occur. There may be absence of the entire arm long bones with phocomelia. The scaphoid and the trapezium may be absent.
2.   **Amniotic Fluid:** Generally normal, but may be decreased with some etiologies.

3.   **Placenta:** Normal.
4.   **Measurement Data:** Abdomen and head measurements are normal.
5.   **When Detectable:** Early second trimester.

Pitfalls   One arm may lie behind the trunk, so it cannot be seen.

Differential Diagnosis   Osteogenesis imperfecta—usually affects lower limbs more than arms.

Where Else to Look
1.   With Holt-Oram syndrome perform fetal echocardiography looking for VSD, ASD, and pulmonic stenosis.
2.   Radial ray problems can be a feature of the VACTERL complex, so look for heart anomalies, kidney deformities, spina bifida, hemivertebra, and gut atresia.
3.   Trisomy 18 can present with radial ray problems, so look for IUGR, cardiac anomalies, and choroid plexus cysts.
4.   Valproic acid can result in radial ray defects—Look at the face for cleft palate and the spine for myelomeningocele if there is an appropriate history.

PREGNANCY MANAGEMENT

Investigations and Consultations Required   Fetal karyotype should be considered especially if other malformations are detected. A careful history is essential to assess for presence of limb or cardiac abnormalities in the parents or previous children. History also should include information regarding consanguinity because many of the disorders are autosomal recessive. Any potential teratogen exposure, specifically valproic acid, should be ascertained.

Both amniocentesis and cordocentesis should be performed. Fetal hematologic status must be assessed to exclude TAR, Fanconi's anemia, and Aase syndrome. Amniotic fluid cultures should be established to look for chromosome breakage (Fanconi's anemia) or premature centromere splitting (Roberts' syndrome). Fetal echocardiography should be performed, as cardiac defects are associated with a number of the possible etiologic conditions.

Other consultations should be based on the presumptive diagnosis and the need for neonatal medical or surgical therapy.

Fetal Intervention   None is indicated.

Monitoring   Ultrasound examinations every 3 to 4 weeks should be performed to assess amniotic fluid status.

Pregnancy Termination Issues   Unless a precise diagnosis has been established prenatally, the method of termination should provide an intact fetus for a complete morphologic and radiologic examination.

Delivery   The complex nature of these multiple malformation conditions requires that delivery and neonatal management occur in a tertiary center. In cases of TAR and Fanconi's anemia with platelet counts less than 50,000/mm³, consideration must be given to elective cesarean section or platelet transfusion just prior to elective induction of labor.

NEONATOLOGY

Resuscitation   In general, any special issues for resuscitation are determined by the associated or underlying etiology of the skeletal defect.

Transport   Referral to a tertiary perinatal center following birth is indicated for definitive diagnosis, particularly if cardiac or chromosomal abnormalities are suspected.

Testing and Confirmation   In general, careful physical examination, blood cell morphology, extremity radiographs, echocardiogram, and chromosomal analysis, if there are other dysmorphic features, complete the basic evaluation.

Nursery Management   The primary issue is a definitive etiologic diagnosis. Long-term prognosis is determined by the associated or underlying etiology. Palliative procedures are possible to create a prehensile grasp.

BIBLIOGRAPHY

Auerbach AD, Sagi M, Adler B: Fanconi anemia: prenatal diagnosis in 30 fetuses at risk. *Pediatrics* 1985; 76:794-800.

Brons JTJ, Van Geijn HP, Wladimiroff JW et al: Prenatal ultrasound diagnosis of the Holt-Oram syndrome. *Prenat Diagn* 1988; 8:175-181.

Brons JTJ, Van Der Harten HJ, Van Geijn HP et al: Prenatal ultrasonographic diagnosis of radial-ray reduction malformations. *Prenat Diagn* 1990; 10:279-288.

Donnenfeld AE, Wiseman B, Lavi E et al: Prenatal diagnosis of thrombocytopenia absent radius syndrome by ultrasound and cordocentesis. *Prenat Diagn* 1990; 10:29-35.

Luthy DA, Mack L, Hirsch J et al: Prenatal ultrasound diagnosis of thrombocytopenia with absent radii. *Am J Obstet Gynecol* 1981; 141:350-352.

Meizner I, Bar-Ziv J, Barki Y et al: Prenatal ultrasonic diagnosis of radial-ray aplasia and renal anomalies (acrorenal syndrome). *Prenat Diagn* 1986; 6:223-225.

Varaiter M, Winter RM: *Oxford dysmorphology database.* Oxford, England. Oxford University Press, 1993.

Wood VE: Congenital thumb deformities. *Clin Orthop* 1985; 195:7-25.

Ylagan LR, Budorick NE: Radial ray aplasia in utero: a prenatal finding associated with valproic acid exposure. *J Ultrasound Med* 1994; 13:408-411.

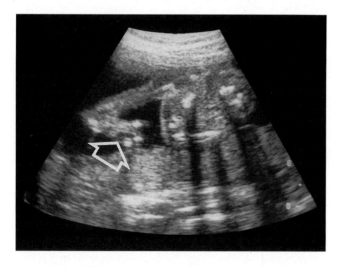

Radial-ray anomaly. View of the humerus, forearm, and hand. Note that the forearm (*arrow*) is very short and that the hand is deformed.

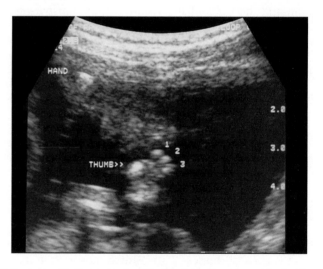

Deformed hand in the same patient. The thumb is rudimentary and the first finger is missing.

8.15 Thanatophoric Dwarfism (Dysplasia)

EPIDEMIOLOGY/GENETICS

Definition Thanatophoric dysplasia is the most common lethal short-limbed skeletal dysplasia and is characterized by micromelia, narrow thorax, and a relatively large head.

Epidemiology 1 out of 40,000 live births.

Embryology Thanatophoric dysplasia has characteristic radiographic findings including "telephone-receiver"–shaped femurs and short ribs. Cloverleaf skull is an uncommon feature.

Inheritance Patterns Most cases are sporadic and probably represent new dominant mutations.

Prognosis Thanatophoric dysplasia is invariably fatal, usually shortly after birth.

SONOGRAPHY

Findings
1. **Fetus**
   a. Very short limbs with telephone-receiver–shaped femurs are seen. There is a rhizomelic pattern to the limb shortening.
   b. A very small chest expands into a bell-shaped abdomen.
   c. The hands have a trident shape with short, stubby fingers that are widely separated. Redundant soft tissue surrounds the limb bones.
   d. A cloverleaf deformity (Kleebattschädel), in which there is a bulge off the top of the head, is occasionally seen. Hydrocephalus may occur.
   e. The intravertebral distance is shortened and the spine is short.
2. **Amniotic Fluid:** Very severe polyhydramnios is always seen.
3. **Placenta:** Normal.
4. **Measurement Data:** Large abdomen and head. Very small chest and bones.
5. **When Detectable:** About 14 weeks

Pitfalls

Differential Diagnosis
1. Achondrogenesis—Some varieties are indistinguishable from thanatophoric dwarfism. In the most typical form, the spine is echopenic.
2. Achondroplasia—The sonographic features are indistinguishable, but all of the findings are seen at a later date. Before 20 to 24 weeks the sonographic appearances are within normal limits.

Where Else To Look This is a generalized process, involving most structures.

PREGNANCY MANAGEMENT

Investigations and Consultations Required Fetal echocardiography, to detect congenital heart defects may assist in establishing a precise diagnosis. A neonatologist should be consulted to plan perinatal management.

Monitoring Supportive psychological care for the family is necessary in localities where late termination is not an option. No obstetric intervention should be done for fetal indications.

Pregnancy Course Nearly 75% of cases of thanatophoric dysplasia will be complicated by severe polyhydramnios.

Pregnancy Termination Issues An intact fetus must be delivered for confirmation of the prenatal diagnosis. As with other skeletal dysplasias, a complete postmortem evaluation of the fetus, including radiologic, morphologic, biochemical, and molecular studies should be performed by individuals with extensive experience in skeletal dysplasias.

Delivery Cesarean section is contraindicated except for dystocia. Cephalocentesis is appropriate to facilitate delivery in those cases with severe hydrocephalus.

NEONATOLOGY

Resuscitation When the diagnosis is known prior to delivery, a prenatal decision for nonintervention, made after discussion with the family, is appropriate. If the diagnosis is uncertain, resuscitation and ventilatory support are appropriate to allow time for diagnostic evaluation and parental adaptation.

Transport Referral to a tertiary perinatal center is appropriate for confirmation of a diagnosis. Mechanical ventilatory support is often required during the transport.

Testing and Confirmation Postnatal skeletal radiographs and careful physical examination will establish the diagnosis.

Nursery Management Confirmation of the diagnosis, comfort care for the infant and counselling and support of the family are the primary goals. Provision of mechanical life support in the interim is appropriate though withdrawal of support may subsequently become a problem.

BIBLIOGRAPHY
Chervenak FA, Blakemore KJ, Isaacson G et al: Antenatal sonographic findings of thanatophoric dysplasia with cloverleaf
skull. *Am J Obstet Gynecol* 1983; 146:984-985.
Cremin BJ, Shaff MI: Ultrasonic diagnosis of thanatophoric
dwarfism in utero. *Radiology* 1977; 124:479-480.

Elejalde BR, de Elejalde MM: Thanatophoric dwarfism: fetal manifestations and prenatal diagnosis. *Am J Med Genet* 1985;
22:669-683.
Martinez-Frias ML, Ramos-Arroyo MA, Salvador J: Thanatophoric
dysplasia: an autosomal dominant condition? *Am J Med Genet
1988*; 31:815-820.

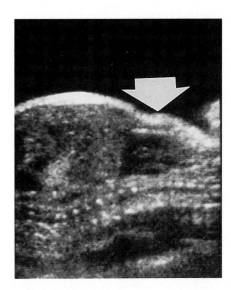

Thanatophoric dysplasia. Sagittal view of the chest and abdomen. Note the small size of the chest and relatively large abdomen. There is severe polyhydramnios.

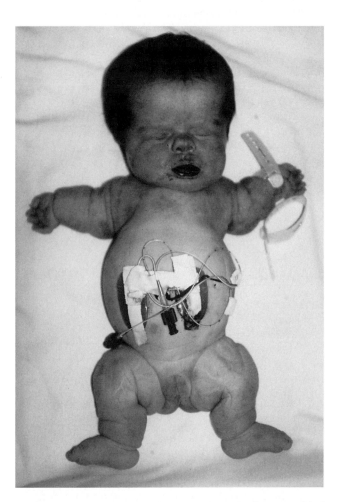

Newborn with thanatophoric dysplasia. Note rhizomelic shortening of limbs and relative macrocephaly.

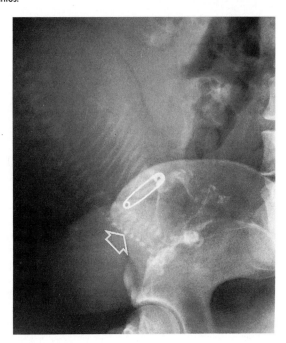

In utero radiograph showing the abnormal vertebrae. There is platyspondyly (*arrow*).

9 Infections

9.1 Cytomegalic Inclusion Disease

EPIDEMIOLOGY/GENETICS

Definition   Cytomegalovirus (CMV) is a large, enveloped DNA herpes virus. Adult infection is frequently asymptomatic, but fetal infection may cause severe damage. Cytomegalovirus is transmitted by way of secretions and sexual contact and transplacentally.

Epidemiology   About 1% to 3% of newborns excrete CMV, but only about 5% will show clinical symptoms in the newborn period. Approximately 1% of pregnant women are infected with CMV infection. Primary maternal infection, in pregnancy, poses the greatest risk to the fetus—30% of fetuses become infected. Transmission of virus in the first half of pregnancy is associated with more severe disease.

Embryology   Cytomegalovirus kills infected cells. Symptoms of severe congenital infection include intrauterine growth retardation (IUGR), hemolytic anemia, pneumonitis, hepatitis, thrombocytopenia, and intracranial calcifications. Microcephaly is frequent and hydrocephaly is uncommon.

Inheritance Patterns   Not genetic.

Screening   Primary maternal infection can be documented by seroconversion for immunoglobulin G (IgG) antibodies to the CMV in women known to have a negative titer prior to pregnancy. For women with a positive IgG during pregnancy, a presumptive diagnosis of primary infection can be made on the basis of a positive immunoglobulin M (IgM) titer, which may persist for up to 4 months after infection. A high false-positive rate for IgM is found when certain immunofluorescent assays are used.

Prognosis   Approximately 95% of infants who secrete CMV at birth are asymptomatic, but of those who show symptoms, 80% will have central nervous system (CNS) sequelae and 30% will die. Asymptomatic survivors may still manifest visual defects, neurological problems, and deafness later in life. Early pregnancy infection usually results in a more severe outcome. There is a high incidence of morbidity in survivors.

Sensorineural hearing loss	50%
Microcephaly	70%
Mental retardation	61%
Cerebral palsy	35%
Chorioretinitis or optic atrophy	22%
Dental enamel defects	40%

Late-occurring sequelae in clinically inapparent infection:

Sensorineural hearing loss	10%–25%
Chorioretinitis	1%
Microcephaly usually with mental retardation	2%
Dental enamel defects	5%

SONOGRAPHY

Findings

1. **Fetus**
   a. Calcification occurs in a number of sites—
      i. Echogenic masses in the fetal abdomen and liver; "echogenic bowel" should be as echogenic as neighboring bone;
      ii. Calcification in the lateral borders of the lateral ventricles is diagnostic of CMV;
      iii. Branching linear calcifications in the basal ganglia.
   b. Nonimmune hydrops due to anemia—pleural and pericardial effusions, ascites, hepatosplenomegaly;
   c. Microcephaly and ventriculomegaly individually or together;
   d. Cardiomegaly, tachyarrhythmia, and bradyarrhythmia;
   e. Hydronephrosis (usually unilateral).

2. **Amniotic Fluid:** Polyhydramnios is seen with nonimmune hydrops, and oligohydramnios with IUGR.

3. **Placenta:** Placentomegaly will occur in association with hydrops or as an isolated finding.

4. **Measurement Data:** Intrauterine growth retardation may occur at an early age.

5. **When Detectable:** Cytomegalovirus has been detected as early as 20 weeks.

Pitfalls   The fetus may appear normal, yet be infected.

Differential Diagnosis
1. Echogenic gut areas are also seen as a normal variant, in trisomy 21, with cystic fibrosis, and following ingestion of intraamniotic blood.
2. All of the other causes of nonimmune hydrops.
3. Microcephaly may also be familial or related to vascular causes.

Where Else to Look   A detailed survey of the entire fetus, except for the limbs, is required.

PREGNANCY MANAGEMENT

Investigations and Consultations Required
1. Maternal viral titers should be performed with appropriate confirmatory studies, when a positive IgM is found. Amniotic fluid culture is the most reliable diagnostic test. Polymerase chain reaction (PCR) molecular testing may increase the reliability of amniotic fluid evaluations for CMV infections.
2. Consultations with a neonatologist may be appropriate to plan delivery management, depending on the severity of the structural malformations.
3. Computed axial tomography (CAT) scanning is helpful in confirming intracranial or liver calcification.

Fetal Intervention   Fetal blood sampling can detect thrombocytopenia, anemia, and CMV-specific IgM in fetal serum (see Table 9-1).

Monitoring   The severity of the CNS effects of CMV cannot be assessed, except in the case of severe hydrocephalus. To prevent further damage from hypoxic causes, fetal evaluation and monitoring may be appropriate in selected cases. Sonograms should be performed every 2 to 3 weeks because nonimmune hydrops may develop.

Pregnancy Course   The presence of IUGR or severe hydrocephalus may require that decisions are made with the family regarding the desirability and type of obstetric intervention to be instituted.

Pregnancy Termination Issues   If a precise diagnosis has been established, there are no special recommendations regarding pregnancy termination.

Delivery   In the presence of severe hydrocephalus resulting in dystocia, consideration should be given to cephalocentesis. Cases diagnosed on the basis of IUGR or mild ventriculomegaly should be managed as normal pregnancies to prevent any further CNS damage.

NEONATOLOGY

Resuscitation   No specific issues, other than blood and body fluids precautions, need to be observed by those having direct contact.

Transport   Referral to a tertiary perinatal center is indicated for treatment of respiratory distress, severe anemia, or hydrops. The infant may require ventilatory assistance in transit.

Testing and Confirmation   Cytomegalovirus can be isolated from urine or saliva within the first 3 weeks of life. Rapid diagnosis using monoclonal antibodies for CMV or PCR is available. After that, positive serum titers may suggest antenatal infection.

Diagnosis is best confirmed by virus recovery from urine or secretions. Specific antibodies can be identified.

Nursery Management   Supportive and symptomatic care only once the diagnosis has been confirmed.

Table 9.1-1   RISK OF FETAL ABNORMALITIES WITH MATERNAL CMV INFECTION

At Onset Of Pregnancy			At Birth	Final Outcome
		(4)*	5%–15% congenitally infected babies are symptomatic	10% normal
CMV seronegative at conception	1%–4% pregnant women develop primary CMV	40% of babies born to mothers with primary CMV are congenitally infected		60% die with sequelae (2.4)*
				30% die within 2 years (1.2)*
(10,000)*	(100)*	(40)*	85%–95% congenitally infected babies are asymptomatic	5%–15% survive with sequelae (2.5)*
		(36)*		85%–95% normal
CMV seropositive at conception	Recurrent CMV	0.5%–1.5% of all babies born to seropositive mothers are congenitally infected	Almost all babies are asymptomatic at birth	1%–15% survive with sequelae (1–15)*
				85%–99% are normal
(10,000)*	(7)*	(50–150)*	(50–150)*	

*Estimated number of affected babies in 10,000 pregnant women are followed (seropositive and seronegative respectively).
CMV, cytomegalovirus.

Blood and body fluid precautions need to be observed during hospital stay and direct contact by pregnant women should be avoided.

No specific treatment is available for congenitally acquired infection as organ damage has already occurred. Ganciclovir may be of use in postnatally acquired infection.

BIBLIOGRAPHY

Bale J, Murph J: Congenital infections and the nervous system. *Pediatr Neurol* 1992; 39:669-690.

Drose JA, Dennis MA, Thickman D: Infection in utero: US findings in 19 cases. *Radiology* 1991; 178:369-374.

Estroff JA, Parad RB, Teele RL et al: Echogenic vessels in the fetal thalami and basal ganglia associated with cytomegalovirus infection. *J Ultrasound Med* 1992; 11:686-688.

Fakhry J, Khoury A: Fetal intracranial calcifications—the importance of periventricular hyperechoic foci without shadowing. *J Ultrasound Med* 1991; 10:51-54.

Forouzan I: Fetal abdominal echogenic mass: an early sign of intrauterine cytomegalovirus infection. *Obstet Gynecol* 1992; 80:535-537.

Freij BJ, Sever JL: Herpesvirus infections in pregnancy: risks to embryo, fetus, and neonate. *Clin Perinatol* 1988; 15:203-231.

Grose C, Itani O, Weiner C: Prenatal diagnosis of fetal infection: advances from amniocentesis to cordocentesis—congenital toxoplasmosis, rubella, cytomegalovirus, varicella virus, parvovirus, and human immunodeficiency virus. *Pediatr Infect Dis J* 1989; 8:459-68.

Grose C, Weiner CP: Prenatal diagnosis of congenital cytomegalovirus infection: two decades later. *Am J Obstet Gynecol* 1990; 163:447-450.

Hohlfeld P, Vial Y, Maillard-Brignon C et al: Cytomegalovirus fetal infection: prenatal diagnosis. *Obstet Gynecol* 1991; 78:615-618.

Kumar ML, Nankervis GA, Jacobs IB et al: Congenital and postnatally acquired cytomegalovirus infections: long-term follow-up. *J Pediatr* 1984; 104:674-679.

Lynch L, Daffos F, Emanuel D et al: Prenatal diagnosis of fetal cytomegalovirus infection. *Am J Obstet Gynecol* 1991; 165:714-718.

Monteagudo A, Matera C, Marks F et al: In utero sonographic diagnosis of congenital cytomegalovirus infection. *Soc Perinatal Obstet—Tenth Annual Mtg.* Houston, TX. Jan 17-23, 1990: 326 (abstract).

Pass RF, Stagno S, Myers GJ: Outcome of symptomatic congenital cytomegalovirus infection: results of long-term longitudinal follow-up. *Pediatrics* 1980; 66:758-762.

Stagno S, Whitley RK: Herpesvirus infections of pregnancy. Part I: cytomegalovirus and Epstein-Barr virus infections. *N Engl J Med* 1985; 313:1270-1274.

Stagno S, Pass RF, Could G et al: Primary cytomegalovirus infection in pregnancy: incidence, transmission to fetus, and clinical outcome. *JAMA* 1986; 256:1904-1908.

Twickler DM, Perlman J, Maberry MC: Congenital cytomegalovirus infection presenting as cerebral ventriculomegaly on antenatal sonography. *Am J Perinatol* 1993; 10:404-406.

Weiner CP, Grose C: Prenatal diagnosis of congenital cytomegalovirus infection by virus isolation from amniotic fluid. *Am J Obstet Gynecol* 1990; 163:1253-1255.

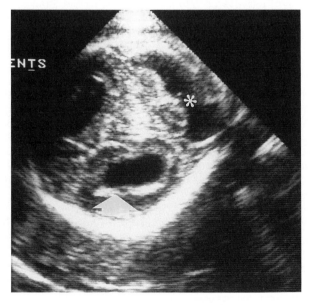

Microcephaly with ventriculomegaly due to cytomegalovirus (CMV). Note the large cisterna magna suggesting atrophy (*asterisk*). The border of the lateral ventricle (*arrow*) is most echogenic because it is calcified. Calcification in this area is typical of CMV.

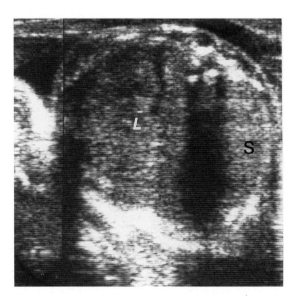

The liver (*L*) and spleen (*S*) are enlarged due to cytomegalovirus.

9.2 PARVOVIRUS
FIFTH DISEASE

EPIDEMIOLOGY/GENETICS

Definition   Parvovirus is a single-stranded DNA virus that causes erythema infectiosum (fifth disease) in children and adults. Infected individuals may be asymptomatic.

Epidemiology   Congenital infection rates vary depending on the prevalence in the community. Approximately 50% to 75% of adult women are immune. The risk for congenital infection from an infected mother is between 10% and 20% and is highest in the first and second trimesters.

Embryology   Parvovirus destroys host cells, particularly red blood cell precursors, and has an affinity for rapidly dividing cells. Congenital infection can cause hydrops fetalis, with resultant stillbirth, or neonatal death. Associated findings include hepatosplenomegaly, polyhydramnios, and liver disease. Transplacental transmission can occur any time during pregnancy.

Inheritance Patterns   Not genetic.

Screening   Maternal serum alpha-fetoprotein (MSAFP) may be elevated due to hydrops.

Prognosis   There is a 10% risk for fetal death due to hydrops from severe fetal anemia. The risk of fetal death in utero is 17% before 20 weeks and 6% after 20 weeks, if the fetus is infected. Most infected women, however, give birth to apparently normal babies.

SONOGRAPHY

Findings
1.   **Fetus**
   a. Ascites is usually the presenting finding.
   b. Other findings of hydrops—pleural effusion, pericardial effusion, and skin thickening—develop later.
   c. There is cardiomegaly and decreased movement in severe cases.
   d. Hepatosplenomegaly may be seen.
2.   **Amniotic Fluid:** Normal amniotic fluid is usual.
3.   **Placenta:** Placentomegaly may develop.
4.   **Measurement Data:** Growth is reported as normal.
5.   **When Detectable:** Hydrops develops between 3 and 13 weeks after maternal infection.

Pitfalls   Pseudopericardial effusion and pseudoascites due to fat deposits may mimic hydrops.

Differential Diagnosis   Numerous other causes of hydrops exist. Ask for a history of maculopapular rash and arthralgia.

Where Else to Look   Look for other causes of hydrops, for example, heart problems, chromosomal abnormalities, CMV, and syphilis.

PREGNANCY MANAGEMENT

Investigations and Consultations Required
1.   Maternal serum titers for infectious agents should be performed.
2.   Evaluation should be done to exclude other causes of both immune and nonimmune hydrops, including assessment of fetal hematologic status by percutaneous umbilical blood sampling (PUBS). Fetal blood sampling can detect anemia and IgM-specific antibody to human parvovirus. Southern blotting can detect parvovirus DNA in fetal tissue samples.

Fetal Intervention   Because the major fetal manifestation of parvovirus infection is anemia, treatment by in utero transfusions is appropriate when a presumptive diagnosis of parvovirus infection is made in the fetus with hydrops. Although spontaneous resolution has been reported, the presence of a severe anemia (hematocrit of less than 25%) in a hydropic fetus, warrants transfusion.

Monitoring   Hydrops has been reported as developing between 3 and, in one instance, 13 weeks following exposure. Weekly sonograms up to 13 weeks, after well-documented exposure, are desirable. Following transfusion, weekly sonographic evaluations is appropriate to monitor resolution of the hydrops. Because of the self-limited nature of the disease, repeat transfusions may not be necessary.

Pregnancy Course   No specific obstetric complications are to be expected if the hydrops resolves.

Pregnancy Termination Issues   There should be no indication for termination, but if this option is chosen careful pathologic examinations must be performed to confirm the diagnosis.

Delivery   The site for delivery will depend on the clinical condition of the fetus. The presence of hydrops or a recent transfusion should be indication for delivery in a tertiary center. Those fetuses in which resolution of hydrops has occurred require no special delivery precautions.

NEONATOLOGY

Resuscitation   Respiratory depression and distress is likely if hydrops or severe anemia present. The neonatologist must be prepared to remove serous fluid collections (pleural, pericardial, peritoneal).

Transport   Neonatal transport is indicated for treatment of respiratory distress, severe anemia, or hydrops. The infant may require ventilatory assistance in transit.

Nursery Management

1. Transfusion—Approach the management as if the neonate has nonimmune hydrops. Indications for replacement transfusion are a hematocrit of less than 36% with symptoms and of less than 32% irrespective of symptoms. Use high hematocrit (75% or greater) packed red blood cells.
2. Treatment of hydrops—Mobilize the anasarca, interstitial, and serosal fluid collections by direct removal or forced diuresis along with infusion of plasma proteins. Peritoneal dialysis is rarely needed. Respiratory support may be required with severe hydrops.

BIBLIOGRAPHY

Anderson LJ, Hurwitz ES: Human parvovirus B19 and pregnancy. *Clin Perinatol* 1988; 15:273-286.

Bale J, Murph J: Congenital infections and the nervous system. *Pediatr Neurol* 1992; 39:669-690.

Grose C, Itani O, Weiner C: Prenatal diagnosis of fetal infection: advances from amniocentesis to cordocentesis—congenital toxoplasmosis, rubella, cytomegalovirus, varicella virus, parvovirus, and human immunodeficiency virus. *Pediatr Infect Dis J* 1989; 8:459-468.

Humphrey W, Magoon M, O'Shaughnessy R: Severe nonimmune hydrops secondary to parvovirus B-19 infection: spontaneous reversal in utero and survival of a term infant. *Obstet Gynecol* 1991; 78:900-902.

Kumar ML: Human parvovirus B19 and its associated diseases. *Clin Perinatol* 1991; 18:209-225.

Pryde PG, Nugent CE, Pridjian G et al: Spontaneous resolution of nonimmune hydrops fetalis secondary to human parvovirus B19 infection. *Obstet Gynecol* 1992; 79:859-861.

Rodis JF, Quinn DL, Gary GW Jr et al: Management and outcomes of pregnancies complicated by human B19 parvovirus infection: a prospective study. *Am J Obstet Gynecol* 1990; 163:1168-1171.

Sahakian V, Weiner CP, Naides SJ et al: Intrauterine transfusion treatment of nonimmune hydrops fetalis secondary to human parvovirus B19 infection. *Am J Obstet Gynecol* 1991; 164:1090-1091.

Sheikh AU, Ernest JM, O'Shea M: Long-term outcome in fetal hydrops from parvovirus B19 infection. *Am J Obstet Gynecol* 1992; 167:337-341.

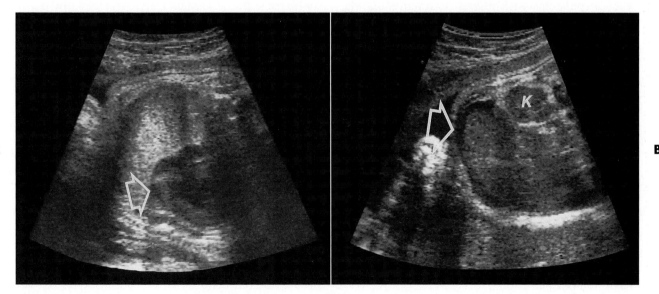

Early hydrops due to parvovirus. **A**, A small pericardial effusion can be seen around the heart (*arrow*). **B**, A small amount of ascites is present around the liver (*arrow*). *K*, kidney.

9.3 CONGENITAL SYPHILIS

EPIDEMIOLOGY/GENETICS

Definition Syphilis is a sexually transmitted infection caused by the spirochete, treponema pallidum, which can damage the developing fetus.

Epidemiology Common. The prevalence of infection is dependent upon the population being studied. The infection rate is on the rise in the United States. In 1986, the incidence was approximately 1 per 100,000 newborn infants. New maternal cases tend to be found in young women from a lower socioeconomic background who little or no prenatal care. The rate of congenital infection correlates to the duration of maternal infection and degree of spirochetemia. The greatest risk occurs with recent onset or current secondary syphilis as both are associated with the greatest load of organisms.

Embryology Treponema pallidum can cross the placenta and infect the developing fetus at any time during pregnancy. Clinical manifestations include characteristic skin and osseous lesions (seen in 90% of infants with untreated congenital syphilis), meningeal inflammation, nephritis, and hepatosplenomegaly. Features become apparent after 18 to 20 weeks gestation when immunocompetence of the fetus is established. Over 50% of pregnancies with untreated syphilis spontaneously abort or result in stillbirth.

Inheritance Patterns Not genetic.

Prognosis Varies with the amount of fetal damage and the timing of treatment. Infants can appear normal at birth and develop signs of infection later in life. Mental retardation, blindness, and sensorineural deafness all occur as the result of fetal infection.

SONOGRAPHY

Findings
1. **Fetus:** Hepatosplenomegaly (above the 90th percentile for size in longitudinal view) is the first, and often, the only finding. In severe cases there is fetal hydrops (pleural effusion, ascites, pericardial effusion, and skin thickening).
2. **Amniotic Fluid:** Polyhydramnios is a late finding.
3. **Placenta:** Placentomegaly occurs, but is uncommon in the early stages of the disease.
4. **Measurement Data:** Growth is normal.
5. **When Detectable:** First detected at about 24 weeks.

Differential Diagnosis
1. Look for other causes of hydrops.
2. Isolated hepatosplenomegaly may be due to other infectious causes such as CMV.

Where Else to Look Look at the maternal liver for stigma of syphilis.

PREGNANCY MANAGEMENT

Investigations and Consultations Required Maternal serologic testing should include not only nonspecific tests such as Venereal Disease Research Laboratory test for syphilis (VDRL) or rapid plasmin reagin (RPR), but also a specific treponemal test such as fluorescent treponemal antibody absorption test (FTA-ABS). If hydrops is present, a complete evaluation as outlined in Chapter 12.2 should be performed.

Fetal Intervention Fetal intervention is contraindicated if a diagnosis of congenital syphilis is established.

Monitoring Antibiotic therapy should be instituted at once for maternal treatment. The effects of fetal infection, however, are not reversible. Fetal assessment modalities are not appropriate once a diagnosis has been established.

Pregnancy Course As in other cases of hydrops, polyhydramnios is a commonly associated finding. The incidence of stillbirth is high.

Pregnancy Termination Issues If a precise diagnosis has been established, no special precautions are necessary. If a diagnosis has not been made in a fetal demise, amniotic fluid should be obtained prior to termination for dark-field evaluation looking for spirochetes. Complete gross and microscopic examinations of the fetus and placenta are necessary to confirm the diagnosis.

Delivery The dismal prognosis for these infants will not be altered by aggressive management. The site of delivery should be one chosen by the patient in consultation with her physician.

NEONATOLOGY

Resuscitation There are usually no specific resuscitation issues for the majority of congenital syphilis cases. However, if there is prenatal evidence of congenital syphilis, there is a high likelihood that the infant will experience difficulty with the onset of cardiorespiratory adaptation. Infrequently, aspiration of serous fluid accumulation—pleural or peritoneal—may be necessary to facilitate breathing, and anemia may be of such severity as to cause difficulty.

Blood and body fluid precautions are important as both may be highly contagious in severe cases of congenital syphilis.

Transport   Transfer to a tertiary perinatal center is indicated for extreme prematurity, uncertain diagnosis, or severe organ involvement such as peritonitis, nephrotic syndrome, or hydrops.

Testing and Confirmation   Clinical features may be present at birth. Radiographic studies will demonstrate the osseous lesions. Testing for treponemal-specific IgM antibodies confirms the diagnosis. Diagnosis should be confirmed by serologic testing including serum and cerebrospinal fluid (CSF) VDRL, serum IgM FTA-ABS, dark-field examination of skin lesions, body fluids, nasal secretions, and long-bone radiographs. Other evaluations should be directed toward determining the extent and severity of organ involvement.

Nursery Management   Neonatal manifestations presenting in the first several days in overt cases include hepatosplenomegaly—91%; anemia—64%; jaundice—49%; periostitis—37%; skin rash—31%; CSF abnormalities—44%. Hydrops, peritonitis, and nephrotic syndrome are infrequent to rare clinical findings. Most neonatal cases have serologic evidence only.

The recommended antibiotic therapy is aqueous penicillin G 50,000 U/kg daily for 10 days. In addition, other therapy such as transfusion, cardiorespiratory support, phototherapy for hyperbilirubinemia should be determined by type and severity of organ involvement.

BIBLIOGRAPHY

Barton JR, Thorpe EM Jr, Shaver DC et al: Nonimmune hydrops fetalis associated with maternal infection with syphilis. *Am J Obstet Gynecol* 1992; 167:56-58.

Centers for Disease Control: Congenital syphilis. *Morbid Mortal Week Rep* 1989; 38:825.

Hira SH, Ganapati JB et al: Early congenital syphilis: clinico-radiologic features in 202 patients. *Sex Trans Dis* 1985; 12:177.

Minkoff HL: Preventing fetal damage from sexually transmitted diseases. *Clin Obstet Gynecol* 1991; 34:336-344.

Nathan L, Twickler DM, Peters MT et al: Fetal syphilis: correlation of sonographic findings and rabbit infectivity testing of amniotic fluid. *J Ultrasound Med* 1993; 12:97-101.

Raafat NA, Birch AA, Altieri LA et al: Sonographic osseous manifestations of fetal syphilis: a case report. *J Ultrasound Med* 1993; 12:783-785.

Rawstron SA, Jenkins S, Blanchard S et al: Maternal and congenital syphilis in Brooklyn, NY: epidemiology, transmission, and diagnosis. *Am J Dis Child* 1993; 147:727-731.

Wendel GD: Gestational and congenital syphilis. *Clin Perinatol* 1989; 15:287.

9.4 TOXOPLASMOSIS

EPIDEMIOLOGY/GENETICS

Definition   An infection by the parasite, toxoplasma gondii. There are three forms: the tachyzoite or obligate intracellular form, the tissue cyst, and the oocyst found only in cats. Infection in adults occurs from ingestion of raw meats or contact with cat feces. Fetal transmission is transplacental.

Epidemiology   Occurrence differs widely with different populations and climates. An estimated 3000 congenitally infected births occur each year in the United States. Exact infection rates for exposed fetuses are unknown, but may be as high as 40%. It is estimated that over 75% of infected fetuses are unaffected and 10% have severe disease. The risk for severe disease is greatest in first and second trimester infection; congenital infection is more likely to be acquired in the third trimester. Fetal infection only occurs with primary maternal infection.

Embryology   Tachyzoites proliferate and destroy fetal cells. Severe congenital infection results in chorioretinitis, microcephaly, hydrocephaly, intracranial calcifications, thrombocytopenia, anemia, and hydrops fetalis. More severe disease is generally associated with early pregnancy transmission.

Inheritance Patterns   Not genetic.

Screening   A precise diagnosis is established if there is the appearance of IgG antibodies in a woman who has been previously seronegative. An initial low level of IgG should be repeated in 3 weeks and the paired samples tested in parallel. A fourfold rise in titer is indicative of recent infection. In the patient with an initial high titer (≥ 1024), assessment of specific IgM should be done to differentiate recent from old infection.

Prognosis   Most congenital infections are asymptomatic. The mortality rate, including stillbirth, is 12% for those with severe disease. Ocular and CNS abnormalities are seen in about 80% of infants who show severe infection. Apparently asymptomatic infants are at risk for the later development of mental retardation, deafness, and ocular problems.

SONOGRAPHY

Findings
1. **Fetus**
    a. Random calcification in the brain is seen usually as echogenic areas.
    b. Hepatosplenomegaly with intrahepatic echogenic densities occurs.
    c. Cranial ventriculomegaly occurs, starting in the occipital horns.
    d. Ascites seen as pleural and pericardial effusions are seen either separately or together. Full-blown hydrops may develop.
2. **Amniotic Fluid:** Polyhydramnios may occur with hydrops.
3. **Placenta:** Placentomegaly with occasional increase in density is seen.
4. **Measurement Data:** Hepatosplenomegaly may cause abdominal circumference increase. Normal tables for liver and spleen size exist.
5. **When Detectable:** Reported as being first detected in second trimester.

Differential Diagnosis   Similar to CMV, but with different patterns of calcification. The calcification is randomly distributed. Microcephaly has not been reported with toxoplasmosis.

Where Else to Look   A generalized disease, so all organs need to be examined.

PREGNANCY MANAGEMENT

Investigations and Consultations Required   The work-up should include maternal serum analysis for viral-specific IgG and IgM for common viral infections. Previous studies have documented the reliability of PUBS at 20 to 22 weeks for the prenatal diagnosis of toxoplasmosis. Detection of toxoplasma specific IgM and isolation of the parasite by mouse inoculation are the primary diagnostic tests. Nonspecific signs of fetal infection, such as elevated liver enzymes, low platelet counts, and high eosinophil counts provide additional diagnostic information. More recently a polymerase chain reaction assay has been developed and may allow reliable detection of infection from an amniotic fluid sample.

Fetal Intervention   No specific interventions are indicated. Aggressive maternal treatment with pyrimethamine and sulfadiazine has been shown to be beneficial in the fetus with asymptomatic infection. It is not known whether there is any benefit in the fetus with sonographically detectable abnormalities.

Monitoring   Sonographic monitoring for the development of severe hydrocephalus should be done every few weeks to plan delivery management.

Pregnancy Course   The development of severe hydrocephalus may require a decision between cephalocentesis and cesarean section.

Pregnancy Termination Issues   If a precise microbiological diagnosis has been established, no special precautions are necessary. If not, an intact fetus is necessary for full evaluation by an individual with special expertise in fetal neuropathology.

Delivery The presence of severe hydrocephalus requires an informed decision by the parents regarding either cephalocentesis or cesarean section. In cases without hydrocephalus, delivery management should not be altered as the degree of CNS damage cannot be ascertained by ultrasound examination. In all circumstances, delivery should take place in a tertiary center.

NEONATOLOGY

Resuscitation No specific measures other than infection precautions for the resuscitation team (maternal and fetal blood and body fluids).

Hydrocephalus or hydrops fetalis may predispose to perinatal asphyxia resulting in need for resuscitation. Removal of pleural or peritoneal fluid may be necessary to facilitate lung expansion.

Transport Referral to a tertiary perinatal center is indicated for treatment of respiratory distress, CNS disorders, or hydrops. The infant may require ventilatory assistance in transit.

Testing and Confirmation Infection can be confirmed by detection of antitoxoplasma IgM, the persistence of antitoxoplasma IgG in the infant's serum, or the detection of parasites in tissues, blood, or CSF. Confirm diagnosis with serologic testing and CNS diagnostic imaging.

Nursery Management Cerebrospinal fluid findings of lymphocytosis and elevated protein may be found in otherwise asymptomatic infants.

Neonatal manifestations:

Low birthweight (<2500 g)	28%
Hepatomegaly	37%
Splenomegaly	40%
Jaundice	42%
Petechiae/purpura	10%
Pneumonia	12%
Cataracts	2%
Chorioretinitis	90%
Microcephaly	10%
Hydrocephaly	20%
Intracranial calcifications	38%

Two clinical syndromes:
1. Generalized disease—jaundice, anemia, visceral involvement, birth to 1 month.
2. Neurologic disease—seizures, meningoencephalitis, after 1 month.

Treatment is both nonspecific—directed at symptoms of jaundice, anemia, respiratory distress; and specific—antimicrobial, pyrimethamine, and sulfadiazine.

Ninety percent survivors of neonatal clinical disease have serious neurologic sequelae: mental retardation, seizures, cerebral palsy, visual impairment, hydrocephalus, microcephaly, and sensorineural deafness.

Asymptomic disease in the neonatal period progresses to clinical disease as late as 9 to 10 years of age with chorioretinitis and neurologic manifestations.

BIBLIOGRAPHY

Bale J, Murph J: Congenital infections and the nervous system. *Ped Neurol* 1992; 39:669-690.

Carter AO, Frank JW: Congenital toxoplasmosis: epidemiologic features and control. *Can Med Assoc J* 1986; 135:618-623.

Daffos F, Forestier F, Capella-Pavlovksy M et al: Prenatal management of 746 pregnancies at risk for congenital toxoplasmosis. *N Engl J Med* 1988; 318:271-275.

Desmonts G, Convreur J: Congenital toxoplasmosis: a prospective study of 378 pregnancies. *N Engl J Med* 1974; 290:1110-1116.

Desmonts G, Convreur J: Toxoplasmosis: epidemiologic and serologic aspects of perinatal infection. In: Drugman S, Gershon AA (eds): *Infections of the fetus and newborn infant.* New York. Alan R. Liss, 1975.

Grose C, Itani O, Weiner C: Prenatal diagnosis of fetal infection: advances from amniocentesis to cordocentesis—congenital toxoplasmosis, rubella, cytomegalovirus, varicella virus, parvovirus, and human immunodeficiency virus. *Pediatr Infect Dis J* 1989; 8:459-468.

Hohlfeld P, MacAleese J, Capella-Pavlovski M et al: Fetal toxoplasmosis: ultrasonographic signs. *Ultrasound Obstet Gynecol* 1991; 1:241-244.

Lee RV: Parasites and pregnancy: the problems of malaria and toxoplasmosis. *Clin Perinatol* 1988; 15:351-363.

Sever JL, Ellenberg JH, Ley AC et al: Toxoplasmosis: maternal and pediatric findings in 23,000 pregnancies. *Pediatrics* 1988; 82:181-192.

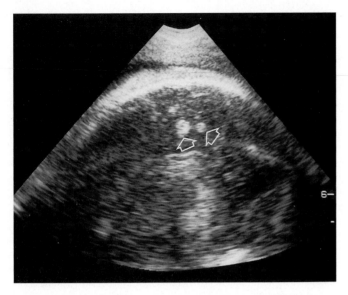

Intracranial calcifications due to toxoplasmosis (*arrows*). They are randomly located throughout the brain.

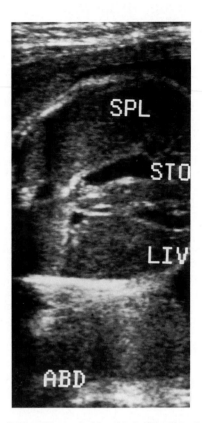

Massive spleen (*SPL*) and less marked liver (*LIV*) enlargement due to toxoplasmosis. The stomach is squashed between the two enlarged organs. *STO*, stomach; *ABD*, abdomen.

9.5 VARICELLA INFECTION
VARICELLA-ZOSTER VIRUS

EPIDEMIOLOGY/GENETICS

Definition   Varicella-zoster is a DNA herpes virus. Primary infection causes chickenpox and may lead to latency of the virus in sensory dorsal-root ganglia. Reactivation of the virus later in life causes shingles.

Epidemiology   The incidence of varicella-zoster infection during pregnancy is 1 to 5 out of 10,000 births (1989). The risk to the fetus of congenital infection differs during the course of pregnancy, but is low. Of these, less than 5% will have congenital abnormalities. Observed M:F ratio is 1:4 for severe disease.

Embryology   The virus is transmitted transplacentally. It is neurotropic and denervates fetal structures. The most severe features are associated with first trimester infection and include focal cutaneous ulcerations with scarring, reduction deformity of limbs, microphthalmia, microcephaly, and other CNS abnormalities.

Inheritance Patterns   Not genetic.

Prognosis   Prognosis is dependent upon the timing and severity of infection, with most infected infants being asymptomatic. As many as one third of severely infected infants, die in the newborn period. When only skin scarring is present, the prognosis is good.

SONOGRAPHY

Findings
1. **Fetus**
    a. Ascites—Pleural effusion and other features of hydrops may occur.
    b. Liver—There may be echogenic foci related to calcification. These have been found at autopsy in other organs.
    c. Club feet and malpositioned limbs may occur.
    d. Decreased fetal motion with a limb fixed in position adjacent to the fetal trunk is seen.
    e. Hydrocephalus or meningocele has been found.
2. **Amniotic Fluid:** Polyhydramnios is common.
3. **Placenta:** Normal.
4. **Measurement Data:** Intrauterine growth retardation may occur.
5. **When Detectable:** 3 to 12 weeks after maternal exposure.

Pitfalls   Over-diagnosis of calcification due to a sonographic system that enhances echogenicity.

Differential Diagnosis   Cytomegalovirus and toxoplasmosis also give intraorgan calcification.

Where Else to Look   Look for calcification in all organs. See if all limbs move as limb adherence to the trunk is a known complication.

PREGNANCY MANAGEMENT

Investigations and Consultations Required   Maternal viral titers for common viral infections should be performed. Invasive testing should await the results of this testing. Because the sensitivity and specificity of fetal IgM, amniotic fluid culture, and PCR assay of chorionic villi are all unknown, the presence of suggestive sonographic features and evidence of recent maternal infection (clinical and serologic) may be sufficient for a presumptive diagnosis of the congenital varicella syndrome.

Monitoring   Sonographic monitoring for the detection of ventriculomegaly is appropriate. Sonographic evidence of CNS damage suggests a dismal prognosis and a nonaggressive approach to pregnancy management and delivery should be discussed with the family.

Pregnancy Course   The development of severe hydrocephalus and polyhydramnios has been reported and may complicate delivery management.

Pregnancy Termination Issues   The difficulty in establishing a precise diagnosis prenatally may warrant a nondestructive approach to pregnancy termination in those cases without classic sonographic features of the congenital varicella syndrome.

Delivery   Those cases without evidence of CNS involvement should be managed in standard fashion for uninfected pregnancies. Those fetuses with severe ventriculomegaly are candidates for cephalocentesis or no electronic monitoring during pregnancy.

NEONATOLOGY

Resuscitation   No specific issues.

Transport   Referral to a tertiary perinatal center is indicated if the infant is symptomatic or the diagnosis is uncertain.

Testing and Confirmation   Anti–varicella-zoster antibodies may persist after birth. Evaluation of CNS and ophthalmic involvement is required.

Nursery Management   Delineation of extent of organ involvement and supportive care are the principal components of management. Isolation of infants with structural defects secondary to varicella is not necessary as the virus is not shed.

BIBLIOGRAPHY

Bale J, Murph J: Congenital infections and the nervous system. *Pediatr Neurol* 1992; 39:669-690.

Grose C, Itani O, Weiner C: Prenatal diagnosis of fetal infection: advances from amniocentesis to cordocentesis—congenital toxoplasmosis, rubella, cytomegalovirus, varicella virus, parvovirus, and human immunodeficiency virus. *Pediatr Infect Dis J* 1989; 8:459-468.

Paryani SJ, Arvin AM: Intrauterine infection with varicella-zoster virus after maternal varicella. *N Engl J Med* 1986; 314:1542-1546.

Pretorius DH, Hayward I, Jones KL et al: Sonographic evaluation of pregnancies with maternal varicella infection. *J Ultrasound Med* 1992; 11:459-463.

Stagno S, Whitney RJ: Herpesvirus infections of pregnancy. Part II. Herpes simplex virus and varicella-zoster virus infections. *N Engl J Med* 1985; 313:1327-1330.

Williamson AP: The varicella-zoster virus in the etiology of severe congenital defects: a survey of eleven reported instances. *Clin Pediatr* 1975; 14:553-555.

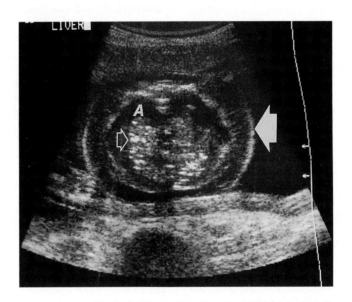

Transverse view of the fetal abdomen. There is much skin thickening (*arrow*). Fetal ascites (*A*) surrounds the liver (*open arrow*). The liver contains numerous calcific foci.

10 Drugs

10.1 Fetal Alcohol Syndrome

EPIDEMIOLOGY/GENETICS

Definition Fetal alcohol syndrome (FAS) is a characteristic pattern of physical malformations including growth and mental retardation seen in the offspring of chronic alcoholic women.

Epidemiology The incidence of FAS varies with the population being studied, with estimates ranging from 1 out of 1000 to as high as 1 out of 100 in some Native American populations. The risk for a chronic alcoholic mother to have a child with FAS is between 20% and 40%, but effects on mental development have been reported with exposures of greater than two drinks per day (M1:F1).

Embryology Alcohol and its metabolites easily cross the placenta. Alcohol causes cell death and inhibits cell growth. The diagnostic criteria for FAS include prenatal or postnatal growth retardation, a characteristic face (midface hypoplasia, epicanthal folds, smooth philtrum with thin upper lip, and ear malformations), and central nervous system (CNS) involvement. Associated abnormalities include cardiovascular defects (70%), microcephaly (80%), microphthalmia, genitourinary tract malformations (10%), and skeletal abnormalities. Spina bifida and cleft lip/palate have also been reported.

Inheritance Patterns Not genetic.

Prognosis Dependent upon the timing and amount of alcohol exposure. The average IQ of children with FAS is about 65. In addition to mental retardation, many children have serious behavioral disturbances.

SONOGRAPHY

Findings
1. **Fetus:** Most fetuses with FAS appear normal sonographically. Sonographically visible congenital anomalies include:
    a. Cardiac malformations such as ventricular septal defect (VSD), atrial septal defect (ASD), double-outlet right ventricle, pulmonary atresia, dextrocardia and tetralogy of Fallot;
    b. CNS anomalies including microcephaly and neural tube defects;
    c. Facial abnormalities such as micrognathia, cleft palate and lip, and hypoplastic maxilla;
    d. Truncal and skeletal anomalies including diaphragmatic hernia, pectus excavatum, and cervical vertebral malformations;
    e. Genitourinary malformations such as hypoplastic external genitalia.
2. **Amniotic Fluid:** Oligohydramnios may be seen accompanying intrauterine growth retardation (IUGR).
3. **Placenta:** Normal
4. **Measurement Data:** Intrauterine growth retardation is a common feature of this disorder.
5. **When Detectable:** Most features are not detectable until late second trimester, when the findings may be subtle.

Pitfalls This is a syndrome affecting multiple organ systems and any one anomaly may have alternate etiologies.

Differential Diagnosis The two features of the FAS most likely to cause confusion with other entities are congenital heart defects and IUGR.

PREGNANCY MANAGEMENT

Investigations and Consultations Required
1. Chromosome studies and toxoplasmosis, other, rubella, cytomegalovirus, and herpes simplex virus (TORCH) titers should be done.
2. An evaluation for maternal medical disorders, including phenylketonuria (PKU), should be done.
3. A history of maternal drug exposure should be obtained.
4. A fetal echocardiogram should be performed.
5. Consultation with a neonatologist is necessary to plan perinatal management.

Monitoring With IUGR, serial ultrasound examinations to monitor growth and appropriate fetal assessment modalities are the major additions to standard obstetric care.

Pregnancy Course   The presence of prenatal growth deficiency in these infants is likely to present as IUGR in the third trimester.

Pregnancy Termination Issues   The lack of a precise risk figure for FAS makes pregnancy termination a controversial issue. The subtle features of FAS are not likely to be seen in a fetus except by a very experienced dysmorphologist.

Delivery   Except in circumstances when neonatal withdrawal is likely to be a complication, there is no specific need for delivery in a tertiary center.

NEONATOLOGY

Resuscitation   There may be a slight increased risk for fetal distress and a low one-minute Apgar score in FAS infants. No special resuscitation measures are required.

Transport   Referral to a tertiary center in the neonatal period is indicated only if a major CNS or cardiac malformation is present.

Testing and Confirmation   Careful assessment for cardiac or CNS malformations is important when FAS is suspected and prenatal evaluation has not been done.

Nursery Management   An alcohol withdrawal syndrome with tremors, agitation, metabolic acidosis, hypoglycemia, and seizures has been described in newborns who are born to severely alcoholic mothers who are intoxicated at the time of delivery.

BIBLIOGRAPHY

Abel EL: Fetal alcohol effects: advice to the advisors. *Alcohol Alcohol* 1985; 20:189-193.

Abel EL, Sokol RJ: Incidence of FAS and economic impact of FAS-related anomalies. *Drug Alcohol Depend* 1987; 19:51-70.

Eliason MJ, Williams JK: Fetal alcohol syndrome and the neonate. *Perinat Neonatal Nurs* 1990; 3:64-72.

Ernhart CB, Sokol RJ, Martier S et al: Alcohol teratogenicity in the human: a detailed assessment of specificity, critical period, and threshold. *Am J Obstet Gynecol* 1987; 156:33-39.

Hill RM, Hegemier S, Tennyson LM: The FAS: a multihandicapped child. *Neurotoxicology* 1989; 10:585-595.

Jones KL: Fetal alcohol syndrome. *Pediatr Rev* 1986; 8:122-126.

Koren G, Edwards MB, Miskin M: Antenatal sonography of fetal malformations associated with drugs and chemicals: a guide. *Am J Obstet Gynecol* 1987; 156:79-85.

Little BB, Snell LM, Rosenfeld CR et al: Failure to recognize FAS in newborn infants. *Am J Dis Child* 1990; 144:1142-1146.

Russell M: The impact of alcohol-related birth defects (ARBD) on New York State. *Neurobehav Toxicol* 1980; 2:277.

Streissguth AP, Aase JM, Clarren SK et al: Fetal alcohol syndrome in adolescents and adults. *JAMA* 1991; 265:1961-1967.

Sulaiman ND, Florey CD, Taylor DJ et al: Alcohol consumption in Dundee primigravidas and its effects on outcome of pregnancy. *Br Med J* 1988; 296:1500-1503.

Walpole I, Zubrick S, Pontre J: Confounding variables in studying the effects of maternal alcohol consumption before and during pregnancy. *J Epidemiol Community Health* 1989; 43:153-161.

Werler MM, Lammer EJ, Rosenberg L et al: Maternal alcohol use in relation to selected birth defects. *Am J Epidemiol* 1991; 134:691-698.

10.2 ANTISEIZURE DRUGS
PHENYTOIN, CARBAMAZEPINE, VALPROIC ACID, AND PHENOBARBITAL

EPIDEMIOLOGY/GENETICS

Definition   A variety of medications are used to control seizures with the four most common being phenytoin (Dilantin), phenobarbital, carbamazepine (Tegretol), and valproic acid (Depakote). These drugs are used either alone or in combination with each other, and each has been implicated as a potential teratogen.

Epidemiology   All epileptic women have an overall twofold to threefold increase in the risk for congenital anomalies in their offspring, with cleft lip, with or without cleft palate, and cardiovascular abnormalities being most common. A specific syndrome is associated with phenytoin use consisting of a characteristic facies, microcephaly, digital and nail hypoplasia, and growth and mental delay. A similar phenotype is seen in infants exposed to carbamazepine during pregnancy. In addition, valproic acid and carbamazepine have been associated with a 1% risk for spina bifida. An overall risk for a "fetal anticonvulsant syndrome" may be about 10%.

Embryology   Teratogenicity of several anticonvulsants has been associated with the activity of the enzyme epoxide hydrolase. This enzyme activity is inherited in an autosomal recessive pattern, with homozygotes for decreased activity being at the greatest risk for congenital abnormalities.

Inheritance Patterns   Not genetic.

Prognosis   Over 90% of all women with epilepsy have normal babies. Prognosis is dependent upon the type of involvement and the severity of the developmental delays.

SONOGRAPHY

Findings
1.   **Fetus:** Ultrasonographically visible side effects of anticonvulsants include the following.
   a. CNS abnormalities—microcephaly and, rarely, holoprosencephaly. Myelomeningocle and Arnold-Chiari malformation are seen with valproic acid.
   b. Facial anomalies—ocular hypertelorism, cleft lip and/or palate, short nose, and broad nasal bridge.
   c. Skeletal malformations—hypoplasia of the distal phalanges, digitalized thumb, hip dislocation, short webbed neck, rib, or sternal anomalies.
   d. Cardiac anomalies—VSDs and pulmonary and aortic valvular stenoses.
   e. Genitourinary abnormalities—ambiguous genitalia and rare renal malformations.
2.   **Amniotic Fluid:** Oligohydramnios may be associated with IUGR.
3.   **Placenta:** Normal.
4.   **Measurement Data:** Mild to moderate IUGR is a common feature with or without associated antenatally detectable anomalies.
5.   **When Detectable:** Most associated anomalies are subtle and not detectable until well into the second trimester.

Pitfalls   Myelomeningocele associated with valproic acid may be small and at a sacral level.

Differential Diagnosis   The two malformations most commonly associated with these medications that will cause a management dilemma are congenital heart defects and myelomeningocele. Because of the relatively low incidence of the findings in patients exposed to antiepileptic medications, a careful search for other etiologies must be made.

PREGNANCY MANAGEMENT

Investigations and Consultations Required
1.   Other etiologies such as chromosome abnormalities should be excluded.
2.   There is preliminary evidence that measurement of epoxide hydrolase activity in amniotic fluid may predict those fetuses at greatest risk for the fetal hydantoin syndrome. Unfortunately, this work remains experimental, and should not, at the present time, be used for clinical management.

Monitoring   The obstetric management should be based on the specific type of malformation seen. In the absence of structural malformations, standard obstetric care should be performed.

Pregnancy Course   No specific obstetric complications are to be expected, although mild prenatal growth deficiency may be a feature in some cases.

Pregnancy Termination Issues   Pregnancy termination, if chosen, must be done in such a way to provide an intact fetus. The subtle features that are seen with exposure to these drugs require that a trained dysmorphologist and fetal pathologist evaluate the fetus.

Delivery   In the absence of structural malformations, delivery does not need to occur in a tertiary center. Delivery management of the fetus with a malformation will be as outlined in previous chapters discussing that specific abnormality.

A small risk of intracranial hemorrhage with fetal hydantoin exposure in the fetus has been reported and, therefore, the recommendation that vitamin K is given to the mother early in labor. Hydantoin is known to depress liver production of K-dependent coagulation factors.

NEONATOLOGY

Resuscitation   No antiepileptic agent has been reported to produce fetal depression or delay in onset of respirations. As all are teratogenic, the management at birth will be dictated by the specific defect manifested by the infant. (See Chapters 2.14, 3, and 7.1—Myelomeningocoele, Cardiac Defects, and Cleft Lip and/or Palate).

Transport   Referral to a tertiary center is not indicated for antenatal exposure only, but is indicated for diagnosis and management of major organ anomalies. Referral to a multidisciplinary program for orofacial abnormalities is indicated for infants having a cleft lip and/or palate.

Nursery Management   If cleft lip and/or palate is present, care is directed toward establishing an appropriate feeding technique and initiating a plan for repair and rehabilitation.

If intrapartum vitamin K was not given to the mother, it is important that the infant receives it immediately after birth and that close monitoring for intracranial hemorrhage is done.

Once a specific organ defect is identified, care requirements are based on the diagnosis.

Carbamazepine has been associated with postnatal growth failure and development delay, therefore, careful monitoring for both should continue through infancy and early childhood.

BIBLIOGRAPHY

Buehler BA, Delimont D, Van Waes M et al: Prenatal prediction of risk of the fetal hydantoin syndrome. *N Engl J Med* 1990; 332:1567-1572.

Hanson JW, Buehler BA: Fetal hydantoin syndrome: Current status. *J Pediatr* 1982; 101:816-818.

Hanson JW, Myrianthopoulos NC, Harvey MA et al: Risks to the offspring of women treated with hydantoin anticonvulsants, with emphasis on the fetal hydantoin syndrome. *J Pediatr* 1976; 89:662-668.

Jones KL, Lacro RV, Johnson KA et al: Pattern of malformations in the children of women treated with carbamazepine during pregnancy. *N Engl J Med* 1989; 320:1661-1666.

Koren G, Edwards MB, Miskin M: Antenatal sonography of fetal malformations associated with drugs and chemicals: a guide. *Am J Obstet Gynecol* 1987; 156:79-85.

Rosa FW: Spina bifida in infants of women treated with carbamazepine during pregnancy. *N Engl J Med* 1991; 324:674-677.

Weinbaum PJ, Cassidy SB, Vintzileos AM et al: Prenatal detection of a neural tube defect after fetal exposure to valproic acid. *Obstet Gynecol* 1986; 67:31S-37S.

10.3 ILLEGAL DRUGS
COCAINE, HEROIN

EPIDEMIOLOGY/GENETICS

Definition   Cocaine and heroin are commonly abused drugs that are both a CNS stimulant and a local anesthetic. As drugs of abuse, they can be sniffed, injected intravenously, or smoked.

Epidemiology   Drug use is dependent upon population. Teratogenic effects in exposed fetuses are probably uncommon.

Embryology   Cocaine and heroin cause a transient rise in maternal blood pressure, placental vasoconstriction, and interruptions of blood flow to the fetus. Vascular hypotension, with vascular constriction and disruption of blood flow has been proposed as a possible mechanism for the teratogenic effects of cocaine and heroin. A small increase in urogenital anomalies, craniofacial defects, cardiovascular abnormalities, and CNS disruptions has been reported with exposure. Additional abnormalites have included limb-reduction defects, ocular defects, and IUGR. Heroin decreases cell multiplication and is associated with IUGR.

Inheritance Patterns   Not genetic.

Prognosis   The most significant effects associated with cocaine and heroin use appear to be adverse pregnancy outcomes and include placental abruption, stillbirth, and premature birth. The exact risk for congenital malformations in a pregnancy exposed to cocaine or heroin is unknown, but is probably low.

SONOGRAPHY

Findings
1.   **Fetus:** Most fetuses are normal. Antenatal sonographic findings in the fetus involve multiple organ systems. The following findings have been reported as associated with illegal drug usage. The quality of documentation for these associations is variable.
  a. CNS-acquired anomalies including cerebral infarctions or hemorrhage, porencephaly, hydrocephalus and hydranencephaly. Congenital malformations include microcephaly; midline abnormalities, such as agenesis of the corpus callosum; septooptic dysplasia; schizencephaly; encephalocele; and teratoma.
  b. Genitourinary and cardiac malformations.
  c. Limb-reduction abnormalities with limb shortening or amputation.
  d. Intestinal atresia and perforation with meconium peritonitis.
  e. Spontaneous abortion.
  f. Occasional facial anomalies such as cleft palate and lip.
2.   **Amniotic Fluid:** IUGR, and premature rupture of membranes (PROM) are often seen in cocaine and heroin abusers, so oligohydramnios may be found.
3.   **Placenta:** Placental abruption is more common in cocaine abusers. A hematoma may be seen in a marginal location; a retroplacental location; a preplacental location; an intraamniotic location; or in an intraplacental location.
4.   **Measurement Data:** Symmetric growth retardation is a common finding.
5.   **When Detectable:** Depends upon the severity of the anomaly and the frequency of substance abuse.

Pitfalls   Multisubstance abuse is common and the simultaneous use of other drugs such as heroin and cocaine, cigarettes, and alcohol or the presence of congenital infections must always be considered as alternate etiologies for congenital anomalies.

PREGNANCY MANAGEMENT

Investigations and Consultations Required   The presence of a structural malformation should prompt chromosome studies and fetal echocardiography to exclude associated cardiac malformations. Other consultations should be based on the specific malformations detected. The neonatology staff should be made aware of the potential for neonatal withdrawal.

Monitoring   No specific change in standard obstetric care is required, unless IUGR complicates the pregnancy. Pregnancy management should be coordinated by a perinatologist.

Pregnancy Course   The increased risk of placental abruption in patients using cocaine may be the major risk to fetal well-being. Intrauterine growth retardation also occurs more commonly in these patients.

Pregnancy Termination Issues   Should pregnancy termination be chosen because of a fetal malformation, delivery of an intact fetus is essential to establish a precise diagnosis.

Delivery   The significant risk associated with maternal and neonatal withdrawal requires that delivery occur in a tertiary center.

NEONATOLOGY

Resuscitation   An increased incidence of fetal distress is associated with maternal cocaine use precipitating preterm labor and placental abruption. No special resuscitative measures are required, although acute volume expansion may be needed if there is an abruption.

Transport   Referral to a tertiary center is required for management of problems associated with prematurity or structural defects resulting from vascular disruptions.

Nursery Management   The gestational age at delivery and the presence of anomalies resulting from vascular disruptions determine the neonatal management problems and care needed. There appears to be an increased risk for early onset necrotizing enterocolitis in larger infants with maternal cocaine exposure.

BIBLIOGRAPHY

Chasnoff IJ, Burns WJ, Schnoll SH et al: Cocaine use in pregnancy. *N Engl J Med* 1985; 313:666-669.

Chavez GF, Mulinare J, Cordero JF: Maternal cocaine use during early pregnancy as a risk factor for congenital urogenital urogenital anomalies. *JAMA* 1989; 262:795-798.

Cohen HL, Sloves JH, Laungani S et al: Neurosonographic findings in full-term infants born to maternal cocaine abusers: visualization of subependymal and periventricular cysts. *J Clin Ultrasound* 1994; 22:327-333.

Dominguez R, Aguirre Vila-Coro A, Slopis JM et al: Brain and ocular abnormalities in infants with in utero exposure to cocaine and other street drugs. *Am J Dis Child* 1991; 145:688-695.

Hall TR, Zaninovic A, Lewin D et al: Neonatal intestinal ischemia with bowel perforation: an in utero complication of maternal cocaine abuse. *Am J Roentgenol* 1992; 158:1303-1304.

Heier LA, Carpanzano CR, Mast J et al: Maternal cocaine abuse: the spectrum of radiologic abnormalities in the neonatal CNS. *Am J Neuroradiol* 1991; 12:951-956.

Hollingsworth DR: Drugs and reproduction: maternal and fetal risks. In: Hollingsworth DR, Resnik R (eds): *Medical Counseling Before Pregnancy*. New York. Churchill Livingstone, 1988. pp. 59-63.

Hoyme HE, Jones KL, Dixon SD et al: Prenatal cocaine exposure and fetal vascular disruption. *Pediatrics* 1990; 85:743-747.

Viscarello RR, Ferguson DD, Nores J et al: Limb-body wall complex associated with cocaine abuse: further evidence of cocaine's teratogenicity. *Obstet Gynecol* 1992; 80:523-526.

Volpe JJ: Effect of cocaine use on the fetus. *N Engl J Med* 1992; 327:399-407.

11 Twins

11.1 Acardiac Twin (Acardiac Monster) Holoacardius
Twin Reversed Arterial Perfusion Sequence (TRAP)

EPIDEMIOLOGY/GENETICS

Definition Acardia is a complex malformation associated with monozygotic, monochorionic twins or triplets, in which one twin has a severe abnormality involving malformations of the head and upper body with an absent or rudimentary, nonfunctioning heart.

Epidemiology 1 out of 35,000 births, or 1 out of 100 monozygotic twin pairs.

Embryology Most likely caused by placental, anastomotic, vascular connections between twins leading to reversal of blood flow to one twin. The "perfused" twin receives unoxygenated blood, which results in aplasia or hypoplasia of the heart, head, and upper limbs. The "pump" twin is usually morphologically normal, but may show signs of congestive heart failure (CHF) including hydrops.

Inheritance Patterns Sporadic.

Teratogens None known.

Prognosis All of the perfused twins die. The pump twin has a 50% mortality rate, with death most often caused by heart failure or death of the co-twin.

SONOGRAPHY

Findings
1. **Fetus:** In addition to a normal fetus, a second fetus is seen that has no heart—the "acardiac fetus."
   a. Acardiac twin—This twin obtains its blood supply from the normal pump twin. The acardiac twin either has no head or there is anencephaly with only the base of the brain present. There will be gross skin thickening of the upper trunk and neck areas. Large cystic hygromalike spaces in the skin are seen. An omphalocele may be present. Sometimes the upper limbs are absent. Club feet and absent toes are often seen. Although there are no cardiac pulsations, limb movements are visible.
   b. The pump twin—The normal twin may show signs of hydrops with hepatosplenomegaly, pleu-

ral and pericardial effusions, and skin thickening. The heart may be enlarged with a prominent right atrium.
2. **Amniotic Fluid:** Polyhydramnios is present. No membrane or a thin membrane may be seen between the two fetuses. If a membrane is present, polyhydramnios may develop around the pump twin with oligohydramnios around the acardiac twin. The blood flow in the umbilical arteries can be shown, by color flow Doppler, to be towards the fetal abdomen of the acardiac twin—the reverse of normal. A single umbilical artery is seen in 50% of cases.
3. **Placenta:** Single placenta. Placental thickening may develop if hydrops occurs.
4. **Measurement Data:** Usually normal in the pump twin, but the abdominal circumference may increase in the pump twin if there is impending hydrops due to hepatosplenomegaly.
5. **When Detectable:** At about 11 to 12 weeks by vaginal sonography.

Differential Diagnosis The acardiac twin may be mistaken for a dead anencephalic twin fetus. The skin thickening, absence of the heart, cystic hygroma, and presence of leg movement give the diagnosis away. Misdiagnosis may be associated with significant fetal and maternal risks.

Where Else to Look Look in the normal fetus for signs of hydrops—cardiomegaly, hepatosplenomegaly, pleural effusion, ascites, abnormal Doppler, and so on.

PREGNANCY MANAGEMENT

Investigations and Consultations Required
1. A follow-up ultrasound showing interval growth of the dead twin should establish the diagnosis.
2. The high risk of prematurity mandates a consultation with a neonatologist to discuss management options with the family.

Fetal Intervention A number of therapeutic approaches have been attempted, including maternal digitalization, serial amniocentesis, maternal indomethacin therapy, endoscopic ligation of the umbilical cord, thrombosis of the umbilical artery using the percutaneous placement of a thrombogenic coil or laser therapy, and hysterotomy with selective delivery of the affected twin. For those cases with evidence of cardiac compromise in the pump twin, the endoscopic ligation or the use of a thrombogenic coil theoretically offer the greater likelihood of a favorable outcome. In cases with only polyhydramnios, the use of indomethacin may prolong the pregnancy to improve perinatal outcome.

Monitoring   The extremely high risk of pregnancy complications requires that care is coordinated by a perinatologist and that serial ultrasound examinations are performed every 1 to 2 weeks to assess fetal status.

Pregnancy Course   There is a high risk of polyhydramnios and cardiac failure in the pump twin with a mortality rate of 50% to 75%.

Pregnancy Termination Issues   Should this option be chosen, a complete evaluation of an intact fetus and placenta should be done to confirm the diagnosis.

Delivery   Delivery should occur in a tertiary center because of the high risk of prematurity and of delivering a compromised infant.

NEONATOLOGY

Resuscitation   Anticipate difficulty with spontaneous onset of respiration as well as problems associated with preterm delivery in the pump twin. The team must be prepared to deal with CHF early in the course.

Transport   Transfer to a tertiary center for neonatal intensive care is necessary in the majority of cases.

Respiratory assistance, as well as support of myocardial function with continuous infusion of ionotropic medication, may be required during transport.

Nursery Management   Respiratory support, relief of myocardial stress, reduction of CHF, and correction of perinatal asphyxia are usually needed and therefore, it is necessary to institute measures to accomplish these goals immediately following birth. As most TRAP sequence gestations are delivered prematurely, respiratory distress syndrome may also further complicate the clinical course. Early administration of surfactant replacement therapy may hasten the resolution of the latter.

BIBLIOGRAPHY

Al-Malt A, Ashmead G, Judge N et al: Color-flow and Doppler velocimetry in prenatal diagnosis of acardiac triplet. *J Ultrasound Med* 1991; 10:341-345.

Benson CB, Bieber FR, Genest DR et al: Doppler demonstration of reversed umbilical blood flow in an acardiac twin. *J Clin Ultrasound* 1989; 17:291-295.

Fries MH, Goldberg JD, Golbus MS: Treatment of acardiac-acephalus twin gestations by hysterotomy and selective delivery. *Obstet Gynecol* 1992; 79:601-604.

Langlotz H, Sauerbrei E, Murray S: Transvaginal Doppler sonographic diagnosis of an acardiac twin at 12 weeks gestation. *J Ultrasound Med* 1991; 10:175-179.

McCurdy CM Jr, Childers JM, Seeds JW: Ligation of the umbilical cord of an acardiac-acephalus twin with an endoscopic intrauterine technique. *Obstet Gynecol* 1993; 82:708-711.

Pretorius DH, Leopold GR, Moore TR et al: Acardiac twin: report of Doppler sonography. *J Ultrasound Med* 1988; 7:413-416.

Van Allen MI, Smith DW, Shepard TH: Twin reversed arterial perfusion (TRAP) sequence: a study of 14 twin pregnancies with acardius. *Semin Perinatol* 1983, 7:285-293.

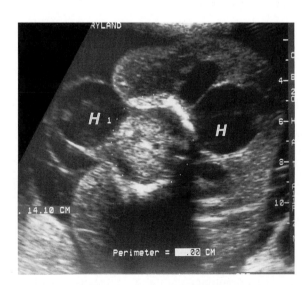

Normal "pump" twin (*open arrow*) alongside the acardiac acephalic twin (*closed arrow*). Note the discrepancy in size between the twins. There is no evidence as yet of hydrops in the pump twin.

Acardiac acephalic twin. There is massive skin thickening around the fetal trunk and several large cystic spaces (*H*) can be seen in the thickened skin resembling cystic hygroma. No fetal head was present although moving lower limbs were seen.

11.2 CONJOINED TWINS

EPIDEMIOLOGY/GENETICS

Definition Conjoined twins refers to incomplete anatomic separation at some location between monozygotic twins. Fusion at the thorax/abdomen (thoracopagus) account for 70% of cases.

Epidemiology The incidence is estimated to be 1 in 33,000 to 1 in 165,000 births, accounting for approximately 1% of monozygotic twins. Of note is the striking female prevalence (75% or greater).

Embryology Conjoined twins are thought to be an incomplete separation of a single embryo. The precise etiology for this event has not been established.

Inheritance Patterns Sporadic, with no increased recurrence risk in subsequent pregnancies.

Prognosis Potential for separation with optimal survival of both infants is directly related to the location of the union, the status of shared vital organs, and the presence of associated organ malformations.

SONOGRAPHY

Findings
1. **Fetus:** Twin fetuses lie adjacent to each other and do not move apart with fetal movement. The twins can be joined at the head (craniopagus), rump (ischiopagus), thorax/abdomen (thoracopagus), or some combination (e.g., cephalothoracopagus). There can be two heads (dicephalus), but all other structures are single.
2. **Amniotic Fluid:** Polyhydramnios is frequent.
3. **Placenta:** Normal. This malformation only occurs with monochorionic, monoamniotic placentation.
4. **Measurement Data:** Normal where the fetus is not joined.
5. **When Detectable:** The syndrome has been detected as early as 9 weeks.

Pitfalls
1. Precise definition of joined areas may be difficult due to fetal lie.
2. Small zones of fusion may permit the twins to rotate 180°; a vertex breech presentation does not exclude the diagnosis.
3. With extreme degrees of fusion, the twins may be mistaken for a singleton.

Differential Diagnosis Two normal fetuses that are relatively immobile and lie adjacent to each other.

Where Else to Look Look in detail at the fusion site, for example, establish with color Doppler whether there is common liver arterial circulation or common cardiac system.

PREGNANCY MANAGEMENT

Investigations and Consultations Required Fetal echocardiography should be performed to assess cardiac structure. Consultations with a pediatric surgeon and a neonatologist are essential to assess prognosis for separation and to plan perinatal management.

Fetal Intervention None is indicated.

Monitoring If the diagnosis is made early, the option of pregnancy termination should be offered to the parents. Serial ultrasound examinations, every 3 to 4 weeks, should be done to monitor growth, to detect fetal hydrops, and to detect fetal demise.

Pregnancy Course Polyhydramnios is a complicating feature in up to 75% of cases. Nearly one third of conjoined twins will be stillborn.

Pregnancy Termination Issues No special considerations are necessary. Delivery by a destructive procedure is appropriate to avoid hysterotomy.

Delivery A planned cesarean delivery with appropriate personnel in attendance should be performed in a tertiary center.

NEONATOLOGY

Resuscitation The onset of respiration may be complicated by the site of attachment, particularly for thoracic and/or abdominally conjoined pairs. A very skilled intubator will be required if mechanical respiratory support is needed. Bag and mask ventilation should be provided to the lesser depressed infant, if mechanically feasible, while an endotracheal tube is placed in the more depressed one initially. Performing chest compressions may not be possible for twins conjoined at the chest.

Transport Transfer to a tertiary center, with comprehensive pediatric diagnostic and surgical capabilities, after stabilization, is important to facilitate evaluation for potential for separation. Provision of a reliable airway, warmth, and intravenous fluids are essential to a safe transport. Frequently, prematurity mandates special care.

Nursery Management The major objective is to establish the proper priority for diagnostic and treatment interventions:
1. establish appropriate cardiorespiratory adaptation;
2. maintain basic support—warmth, nutrition, protection from infection;
3. maintain family confidentiality;
4. plan diagnostic studies for optimum delineation of organ structure, by order of organ importance for survival first and separation potential second.

The timing for surgical separation must be individualized for each conjoined twin pair. The majority experience seems to favor delay beyond the immediate neonatal period in the absence of either a life-threatening anomaly or complication forcing surgical separation on an emergent basis.

SURGERY

Preoperative Assessment   The specific diagnosis of the type of conjoined twins should follow the postnatal resuscitation. An accurate diagnosis of the type of twinning is essential for any perioperative assessment.

There are four types of conjoined twins and subclasses based on a spectrum of malformations. Thoracopagus twins are joined at the sternum, diaphragm, and liver. As such, they face each other. Approximately half the cases have fused gastrointestinal tracts and in an additional 25%, the biliary tract is fused. Thoracopagus twins and variants of this form represent approximately 75% of all conjoined twins. Like most problems of embryogenesis there is a spectrum of fusion defects that characterize thoracopagus twins. The omphalopagus variant involves union from the xiphoid to the umbilicus. This is the most common type of conjoined twins. Sternopagus twins are joined only at the sternum and represent the second variation of thoracopagus twins. Ischiopagus twins are connected from the umbilicus to a fused pelvis and comprise 5% of all forms of conjoined twins. These twins have three or four legs. In addition, ischiopagus twins share a lower gastrointestinal tract. Pygopagus twins are joined both at the lower back and sacrum and therefore the twins are back to back. The incidence of pygopagus twins is approximately 18%. Again there is one rectum and one anus, but usually separate spinal cords. Craniopagus twins are fused at the skull and represent the most rare twin malformation with an incidence of 2%. There are separate brains, but frequently a common venous drainage.

In general, survival rates are better if the twins are allowed to grow and develop. However, emergency separation procedures are indicated if one twin is stillborn or in full cardiac arrest. Associated malformations such as ruptured omphalocele, obstructive uropathy, cloacal exstrophy, imperforate anus, or severe intracardiac defects may also necessitate emergency separation.

A systematic approach to the work-up is predicated on the diagnosis of the twins. In general, priorty is given to the cardiac status in the event that emergency separation is required for deteriorating heart function. Electrocardiography (ECG), echocardiography, and cardiac catheterization are all useful to evaluate the cardiac system. The gastrointestinal tract is best evaluated with a contrast study and the biliary tree should be studied separately with isotopic tracers (DISIDA scans). Excellent hepatopancreaticobiliary detail can be obtained from ultrasonography. Selective angiography is helpful to obtain information about the vascular contribution of liver lobes. Computed tomography (CT) scans are helpful for pelvic and perineal musculature and the bony pelvis architecture. Plain films are helpful for architecture of the extremities. The nervous system is best evaluated using electroencephalography (EEG), CT scan, and magnetic resonance (MR) scans. Contrast studies of both the vagina and urethra are best performed in conjunction with cystoscopy to determine the extent of shared organs of the reproductive and genitourinary tracts (GU). Ultrasound, CT, MR, and intravenous pyelogram (IVP) are all also helpful for the shared components of the GU tract alone.

Ultimately, two separate operative teams consisting of surgeons, anesthesiologists, and nurses should all be aware of the planned procedure preoperatively. A diagram of the anatomy is essential as well as an algorithm of the planned separation. If necessary, multiple rehearsals should be performed of the entire separation and definitive repair. Monitoring apparatus should also be discussed preoperatively.

Operative Indications   All conjoined twins will require separation for long-term survival. In general, survival rates are close to 50% in the first 3 weeks of life, whereas operation during the weeks 4 to 14 approaches a survival rate of 90%. Therefore, most surgical teams prefer to perform separation in the second or third month of life. If necessary, gastrointestinal decompression (colostomy or ileostomy) or genitourinary diversion (pyeloplasty or vesocostomy) may be performed long before definitive repair.

Types of Procedures   The choice of operative procedures depends on the complexity of the malformation. In general, shared organs must be divided such that functional integrity is maintained for each twin. If residual organ function is not possible, then innovative bypass techniques should be considered. Such is the case with the extrahepatic biliary tree. If vascular and anatomic integrity to these structures cannot be maintained, then one twin may require a portoenterostomy for biliary drainage into the gastrointestinal tract. In addition, muscle and bone defects must be covered. Skin can be a major problem and therefore, serious consideration should be given to prior insertion of tissue expanders.

Thoracopagus twins require attention to the heart, pericardium, chest cavity, abdominal wall, and potentially fused abdominal organs. Thoracopagus twins have a spectrum of cardiac defects ranging from two hearts and a shared pericardium to one muscle system for the conjoined twins. Frequently, cardiopulmonary bypass must be employed for this step in the procedure. The liver in these twins usually requires separation and in one quarter of cases a decision must be made about the biliary tree. The gastrointestinal tract is frequently fused at the second portion of the duodenum, again making it a difficult decision to bypass one twin and render the entire extrahepatic biliary system to the other.

Ischiopagus twin separation involves division of a fused pelvis, abdominal wall, and lower gastrointestinal tract. In addition, complex separation of the GU tract is required. Here again following separation a decision is made about who gets what. One twin will have a normal anus and rectum and the other will require reconstruction using the proximal colon. Each twin will require some type of pelvic bone reconstruction, such as an iliac osteotomy, which can be performed at the time of separation or as a secondary procedure. Vertebral body and hip support may also be required and may involve prosthetic parts. For orthopedic and gastrointestinal reasons the anatomy of the pelvis must be restored. The ischiopagus tetrapus variant is easier to reconstruct in contrast to the tripus type of twin. Skin coverage is also a problem with the ischiopagus twins. As expected, inadequate skin coverage may lead to infection, evisceration, and often times sacrifice of the tripus third limb. Preoperative tissue expansion usually takes 8 to 12 weeks for a total of 12 to 20 cm of tissue expansion.

Pygopagus twins require division at the level of the sacrum, spinal canal, rectum, and, on occasion, bladder, vagina, and urethra. Perineal musculature can be a problem for the shared rectum especially if there is a sacral plexus defect, thereby denervating a portion of the levator diaphragm musculature. Skin coverage is usually not a problem for the pygopagus twin separation and closure.

Craniopagus twin separation requires division of the calvaria. Usually there are two whole brains, but a shared venous sinus, despite the use of hypothermic circulatory arrest. Division of this shared venous sinus makes the operative procedure a very high risk for exsanguination. Again the preoperative use of tissue expanders facilitates closure of the scalp for both children.

The twins are subject to life-threatening as well as chronic, debilitating complications. Intraoperative bleeding represents the most insidious life-threatening problem. This complication occurs when large shared hepatic and perineal vessels are emptied in favor of the larger twin thus producing hypovolemic shock in the smaller of the twins. Preoperative recognition of these large low-resistance shunts facilitates prompt separation of these vessels prior to other procedures. This is a potential problem for the thoracopagus variants as well as the ischiopagus twins. Inadequate skin coverage for any of the conjoined twins separation may lead to evisceration and cardiopulmonary collapse in the postoperative period. Infection may occur at any time, especially if prosthetic material becomes infected. Spinal communication at any level may predispose to meningitis. This potention neurological complication can accompany separation of ischiopagus and pygopagus twins.

Surgical Results/Prognosis There is a paucity of morbidity and mortality data for separation of conjoined twins. In general, results are dependent on the complexity of the malformation, the extent of shared organs, and the general condition of the infants at the time of separation. Results are best in situations where there is no life-threatening operative division of shared organs, such as the heart and brain. Therefore, good results are expected for thoracopagus twins (omphalopagus and xiphipagus) who do not share hearts and pygopagus separation. Ischiopagus twin separation involves separation and reconstruction of the gastrointestinal, GU, and reproductive tracts as well as the skeleton. As expected, significant morbidity and long-term disability in all these systems is certainly possible. Craniopagus separation outcome is improved if there is no required venous division and reconstruction.

Ethical and moral decisions abound for all members of the multidisciplinary team, including the parents, at all stages of the evaluation process and actual operative procedure. At each step in the algorithm of the separation of conjoined twins there is the potential for life and death decisions.

BIBLIOGRAPHY

Barth RA, Filly RA, Goldberg JD et al: Conjoined twins: prenatal diagnosis and assessment of associated malformations. *Radiology* 1990; 177:201-207.

Filler RM: Conjoined twins and their separation. *Semin Perinatol* 1986; 10:82-91.

Hoyle RM: Surgical separation of conjoined twins. *Surg Gyn Obstet* 1990; 170:549-562.

Lipsky K: Conjoined twins: psychosocial aspects. *AORN J* 1982; 35:58-61.

Mann MD, Coutts JP, Kaschula RO et al: The use of radionuclides in the investigation of conjoined twins. *J Nucl Med* 1983; 24:479-484.

Miller D, Columbani P, Buck JR et al: New techniques in the diagnosis and operative management of Siamese twins. *J Pediatr Surg* 1983; 18:373-376.

O'Neill JA, Holcomb GW, Schnaufer L et al: Surgical experience with thirteen conjoined twins. *Ann Surg* 1988; 208:299-312.

Ricketts R, Gray SW, Skandalakis JE: Conjoined twins. In: Skandalakis JE, Gray SW (eds): *Embryology for surgeons*. 2nd Ed. Baltimore, MD. Williams & Wilkins, 1994. pp. 1066-1078.

Schnaufer L: Conjoined twins. In: Raffensperger JG (ed): *Swenson's pediatric surgery*. 5th Ed. Norwalk, CT. Appleton & Lange, 1990. pp 969-978.

Votteler TP: Conjoined twins. In: Welch KJ, Randolph JG, Ravitch MM et al (eds): *Pediatric surgery*. 4th Ed. Chicago, IL. Mosby–Year Book, 1986. pp 771-779.

Wong KC, Ohimura A, Roberts TH et al: Anesthesia management for separation of craniopagus twins. *Anesth Analg* 1980; 59:883-886.

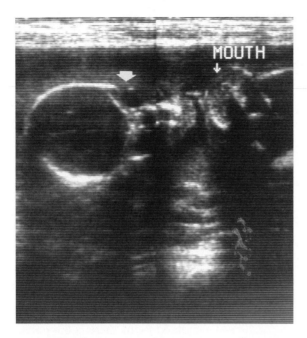

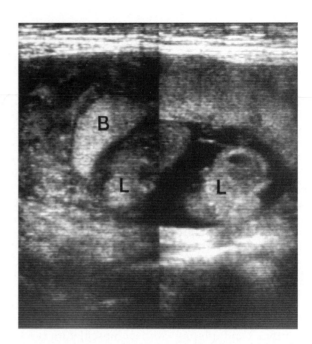

Conjoined twins joined at the thorax (thoracopagus). There were two fetal heads present that faced each other. *Broad arrow*, orbit of A; *small arrow*, mouth of B.

Conjoined twins. Single fetal abdomen with ascites and two livers within it. Although spines were visible in the thorax, caudal regression was present and there was no spine present in the abdomen. *B*, placenta; *L*, liver.

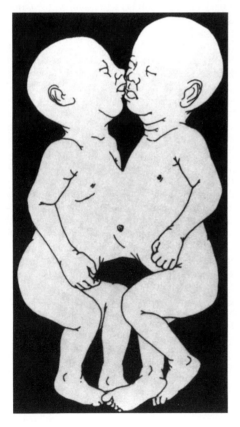

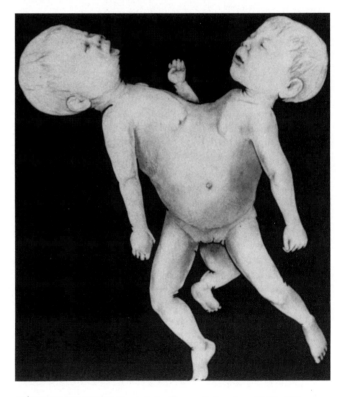

Ischiopagus tripus twins. *Reprinted with permission; from Vottler TP: Surgical separation of conjoined twins. AORN J 1982; pp. 36-38. Copyright © AORN, Inc.*

Thoracoomphalopagus twins. *Reprinted with permission; from Vottler TP: Surgical separation of conjoined twins. AORN J 1982; pp. 36-38. Copyright © AORN, Inc.*

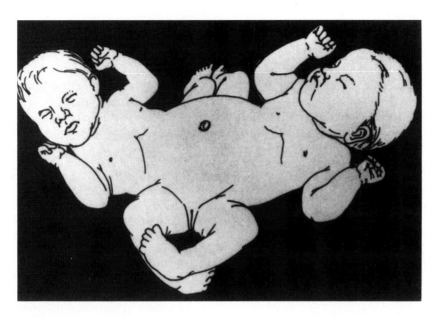

Ischiopagus tetrapus twins. *Reprinted with permission; from Vottler TP: Surgical separation of conjoined twins. AORN J 1982; pp. 36-38. Copyright © AORN, Inc.*

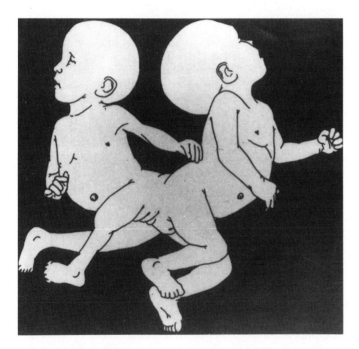

Pygopagus twins. *Reprinted with permission; from Vottler TP: Surgical separation of conjoined twins. AORN J 1982; pp. 36-38. Copyright © AORN, Inc.*

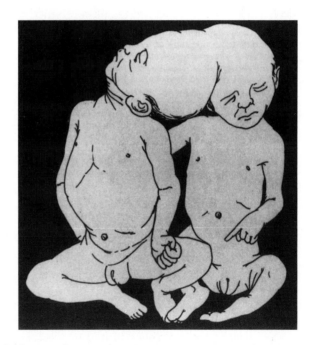

Craniopagus twins. *Reprinted with permission; from Vottler TP: Surgical separation of conjoined twins. AORN J 1982; pp. 36-38. Copyright © AORN, Inc.*

11.3 STUCK TWIN

EPIDEMIOLOGY/GENETICS

Definition "Stuck twin" is described as a diamniotic pregnancy in which one fetus resides against the uterine wall in a severely oligohydramniotic sac, and the co-twin is in a severely polyhydramniotic sac.

Epidemiology This problem complicates up to 8% of twin pregnancies and as many as 35% of monochorionic diamniotic gestations.

Embryology Most cases probably represent the severe end of the twin-twin transfusion syndrome. However, it has been described in dichorionic, and even dizygotic pregnancies. The etiology for these cases remains unknown.

Inheritance Patterns "Stuck twin" is a sporadic event, limited to the present pregnancy.

Prognosis Fetal/neonatal mortality and morbidity rates are high. Fetal death and preterm delivery are the most common complications.

SONOGRAPHY

Findings
1. **Fetus**
   a. On the initial study there is apparently no membrane between the twins, although detailed inspection may show a small portion of a membrane close to the smaller twin. The membrane is actually lying very close to the smaller twin because there is almost no fluid in the smaller sac. The twins are of different sizes. The smaller twin lies adjacent to the uterine border and will not move away from the myometrium if the mother's position is changed, even if the twin is then in a nondependent position—this twin is "stuck."
   b. In most instances, the syndrome is related to twin-twin transfusion syndrome and the large twin may show evidence of hydrops with skin thickening, ascites, pleural effusion, and so on.
2. **Amniotic Fluid:** There will be polyhydramnios around the larger twin and, although not immediately apparent, there is oligohydramnios with little or no fluid in the smaller sac, which will be held "shrink wrapped" against the uterine wall and fetus.
3. **Placenta:** In most instances, a single placenta is present. The syndrome is thought to be related to a shared circulation through the single placenta with excessive blood going to the larger twin and too little blood perfusing the smaller twin, leading to an imbalance in amniotic fluid quantity in the two sacs. Doppler values are abnormal in the cord with little or no diastolic flow in the smaller twin's cord.

4. **Measurement Data:** There is a marked discrepancy in size with the smaller twin almost always at least 2 weeks smaller than the larger twin.
5. **When Detectable:** The syndrome has been reported as early as 15 weeks, but usually develops at about 22 weeks.

Pitfalls Growth discrepancy in diamniotic twins is common, but the amniotic fluid volumes should be only mildly discrepant with intrauterine growth retardation (IUGR) in one dizygotic twin. No polyhydramnios should surround the larger twin.

Differential Diagnosis
1. Diamniotic twins, with IUGR in one twin.
2. Monoamniotic twins, with IUGR in one.
3. Twin-twin transfusion, without stuck twin syndrome.

Where Else to Look
1. Look hard for findings of hydrops in both twins. The donor twin may eventually become the recipient. Early findings of hydrops include hepatosplenomegaly and a small pericardial effusion.
2. Look in the stuck twin for renal anomalies causing oligohydramnios, because not all stuck twins relate to twin-twin transfusion syndrome.
3. Particularly, the stuck twin may show signs of embolization or infarction, after repeated amniocenteses have been performed. Intracranial echogenic areas or hydrocephalus may develop.

PREGNANCY MANAGEMENT

Investigations and Consultations Required Congenital malformations, including chromosome abnormalities resulting in severe IUGR in one fetus, also must be ruled out.

Fetal Intervention Selective termination is contraindicated because the vascular anastomosis between placentas may result in significant damage to, or death of, the surviving fetus. Repeated amniocenteses to drain off the excess amniotic fluid in the sac with polyhydramnios are required. Fluid in this sac should be kept at a low volume. This may require daily or every other day removal of liters of fluid when the diagnosis is first made. Fluid will sometimes spontaneously return to the anhydramniac sac.

Monitoring Frequent monitoring at daily (immediately after therapeutic amniocentesis) or weekly intervals is required in case oligohydramnios returns or hydrops develops. Fetal death is common.

Pregnancy Course: Without the use of repeated amniocenteses, fetal mortality with the stuck twin syndrome is approximately 80%. A survival rate of approximately 80% has been reported if repeated amniocenteses are used.

Pregnancy Termination Issues   If termination is an option, morphologic evaluation of the fetuses and placentas should be done to confirm the diagnosis.

Delivery   The extremely high risk of neonatal complications mandates that delivery occur in a tertiary center.

NEONATOLOGY

Resuscitation   This is an antenatal problem that does not present specific neonatal clinical issues beyond those common to twins in general. Most are born prematurely and therefore, may require assistance with the onset of respiration.

Transport   Transfer to a tertiary perinatal center will be dependent on the degree of prematurity and the concomitant problems of respiratory distress syndrome, as well as other factors.

Nursery Management   As noted above, the management issues are determined by the degree of prematurity and its concomitant problems. Twin-twin transfusion may play a role in the pathogenesis of the in utero course and, if present, requires appropriate intervention in the neonatal period.

BIBLIOGRAPHY

Bruner JP, Rosemond RL: Twin-to-twin transfusion syndrome: a subset of the twin oligohydramnios-polyhydramnios sequence. *Am J Obstet Gynecol* 1993; 169:925-930.

Elliott JP: Amniocentesis for twin-twin transfusion syndrome. *Contemp OB GYN* 1992; Aug:30-47.

Mahony BS, Petty CN, Nyberg DA et al: The stuck twin phenomenon: ultrasonographic findings, pregnancy outcome, and management with serial amniocenteses. *Am J Obstet Gynecol* 1990; 163:1513-1522.

Patten RM, Mack LA, Harvey D et al: Disparity of amniotic fluid volume and fetal size: problem of the stuck twin—US studies. *Radiology* 1989; 172:153-157.

Reisner DP, Mahony BS, Petty CN et al: Stuck twin syndrome: outcome in thirty-seven consecutive cases. *Am J Obstet Gynecol* 1993; 169:991-995.

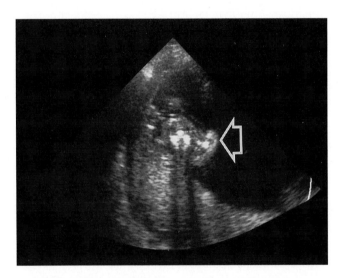

"Stuck" twins. There was polyhydramnios with an apparently monoamniotic pregnancy. The smaller twin was immobile and, with detailed views, a membrane adherent to the smaller twin was seen (*arrow*).

Right side up view. The "stuck" twin (*arrow*) remains adherent to the uterine wall and does not drop into a dependent position.

11.4 TWINS: INTRAUTERINE GROWTH RETARDATION

EPIDEMIOLOGY/GENETICS

Definition   Generally defined as weight less than the tenth percentile. Should be based on a growth chart for twins, not singleton pregnancies.

Epidemiology   Reported to occur in 12% to 47% of twin pregnancies, in contrast to 5% to 7% in singleton pregnancies. The higher rate is thought to be due to competition for available nutrients. However, more commonly a single fetus is growth retarded, which may be due to abnormalities such as the twin-twin transfusion syndrome (TTTS) or some genetic disorders in the growth retarded twin, and not an intrinsic placental problem.

Embryology   Discordancy in fetal growth can result from a nutritional, genetic, chromosomal, infection, or other cause.

Inheritance Patterns   Dizygotic twinning, but not monozygotic, has some genetic component, occurring more often in certain families and more commonly in women of African-American ancestry.

Prognosis   The overall rate of both fetal mortality and neonatal morbidity is significantly increased for the growth retarded fetus. In the TTTS, severe polyhydramnios may result in preterm delivery with increased rates of mortality and morbidity.

SONOGRAPHY

Findings
1.   **Fetus:** One or both twins will be too small for gestational age.
2.   **Amniotic Fluid:** Fluid around the smaller fetus or fetuses will be decreased.
3.   **Placenta:** The placenta related to the smaller twin will be decreased in size.
4.   **Measurement Data:** The abdominal circumference measurement will be decreased and other measurement data (head and limb measurements) may or may not be decreased.
5.   **When Detectable:** Growth retardation in twins may be detected earlier than in singletons.

Pitfalls   If one twin lies anterior to the other, abdominal circumference measurements may be unobtainable.

Differential Diagnosis   The vast majority of the reports indicate IUGR affecting only one twin, and in monozygotic twining many of these cases represent variants of the TTTS. However, discrepancy in placental support is the probable etiology of most discordant IUGR in multiple gestation.

Where Else to Look
1.   Look for evidence of hydrops as in TTTS.
2.   If there is apparently a diamniotic monochorionic pregnancy, make sure that there is not a stuck twin with the amniotic membrane apparently shrink wrapped around the smaller fetus.
3.   A biophysical profile and cord Doppler studies should be performed.

PREGNANCY MANAGEMENT

Investigations and Consultations Required   Intrauterine growth retardation in one of the twins should prompt evaluations of chromosome status of that fetus and a determination of maternal serology for toxoplasmosis, other, rubella, cytomegalovirus, and herpes simplex virus (TORCH) infection, which may present in a discordant manner. Intrauterine growth retardation involving both twins requires a thorough evaluation of the patient for lifestyle factors or underlying medical conditions that cause growth retardation.

Fetal Intervention   Not indicated except in cases of TTTS.

Monitoring   The twin pregnancy with IUGR or growth discordancy is a high risk situation that should be managed by a perinatologist. Nonstress testing (NST) appears to be a good method of fetal assessment and can be used in a fashion similar to that for singleton pregnancies for management of IUGR. Discordant findings on NST indicate the need for additional testing and the biophysical profile appears to be the best alternative.

Pregnancy Termination Issues   Not applicable to this situation.

Delivery   The pregnancy with discordant twins is an extremely high-risk situation requiring delivery and management in a tertiary center.

NEONATOLOGY

Resuscitation   Intrauterine growth retarded twins and the smaller of discordant twins are at very high risk for developing fetal distress during labor and for requiring resuscitation. Two resuscitation teams should be present for every twin delivery. No special techniques are required unless twin-twin transfusion has occurred.

Transport   Referral to a tertiary perinatal center is determined by the degree of postnatal illness and the level of care required.

Nursery Management   The discordant twin with IUGR is at risk for complications of hypoglycemia, respiratory distress, polycythemia, hyperbilirubinemia, and postasphyxial syndromes of organ injury and malfunction. Management is determined by the degree of prematurity, the birth weight, and the presence of complications.

BIBLIOGRAPHY

Blickstein I, Lancet M: The growth discordant twin. *Obstet Gynecol Surv* 1988; 43:509-515.

Bronsteen R, Goyert G, Bottoms S: Classification of twins and neonatal morbidity. *Obstet Gynecol* 1989; 74:98-101.

Naeye RL, Benirschke K, Hagstrom JW et al: Intrauterine growth of twins as estimated from liveborn birth-weight data. *Pediatrics* 1966; 37:409-416.

11.5 TWIN-TWIN TRANSFUSION

EPIDEMIOLOGY/GENETICS

Definition   Twin-twin transfusion syndrome (TTTS) describes a continuum of complications that are seen in monozygotic, monochorionic twins resulting from transplacental vascular communications.

Epidemiology   The incidence of twin-twin transfusion ranges from 5% to 15% of all twin pregnancies. However, the acute, severe form is seen in only approximately 1% of monochorionic gestations.

Embryology   This pregnancy complication results from transplacental arteriovenous communications. Blood is shunted from one twin, the donor, who develops anemia, growth retardation, and oligohydramnios, to the recipient who becomes plethoric, macrosomic, and occasionally hydropic with severe polyhydramnios.

Inheritance Patterns   This is a sporadic event unique to the monozygotic, monochorionic gestation.

Prognosis   Mortality rates of 50% to 100% have been reported. Complications include intrauterine death of one or both fetuses and a high risk of preterm labor. For a surviving twin, there is significant risk of central nervous system and other malformations, now thought to be on the basis of acute hemodynamic and ischemic changes at the time of the death of the co-twin.

SONOGRAPHY

Findings
1. **Fetus**
   a. Monozygotic twins of discrepant size. One twin (the recipient) is larger and one (the donor) smaller than expected by gestational age.
   b. The larger twin may become hydropic—There may be pleural effusion, ascites, pericardial effusion and skin thickening. Hepatosplenomegaly may be present. The stomach and bladder will be larger in the recipient twin.
2. **Amniotic Fluid**
   a. Membrane—The syndrome only occurs if the twins are monochorionic, but there may be two amniotic sacs. The membrane will have only two components.
   b. Fluid—The amniotic sacs may be unequal with the smaller twin having less fluid around it and the larger twin with polyhydramnios (see Stuck Twin, Section 11.3).
3. **Placenta:** With a monochorionic diamniotic pregnancy there is only one placenta and the membrane between the two amniotic cavities is thin because it only has two components. The gender of the two fetuses is the same. The cord of the larger twin will be larger than the cord to the smaller twin.
4. **Measurement Data:** One twin shows evidence of IUGR. As follow-up studies are performed the smaller twin may become the recipient and the growth pattern may reverse. The larger twin may have a spuriously large abdominal circumference if there is ascites.
5. **When Detectable:** The syndrome has been detected at 8 weeks, but is usually seen between 16 and 25 weeks. If it presents in the third trimester, the syndrome develops less rapidly, but significant weight (15%) and hematocrit (7.5g/dl) difference may exist.

Pitfalls
1. Apparent TTTS in monozygotic monoamniotic twins may be diamniotic monozygotic twins with a stuck twin.
2. Oligohydramnios around one twin may not relate to TTTS.
3. Hydrops in twins may occur not related to the TTTS.

Differential Diagnosis   Intrauterine growth retardation is common in all forms of twins without the TTTS.

Where Else to Look
1. Look carefully for diamniotic dizygotic twins. Findings that indicate diamniotic dizygotic twins are:
   a. The "twin peak" sign in the placenta—a portion of placenta pokes into the space between the fused amniotic membranes;
   b. More than two components to the intersac membrane;
   c. Different fetal gender.
   These findings eliminate the possibility of TTTS because they establish a diagnosis of diamniotic dizygotic twins. Two placentas make monozygotic twins unlikely, but not impossible as a succenturiate lobe could be present.
2. Make sure the smaller twin is not stuck by placing the mother in positions that force the smaller twin to fall into a dependent position and look for evidence of a membrane.
3. Look for other causes of hydrops, for example, cardiac causes or infection.

PREGNANCY MANAGEMENT

Investigations and Consultations Required   No additional diagnostic studies are necessary. Because of the high risk of prematurity, a neonatologist should be consulted.

Fetal Intervention   Interventional management is discussed under "Monitoring."

Monitoring Because of the extremely high mortality and morbidity rates, a number of treatment modalities have been attempted, including selective termination, therapeutic amniocentesis, and fetoscopic laser occlusion of fetal vessels. Although no controlled studies exist, the use of aggressive therapeutic amniocentesis (removing sufficient fluid to bring the polyhydramniotic sac down to normal or low-normal volumes) appears to provide the best outcome with the least risk. Therapy must be started before preterm labor develops, if this approach is to be successful. Selective termination is contraindicated because of the significant risk to the surviving twin. Frequent (perhaps, weekly) ultrasound studies are required because of the possible rapid onset of stuck twin syndrome or hydrops. Frequent fetal monitoring with umbilical cord Doppler and biophysical profile, especially amniotic fluid volume estimation, is desirable.

Pregnancy Termination Issues The late onset of this disorder and the potential for treatment generally preclude pregnancy termination as an option.

Delivery Delivery must occur in a tertiary center with full neonatal capabilities.

NEONATOLOGY

Resuscitation With chronic in utero twin-twin transfusion, both infants frequently are depressed at birth and require immediate attention to facilitate the onset of respiration and resolution of birth asphyxia. Two skilled resuscitation teams are required and each must be prepared to deal with the resultant blood and red cell volume problem unique to the respective infant—severe anemia in the donor and severe polycythemia/hypervolemia in recipient. Either one or both twins could present with hydrops.

Transport Transfer of both infants to a tertiary perinatal center is indicated when there is preterm delivery, respiratory distress, or distress secondary to anemia or polycythemia. In utero transfer is the best transfer technique.

Nursery Management Issues of respiratory support, transfusion, cardiac failure, perinatal asphyxia, hypoglycemia, and prematurity are frequently encountered. Partial exchange transfusions, to correct both anemia and polycythemia, are usually safer than simple transfusion and phlebotomy, as there is less stress on circulating blood volume and myocardial function with that approach.

BIBLIOGRAPHY

Achiron R, Rabinovitz R, Aboulafia Y et al: Intrauterine assessment of high-output cardiac failure with spontaneous remission of hydrops fetalis in twin-twin transfusion syndrome: use of two-dimensional echocardiography, Doppler ultrasound, and color flow mapping. *J Clin Ultrasound* 1992; 20:271-277.

Brown DL, Benson CB, Driscoll SG et al: Twin-twin transfusion syndrome: sonographic findings. *Radiology* 1989; 170:61-63.

Elliott JP, Urig MA, Clewell WH: Aggressive therapeutic amniocentesis for treatment of twin-twin transfusion syndrome. *Obstet Gynecol* 1991; 77:537-540.

Klebe JG, Inogomar CJ: The fetoplacental circulation during parturition illustrated by the interfetal transfusion sydrome. *Pediatrics* 1972; 49:112-116.

McCulloch K: Neonatal problems in twins. *Clin Perinatol* 1988; 15:141-158.

Rodis JF, Vintzileos AM, Campbell WA et al: Intrauterine fetal growth in discordant twin gestations. *J Ultrasound Med* 1990; 9:443-448.

Tan KL, Tan R, Tan SH, Tan AM: The twin transfusion sydrome. Clinical observations on 35 affected pairs. *Clin Pediatr* 1979; 18:111-114.

Urig MA, Clewell WH, Elliott JP: Twin-twin transfusion syndrome. *Am J Obstet Gynecol* 1990; 163:1522-1526.

Yamada A, Kasugai M, Ohno Y et al: Antenatal diagnosis of twin-twin transfusion syndrome by Doppler ultrasound. *Obstet Gynecol* 1991; 78:1058-1061.

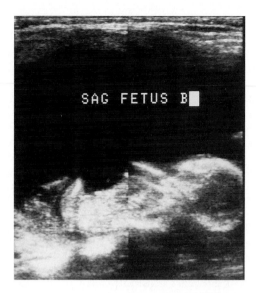

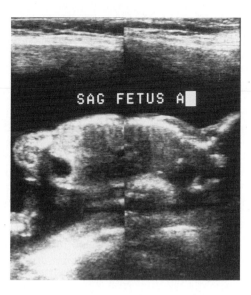

Twin-twin transfusion syndrome. Fetus B is small with little soft tissue. There was moderate polyhydramnios. This was a monoamniotic pregnancy, but the syndrome may develop in monochorionic diamniotic pregnancies.

Fetus A is larger than expected and there is mild skin thickening. Hydrops may occur in more severe examples.

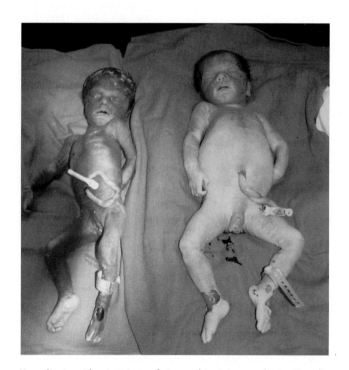

32-week twins with twin-twin transfusion resulting in in utero demise. Note discordant size.

12 Miscellaneous Abnormalities

12.1 CHORIOANGIOMA

EPIDEMIOLOGY/GENETICS

Definition Chorioangiomas are benign vascular tumors of the placenta. They are most commonly encapsulated, round, and intraplacental.

Epidemiology Chorioangiomas are found in approximately 1% of placentas examined at term.

Embryology Chorioangiomas are the most common primary tumor of the placenta.

Inheritance Patterns These tumors are sporadic with no increased risk in future pregnancies.

Prognosis Most chorioangioma are incidental findings. Very rarely, secondary fetal hydrops may develop.

SONOGRAPHY

Findings
1. **Fetus:** Usually the fetus is normal. On rare occasions, severe fetal anemia may develop because the placenta shunts blood and acts as an arteriovenous malformation. Hydrops may develop with skin thickening, ascites, pleural effusion, and other common signs. The earliest signs are hepatosplenomegaly and small pericardial effusions. Pleural effusion, ascites, and skin thickening follow.
2. **Amniotic Fluid:** The amniotic fluid volume is almost always increased if a large mass is present.
3. **Placenta:** A mass is present in the placenta, which will have many arteries within it. The mass usually protrudes into the amniotic cavity and is often located near the cord insertion. Small chorioangiomas occur in about 1% of placenta. Doppler demonstrates arterial flow compatible with arteriovenous malformation.
4. **Measurement Data:** If there is fetal anemia, intrauterine growth retardation (IUGR) is usual. Chorioangiomas are usually not associated with any complications if they are less than 6 cm in diameter.
5. **When Detectable:** Earliest detection reported is at 15 weeks, but chorioangiomas often develop during pregnancy.

Pitfalls
1. Venous flow within a venous lake is usually not visible with Doppler and color flow. Look intently with real time and subtle red cell movement will be seen. Venous lakes may lie at the edge of the placenta and protrude into the amniotic fluid.
2. The chorioangioma may lie alongside the fetus and be mistaken for a fetal mass such as a sacrococcygeal teratoma.

Differential Diagnosis
1. Preplacental hematoma—A mass with a similar appearance to a chorioangioma arising from the placental surface. No flow will be seen on real time or with Doppler.
2. Placental lake on placental surface—The apparent mass will show venous flow on real time and no flow on Doppler.
3. Placental cyst—Cysts arising from the placental surface often have a solid component at the base. A round, thin membrane outlining the echofree component of the cyst will be seen.

Where Else to Look Look at the fetus for IUGR and for evidence of fetal heart failure.

PREGNANCY MANAGEMENT

Investigations and Consultations Required No further investigation is required. Additional consultation will be necessary only if fetal complications develop.

Fetal Intervention None is indicated.

Monitoring Serial ultrasound examinations are essential to detect early signs of fetal hydrops and to monitor fluid volumes. Fetal growth also must be assessed regularly. The development of hydrops should prompt early delivery. In the absence of complications, aggressive intervention is contraindicated as many of these lesions will spontaneously regress.

Pregnancy Course Chorioangiomas are, in rare instances, associated with an increased risk of IUGR, fetal hydrops, and polyhydramnios.

Pregnancy Termination Issues   If pregnancy termination is chosen, an intact fetus and placenta must be delivered to confirm the sonographic diagnosis.

Delivery   In the absence of fetal complications, delivery at a tertiary center is not necessary. Pregnancies with polyhydramnios and/or fetal hydrops are likely to be delivered preterm and should occur at a tertiary center.

NEONATOLOGY

Resuscitation   There are no specific measures required unless fetal anemia and or hydrops fetalis are present (See Chapter 12.2).

Transport   Unless there has been concurrent fetal illness, transfer of the newborn is not indicated.

Nursery Management   There are no special care requirements for the newborn except for the infant who has developed hydrops fetalis (See Chapter 12.2).

BIBLIOGRAPHY

Chazotte C, Girz B, Koenigsberg M et al: Spontaneous infarction of placental chorioangioma and associated regression of hydrops fetalis. *Am J Obstet Gynecol* 1990; 163:1180-1181.

Dao AH, Rogers CW, Wong SW: Chorioangioma of the placenta: report of 2 cases with ultrasound study in 1. *Obstet Gynecol* 1981; 57:46S-48S.

Tonkin IL, Setzer ES, Ermocilla R: Placental chorioangioma: a rare cause of congestive heart failure and hydrops fetalis in the newborn. *Am J Roentgenol* 1980; 134:181-183.

Van Wering JH, Van Der Slikke JW: Prenatal diagnosis of chorioangioma associated with polyhydramnios using ultrasound. *Europ J Obstet Gynecol Reprod Biol* 1985; 19:255-259.

Wolfe BK, Wallace JHK: Pitfall to avoid: chorioangioma of the placenta simulating fetal tumor. *J Clin Ultrasound* 1987; 15:405-408.

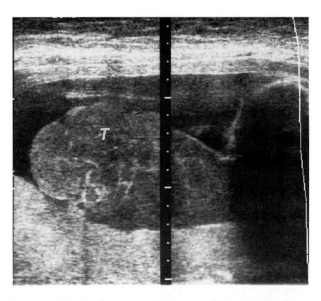

Huge mass arising from the placenta (*T*). Arteries could be seen within the mass using color flow. Despite the large size, no fetal hydrops developed.

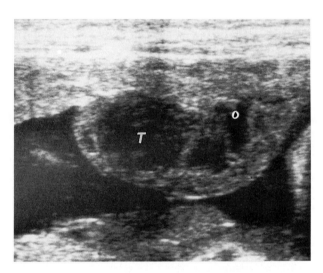

Another example of a chorioangioma (*T*). This mass, which arose from the placenta, had numerous arteries within it visible on real-time and confirmed on color flow.

12.2 Nonimmune Hydrops Fetalis

EPIDEMIOLOGY/GENETICS

Definition   Hydrops fetalis refers to fluid accumulation in serous cavities or edema of soft tissues in the fetus. It is characterized as nonimmune if there is no indication of a fetomaternal blood group incompatibility. Most series include isolated fetal ascites in the definition of hydrops.

Epidemiology   The incidence is approximately 1 in 2500 to 1 in 3500 neonates.

Embryology   The etiologies are diverse and include numerous maternal, fetal, and placental disorders. Table 12.2-1 outlines some of the diverse conditions that have been associated with hydrops fetalis.

Inheritance Patterns   The heterogeneous nature of the etiologic conditions ranges from those that are sporadic to mendelian disorders with a 25% risk of recurrence. In cases for which no etiology can be determined, an empiric risk of recurrence of 5% is appropriate for counselling purposes.

SONOGRAPHY

Findings
1.   Fetus: More than two of the following findings need to be present: Fetal ascites, pleural effusion, pericardial effusion, or skin thickening. Usually, the earliest finding is pericardial effusion.
2.   Amniotic Fluid: Polyhydramnios is commonly seen, depending on the cause of the hydrops.
3.   Placenta: Placentomegaly is often present, depending on the cause of hydrops (for example, Rh disease, chorioangioma).
4.   Measurement Data: Variable, depending on the cause of the hydrops.
5.   When Detectable: Depends on the cause—It can occur at 13 weeks with cystic hygroma.

Pitfalls
1.   Isolated fetal ascites, pericardial effusion, skin thickening, or pleural effusion may have a different prognosis and causation, but may precede hydrops.
2.   Pseudopericardial effusion—The fat pad around the heart may be mistaken for an early pericardial effusion.
3.   Pseudoascites—Apparent small amounts of intraabdominal fluid may represent periabdominal fat or muscle rather than fluid.

Differential Diagnosis   None, if more than two of the four basic components are present. Rh disease, which presents with hydrops, is considered in Chapter 12.3.

It is essential to exclude blood group incompatibility and other conditions for which fetal transfusions would be therapeutic. Likewise, other treatable conditions, such as cardiac arrythmia, must be differentiated before obstetric management plans are formulated.

Where Else to Look   Every structure in the body may be abnormal in association with hydrops. Possible causes include:
1.   Cystic hygroma—The skin thickening will have septation and cystic spaces within.
2.   Cardiac—Many examples of hydrops are due to a cardiac abnormality. Pay particular attention to the heart rhythm and rate because abnormalities of these structures are usually correctable.
3.   Masses, in any site, particularly sacrococcygeal teratoma and cystadenomatoid malformations.

Table 12.2-1   CONDITIONS ASSOCIATED WITH NIHF

CONDITIONS	INDIVIDUAL CONDITIONS
Cardiovascular	Tachyarrhythmia
	Congenital heart block
	Anatomic defects
	Cardiomyopathy
	Myocarditis (Coxsackie virus or CMV)
Chromosomal	Down syndrome (trisomy 21)
	Other trisomies
	Turner's syndrome
	Triploidy
Malformation syndromes	Thanatophoric dwarfism
	Arthrogryposis multiplex congenita
	Osteogenesis imperfecta
	Achondrogenesis
	Neu–Laxova syndrome
	Recessive cystic hygroma
Twin pregnancy	Twin-twin transfusion syndrome
Hematologic	Alpha-thalassemia
	Arteriovenous shunts (e.g., large vascular tumors)
	G6PD deficiency
	Pleural effusion
Respiratory	Diaphragmatic hernia
	Cystic adenoma of the lung
	Mediastinal teratoma
Gastrointestinal	Jejunal atresia
	Midgut volvulus
	Meconium peritonitis
Liver	Polycystic disease of the liver
	Biliary atresia
	Hepatic vascular malformations
Maternal	Severe diabetes mellitus
	Severe anemia
	Hypoproteinemia
Placenta-umbilical cord	Chorioangioma
	Fetomaternal transfusion
	Placental and umbilical vein thrombosis
	Angiomyxoma of the umbilical cord
Medications	Antepartum indomethacin (taken to stop premature labor, causing fetal ductus closure and secondary NIHF)
Infections	CMV
	Toxoplasmosis
	Syphilis
	Congenital hepatitis
	Herpes simplex, type 1
	Rubella
Miscellaneous	Congenital lymphedema
	Congenital hydrothorax or chylothorax
	Sacrococcygeal teratoma

Modified from Holzgreve W, Holzgreve B, Curry CJ: Nonimmune hydrops fetalis: diagnosis and management. *Semin Perinatol* 1985; 9:52-57.
CMV, cytomegalovirus; *G6PD*, glucose-6-phosphate dehydrogenase; *NIHF*, nonimmune hydrops fetalis.

4. Infection—for example, stigma of cytomegalovirus (CMV).
5. Chorioangioma in the placenta.
6. Chromosomal abnormalities, particularly Down syndrome.
7. Twin-twin transfusion syndrome in twins.

PREGNANCY MANAGEMENT

Investigations and Consultations Required   Karyotyping and fetal echocardiography. A protocol for the diagnostic evaluation of the pregnancy complicated by hydrops is outlined in Table 12.2-2. Other consultations will depend on the etiology that is determined.

Fetal Intervention   Intervention should be reserved for those cases in which a precise diagnosis has been established. Intrauterine transfusion has been successful for anemia secondary to parvovirus infection. Shunt placement in cases with primary lung pathology has resulted in resolution of hydrops in a number of reported cases. The most successful form of intervention is the treatment of fetuses with cardiac arrhythmias.

Monitoring   Every attempt must be made to establish a diagnosis. The aggressiveness of the management approach will be highly dependent on the overall prognosis for the fetus. In general, a nonaggressive approach is warranted for idiopathic hydrops as mortality is high and is not improved by early delivery. These high-risk pregnancies should be managed by a perinatologist who is familiar with the diverse etiologies for hydrops. If the cause is unknown, reexamine at frequent intervals, that is, every 2 weeks. A cause may become apparent.

Pregnancy Course   There is a significant risk of polyhydramnios and preeclampsia associated with fetal hydrops. Fetal mortality rates have been reported to range from 75% to 90%.

Pregnancy Termination Issues   Unless a precise diagnosis has been made antenatally, an intact fetus must be delivered for a complete pathologic evaluation.

Delivery   Delivery must occur at a tertiary center because of the complicated neonatal resuscitation likely to be required. The mode of delivery should be based on obstetric indications, but the high risk of "fetal distress" will mean a high rate of cesarean section for fetuses with hydrops.

NEONATOLOGY

Resuscitation   Fetuses with hydrops tolerate labor poorly. They develop asphyxia secondary to the accompanying placental pathology, as well as from the disorder causing the hydrops. Except in very uncommon cases, extensive resuscitation with immediate respiratory support is required. Both thoracentesis and paracentesis may be needed following delivery to permit adequate ventilatory excursions. Manipulation of circulating blood volume, without the capability to monitor both arterial and venous pressure, is fraught with the risk of fetal deterioration.

Transport   Referral to a tertiary perinatal center is mandatory both because of the very high mortality risk and because of the extensive technical support required for diagnostic evaluation and management.

Nursery Management   The management approach is determined by two factors—the effects on cardiorespiratory function of the hydropic state and the underlying etiology. Mobilization of the hydropic fluid without concomitant further hemodynamic compromise is the initial goal. Fluid restriction, diuresis, dialysis, and exchange transfusion have all been used successfully.

If not established prenatally, determining the etiology is imperative both to facilitate therapeutic intervention as well as to provide accurate counseling regarding prognosis and recurrence risk.

BIBLIOGRAPHY

Holzgreve W, Curry CJ, Golbus MS et al: Investigation of nonimmune hydrops fetalis. Am J Obstet Gynecol 1984; 150:805-812.

Holzgreve W, Holzgreve B, Curry CJ: Nonimmune hydrops fetalis: diagnosis and management. Semin Perinatol 1985; 9:52-67.

Hutchinson AA, Drew JH, Yu VY et al: Nonimmunologic hydrops fetalis: a review of 61 cases. Obstet Gynecol 1982; 59:347-352.

Jauniaux E, Van Maldergem L, De Munter C et al: Nonimmune hydrops fetalis associated with genetic abnormalities. Obstet Gynecol 1990; 75:568-572.

Machin GA: Hydrops revisited: literature review of 1,414 cases published in the 1980s. Am J Med Genet 1989; 34:366-390.

McGillivray BC, Hall JG: Nonimmune hydrops fetalis. Pediatr Rev 1987; 9:197-202.

Saltzman DH, Frigoletto FD Jr, Harlow BL et al: Sonographic evaluation of hydrops fetalis. Obstet Gynecol 1989; 74:106-111.

Santolaya J, Alley D, Jaffe R et al: Antenatal classification of hydrops fetalis. Obstet Gynecol 1992; 79:256-259.

Van Maldergem L, Jauniaux E, Fourneau C et al: Genetic causes of hydrops fetalis. Pediatrics 1992; 89:81-86.

Watson J, Campbell S: Antenatal evaluation and management of nonimmune hydrops fetalis. Obstet Gynecol 1986; 67:589-593.

Table 12.2-2   DIAGNOSTIC STEPS IN THE PRENATAL EVALUATION OF NIHF

LEVELS OF INVASIVENESS	DIAGNOSTIC TEST
Noninvasive	Complete blood count and indices
	Hemoglobin electrophoresis
	Kleihauer-Betke stain
	Syphilis (VDRL) and TORCH titers
	Fetal echocardiography
Amniocentesis	Fetal karyotype
	Amniotic fluid viral cultures
	Alpha-fetoprotein
	Specific metabolic tests
Fetal blood sampling	Rapid karyotype
	Hemoglobin chain analysis, if indicated
	Fetal plasma analysis for specific IgM
	Fetal plasma albumin

IgM, immunoglobulin-M; *TORCH,* toxoplasmosis, other, rubella, cytomegalovirus, and herpes simplex virus; *VDRL,* Venereal Disease Research Laboratory [test for syphylis].

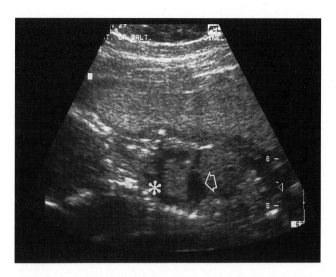

Sagittal view of the fetal trunk. Pleural effusion (*asterisk*) surrounds the fetal lung. Fetal ascites is present (*open arrow*).

12.3 RHESUS INCOMPATIBILITY

EPIDEMIOLOGY/GENETICS

Definition   Rh disease refers to the hemolytic process in the fetus that results from Rh blood group incompatibility between the mother and the fetus.

Epidemiology   Before the advent of passive immunization with Rh immune globulin, erythroblastosis fetalis occurred in approximately 1% of pregnancies. However, the use of Rh immunoglobulin has markedly decreased the incidence of this disorder.

Embryology   The pathophysiology of this condition is a direct result of severe anemia secondary to red cell hemolysis caused by maternal anti-Rh antibodies. These antibodies may be directed at any of the components of the Rh system—c, d, or e are the more common immunizing antigens.

Inheritance Patterns   The genetic component is the inheritance of the "positive" Rh allele. If the father is homozygous, all offspring are positive. If he is heterozygous, there is a 50% risk of an Rh positive fetus. The manifestations in a Rh positive fetus tend to be more severe with each subsequent pregnancy.

Prognosis   In experienced centers intravascular transfusion will result in better than 95% survival rate in non-hydropic fetuses. Survival falls to 80% to 85% in fetuses with hydrops.

SONOGRAPHY

Findings
1.   **Fetus:** Hydrops is seen with severe Rh incompatibility. There is skin thickening, a pleural effusion, a pericardial effusion, and ascites. The liver and spleen are enlarged.
2.   **Amniotic Fluid:** The amniotic fluid volume may be increased.
3.   **Placenta:** The placenta is enlarged with an evenly echogenic texture.
4.   **Measurement Data:** Growth is less than expected, although the trunk circumference may be spuriously large due to hepatosplenomegaly and fetal ascites.
5.   **When Detectable:** The earliest the syndrome has been detected is 16 weeks. With repeated affected infants, the syndrome develops earlier.

Pitfalls   A normal slim echopenic area around the heart may be confused with a pericardial effusion. Pericardial effusions are often not symmetrical.

Differential Diagnosis   There are numerous other causes of hydrops (nonimmune hydrops). For a discussion of the other potential causes see Chapter 12.2.

Where Else to Look   Look for other causes of hydrops: cardiac causes; infectious causes; and chromosomal causes (see Chapter 12.2).

PREGNANCY MANAGEMENT

Investigations and Consultations Required   Maternal antibody screens, and assessment of fetal hematologic status by cordocentesis are the essential components of the workup.

Fetal Intervention   Intravascular transfusions should be performed in a center with significant experience in the management of Rh disease. Transfusion therapy should be instituted when the fetal hematocrit is less than 30%. The procedure involves a simple transfusion of packed red blood cells (70% or greater hematocrit) into the umbilical vein. Paralysis of the fetus with pancuronium (0.3 mg/kg estimated fetal weight intravenously) to prevent fetal movement is preferable.

The final fetal hematocrit should be between 45% and 50%. Repeat transfusions are based on the loss of 1% hematocrit per day, but more frequent transfusions may be necessary initially until the fetal blood volume is essentially all Rh negative red cells (transfused red blood cells).

Monitoring   Once transfusion therapy has been initiated, weekly sonographic evaluations should be performed looking for subtle signs of fetal hydrops. Management must be under the direction of a perinatologist.

Pregnancy Course   In severe cases of hydrops, polyhydramnios may be a late manifestation. Without transfusion, fetal death will occur in cases of severe hydrops.

Delivery   Delivery must occur in a tertiary center. The mode of delivery will depend on the predicted hemoglobin levels. Moderate to severely anemic fetuses may not tolerate labor well and may benefit from elective cesarean section.

NEONATOLOGY

Resuscitation   In general, the majority of fetuses who have been affected by Rh isoimmunization do not experience distress in labor and therefore, do not require assistance with the onset of respiration. Only those with anemia of a profound degree and those with hydrops fetalis are the exception. (See Chapter 12.2 for the specific details of management.)

Transport   Indications for referral to a tertiary perinatal center immediately following birth include: hydrops fetalis, severe anemia (hemoglobin less than 10 g/dl), anticipated need for exchange transfusion in the first 24 hours of life (rise in bilirubin of greater than 1.5 mg/dl per hour). (See Chapter 12.2 for the specific details of management.)

Testing and Confirmation   Other causes of hydrops not associated with anemia, and therefore not treatable by transfusion, must be excluded. The severity of the isoimmunization should be assessed early by obtaining hemoglobin, reticulocyte count, albumin, and fractionated bilirubin concentrations on admission.

Nursery Management   Prompt and efficient cardiorespiratory adaptation is the initial focus of management Restoring adequate oxygen-carrying capacity promptly without hemodynamic stress is important if there is significant anemia. A prehydropic state should be suspected with hypoalbuminemia. Bilirubin accumulation is controllable with phototherapy in mild cases and exchange transfusion in moderate to severe ones. (See Chapter 12.2 for specific details of management.)

BIBLIOGRAPHY

Benacerraf BR, Frigoletto FD Jr: Sonographic sign for the detection of early fetal ascites in the management of severe isoimmune disease without intrauterine transfusion. *Am J Obstet Gynecol* 1985; 152:1039-1041.

Bloom RS: Delivery room resuscitation of the newborn. In: Fanaroff AA, Martin RJ: *Neonatal-perinatal medicine: diseases of the fetus and infant.* St. Louis. Mosby–Year Book, 1992. p. 301.

12.4 VACTERL Association

EPIDEMIOLOGY/GENETICS

Definition   Acronym (VACTERL) for a nonrandom association of birth defects including vertebral anomalies (60%), anal atresia (60%), cardiac defects (60%), tracheoesophageal fistula (85%), renal anomalies (60%), and radial limb abnormalities (65%). Diagnosis is based on the presence of at least three of these defects.

Epidemiology   Very rare (M1:F1).

Embryology   Unknown. May result from a single early defect in fetal blastogenesis or fetal mesoderm formation.

Inheritance Patterns   Sporadic. There is a VACTERL-like syndrome with central nervous system malformations that has autosomal recessive inheritance.

Teratogens   None known. Diabetic embryopathy may result in a similar pattern of malformations.

Prognosis   There is a 75% survival rate. Central nervous system abnormalities are rare and most children have normal intelligence.

SONOGRAPHY

Findings
1. **Fetus**
    a. Polydactyly.
    b. Vertebral anomalies
       i. Caudal regression—shortened spine with absent vertebral bodies, often with scoliosis (see Chapter 2.5).
       ii. Hemivertebra or absent vertebra—These are not easy to detect with ultrasound. There will be an inability to see posterior elements with slight angulation of the spine at the abnormal area. Two or more posterior elements may be fused.
    c. Anal atresia—Anal atresia is rarely diagnosable in utero. Occasionally, dilated large bowel will be visible. The anus can be seen as a small echogenic spot posterior to the genitalia. Absence of this spot may indicate atresia (see Chapter 6.1).
    d. Tracheoesophageal atresia—The stomach will either be small or absent. Polyhydramnios will be present (see Chapter 5.3).
    e. Renal abnormalities—There may be hydronephrosis or multicystic kidney (see Chapter 4.3).
    f. Radial ray problems—The radius may be absent or small with accompanying loss of portions of the hand (see Chapter 8.14).
    g. Congenital heart defects may be found.
2. **Amniotic Fluid:** With gut atresia, polyhydramnios will be present.
3. **Placenta:** Normal placenta.
4. **Measurement Data:** Normal.
5. **When Detectable:** None of the findings are easy to detect, but they should be visible at 16 to 18 weeks.

Differential Diagnosis
1. Many of these findings are also seen with chromosomal anomalies.
2. Multiple malformation syndromes including the Holt-Oram (autosomal dominant) and thrombocytopenia-absent radius syndrome (TAR) may have similar manifestations.
3. The overall good long-term prognosis for infants with VACTERL requires that syndromes, such as Jacho-Levin and other lethal skeletal dysplasias, be excluded before determining an obstetric management plan.

Where Else to Look   A thorough survey of the entire fetus is desirable owing to the fact that the syndrome is so widespread.

PREGNANCY MANAGEMENT

Investigations and Consultations Required   As with all multiple malformation cases, chromosome evaluation is essential, even though VACTERL itself is not associated with a chromosome abnormality. Fetal echocardiography should be performed to delineate the severity of the cardiac defect. A pediatric surgeon should be consulted to discuss surgical management with the family.

Monitoring   In the absence of polyhydramnios no specific changes in obstetric care are required. Serial ultrasounds to detect increasing amniotic fluid volumes are appropriate.

Pregnancy Course   Polyhydramnios may be a complicating factor and may result in preterm labor.

Pregnancy Termination Issues   In order to establish a precise diagnosis, an intact fetus must be delivered, and appropriate morphologic, radiologic, and pathologic examination performed.

Delivery   The site of delivery should be a tertiary center with availability of appropriate medical and surgical specialist to deal with the multiple malformations that are a part of this "syndrome." The mode of delivery should be based on obstetric indications.

NEONATOLOGY

Resuscitation The special management issues at birth are based upon the specific organ defects known to be present. Among the ones included in the VACTERL association, tracheoesophageal fistula and cardiac defects impact on the onset of respiration and early adaptation. Resuscitation and stabilization of cardiorespiratory function measures to be instituted are discussed under these specific defects (see Chapter 5.3 and Chapter 3).

Transport Referral to a tertiary perinatal center with multiple pediatric and surgical subspecialists is always indicated. Care during transport should include the specific measures for each of the defects known or suspected to be present.

Testing and Confirmation A diagnosis can be made at birth. Radiographic studies are recommended to look for associated spinal abnormalities.

Nursery Management Priority in management is determined by the specific malformations known to be present. Therefore, immediate diagnostic evaluation to identify which defects the infant manifests should be instituted. The next step is to coordinate the various surgical interventions. The long-term prognosis is governed by the potential correctibility of the cardiac defect; therefore, prompt accurate diagnosis by echocardiography is essential initially.

Both tracheoesophageal fistula and anal atresia require urgent surgical intervention to alleviate their life-threatening impact once the cardiac defect is determined to be correctible. In general, the vertebral, extremity, and renal defects are not associated with significant dysfunction in the neonatal period and therefore, have lesser influence on the plan of care.

BIBLIOGRAPHY

Czeizel A, Ludanyi I: An aetiological study of the VACTERL-association. *Eur J Pediatr* 1985; 144:331-337.

McGahan JP, Leeba JM, Lindfors KK: Prenatal sonographic diagnosis of VATER association. *J Clin Ultrasound* 1988; 16:588-591.

Weaver DD, Mapstone CL, Yu PL: The VATER association: analysis of 46 patients. *Am J Dis Child* 1986; 140:225-229.

13 Abnormal Sonographic Findings

13.1 AMNIOTIC MEMBRANES

EPIDEMIOLOGY/GENETICS

Definition   A thin echogenic line surrounded on either side by echo-free amniotic fluid.

Epidemiology   Common.

Embryology   See description of membrane types.

SONOGRAPHY

Findings
1.   **Fetus:** Normal, except when the membranes are due to amniotic band syndrome.
2.   **Amniotic Fluid:** Several types of membranes can be seen in the amniotic fluid:
    a. Amniotic bands—thin, curving membranes attached to the fetus. Very difficult to see.
    b. The border of a marginal bleed—This is a relatively thick, slightly curved membrane that ends at the uterine border. It usually starts at the edge of the placenta. When the ultrasound gain control is increased, low level echoes are visible within the area enclosed by the membrane. Old blood may become more or less sonolucent, but because there is proteinaceous material present, the echogenicity is slightly greater than normal amniotic fluid and can be made visible by increasing the gain.
    c. Twin gestational sac membrane—The sac border remains when a blighted ovum occurs with a twin pregnancy. The remaining gestational sac border is smooth, curved and encloses a small space.
    d. Amniotic sheet—If there is a preexisting synechiae, prior to pregnancy, the gestational sac implants on the membrane. This membrane has a double layer, since the amnion and chorion surround the synechiae. A small circle is seen at the amniotic border of the membrane, presumably enclosing the synechiae. Amniotic sheets have, so far, had no pathological significance.
    e. Placental cyst—Placental cysts arise from the amniotic border of the placenta and extend into the amniotic fluid. A solid component may be seen at the placental aspect of the cyst.
    f. Unfused amniotic sac—The amnion and chorion are normally unfused until about 12 to 13 weeks. Occasionally, they remain unfused until as late as 17 weeks. In some patients following amniocentesis, blood is introduced into the space between the amnion and chorion, at the time of amniocentesis. This mishap is associated with prematurity.
    g. Subchorionic lucent space—An echopenic area, just below the placental surface, either represents Wharton's jelly deposition or a venous lake. Low-level echoes will be seen within the suspect area, which will show movement on real-time, if they are due to a venous lake.
3.   **Placenta:** May extend into the base of the membrane with a diamniotic dichorionic pregnancy.
4.   **Measurement Data:** Normal.
5.   **When Detectable:** With a vaginal probe, at about 13 weeks.

Where Else to Look   Look for stigmata of the amniotic band syndrome and the limb-body wall complex.

PREGNANCY MANAGEMENT

Investigations and Consultations Required   In absence of other structural malformations, no additional evaluation is necessary. Additional consultations should be dictated by the specific malformations seen.

Monitoring   No change in standard obstetric management is warranted.

Pregnancy Termination Issues   Not indicated unless severe structural malformation is seen in the fetus.

Delivery   Site is dependent upon presence, or absence, of fetal structural malformation.

BIBLIOGRAPHY

Benacerraf BR, Frigoletto FD Jr: Sonographic observation of amniotic rupture without amniotic band syndrome. *J Ultrasound Med* 1992; 11:109-111.

Burrows PE, Lyons EA, Phillips HJ et al: Intrauterine membranes: sonographic findings and clinical significance. *J Clin Ultrasound* 1982; 10:1-8.

Burton DJ, Filly RA: Sonographic diagnosis of the amniotic band syndrome. *Am J Roentgenol* 1991; 156:555-558.

Finberg HJ: Uterine synechiae in pregnancy: expanded criteria for recognition and clinical significance in 28 cases. *J Ultrasound Med* 1991; 10:547-555.

Herbert WN, Seeds JW, Cefalo RC et al: Prenatal detection of intraamniotic bands: implications and management. *Obstet Gynecol* 1985; 65:36S-38S.

Jeanty P, Lacirica R, Luna SK: Extra-amniotic pregnancy: a trip to the extraembryonic coelom. *J Ultrasound Med* 1990; 9:733-736.

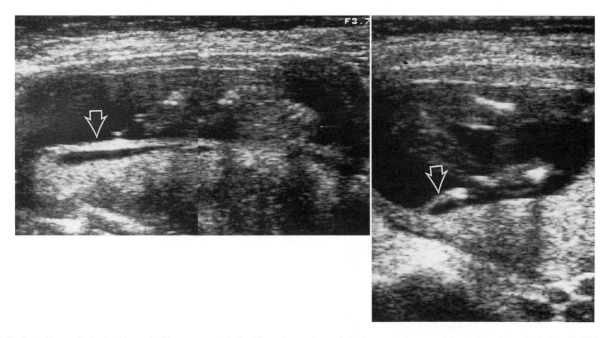

Amniotic sheet. The amniotic sheet has a double component derived from the amnion and chorion, wrapping around a synechiae. On sagittal views (*left*), it can be quite lengthy, but the transverse view (*right*) is short because it ends with a small circle at the site of the synechiae (*arrows*).

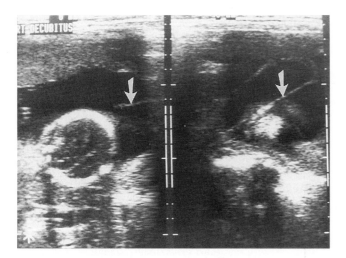

Amniotic band. The thin amniotic band can be seen approaching the fetus and attached to one arm (*arrows*). This type of band follows a disruption of the amnion in the early first trimester.

13.2 Cord Cyst

EPIDEMIOLOGY/GENETICS

Definition   Cyst arising from the cord.

Epidemiology   Rare. No epidemiological survey has been performed.

Embryology   Cysts in the cord may represent a remnant of the primitive allantois present when the cord is formed; cystic expansion of the omphalomesenteric duct, also an embryological remnant; cystic degeneration of Wharton's jelly—the material that surrounds the cord.

Inheritance Patterns   Not recurrent.

Prognosis   If isolated, of no consequence, but associated with fetal and cord abnormalities.

SONOGRAPHY

Findings
1. **Fetus:** None.
2. **Amniotic Fluid:** Normal.
3. **Placenta:** Normal. One or more echo-free cysts are present arising from the cord generally located close to the fetal trunk. Size varies from a few mm to 5 cm.
4. **Measurement Data:** Normal.
5. **When Detectable:** In the second trimester.

Pitfalls   Wharton's jelly can be very prominent and form a thick echopenic area around the cord in some normal individuals.

Differential Diagnosis
1. Cord tumors—will have internal echoes and show flow on color flow.
2. Umbilical artery aneurysm—Nonpulsatile and turbulent flow will be present on color flow Doppler. There may be a calcified wall to the "cyst."
3. Cord pseudocyst—cavity formed by degeneration of Wharton's jelly; there is no epithelial lining. Not distinguishable from allantoic cyst by sonographic appearance if there is only one. Pseudocysts are often multiple and carry a poor prognosis. They are associated with intrauterine growth retardation (IUGR), and chromosomal anomalies.
4. Omphalomesenteric cyst. An enteric lined cyst that connects to the region of the Meckel's diverticulum.
5. Hemangioma of the umbilical cord—densely echogenic cord mass with overall cord edema.
6. Angiomyxoma—mass involving the cord with cystic center but thick irregular echogenic rind. Overall thickening of the cord occurs.
7. Hematoma of the cord. Usually there is a history of an amniocentesis or percutaneous umbilical blood sampling (PUBS). Irregularly shaped mass arising from the cord with internal echoes. Vibrates with cord pulsation.
8. Allantoic cyst. Single often large structure usually located close to the fetal abdomen.

Where Else to Look
1. There is an association with omphalocele and chromosomal anomalies.
2. Urachal cysts are often seen with allantoic cysts. A cyst will be present in the fetal trunk located between the bladder and the umbilicus. The allantoic cyst may appear to communicate with the urachal cyst.

PREGNANCY MANAGEMENT

Investigations and Consultations Required   If an omphalocele, as well as the allantoic cyst, is seen, the fetus should be karyotyped.

Monitoring   Follow-up sonograms are worthwhile. Cord compression by an enlarging allantoic cyst, as evidenced by abnormal Doppler patterns with low diastolic values, has been reported.

Pregnancy Course   Unremarkable.

Delivery   Ensure that the cord is sent for pathological analysis.

BIBLIOGRAPHY
Battaglia C, Artini PG, D'Ambrogio G et al: Cord vessel compression by an expanding allantoic cyst: case report. *Ultrasound Obstet Gynecol* 1992; 2:58-60.

Casola G, Scheible W, Leopold GR: Large umbilical cord: a normal finding in some fetuses. *Radiology* 1985; 156:181-182.

Fortune DW, Ostor AG: Umbilical artery aneurysm. *Am J Obstet Gynecol* 1978; 131:339-340.

Frazier HA, Guerrieri JP, Thomas RL et al: The detection of a patent urachus and allantoic cyst of the umbilical cord on prenatal ultrasonography. *J Ultrasound Med* 1992; 11:117-120.

Ghidini A, Romero R, Eisen RN et al: Umbilical cord hemangioma: prenatal identification and review of the literature. *J Ultrasound Med* 1990; 9:297-300.

Harp J, Rouse GA, De Lange M: Sonographic prenatal diagnosis of allantoic cyst. *JDMS* 1992; 8:28-32.

Iaccarino M, Baldi F, Persico O et al: Ultrasonographic and pathologic study of mucoid degeneration of umbilical cord. *J Clin Ultrasound* 1986; 14:127-129.

Jauniaux E, Campbell S, Vyas S: The use of color Doppler imaging for prenatal diagnosis of umbilical cord anomalies: report of three cases. *Am J Obstet Gynecol* 1989; 161:1195-1197.

Jauniaux E, Moscoso G, Chitty L et al: An angiomyxoma involving the whole length of the umbilical cord: prenatal diagnosis by ultrasonography. *J Ultrasound Med* 1990; 9:419-422.

Jeanty P: Fetal and funicular vascular anomalies: identification with prenatal US. *Radiology* 1989; 173:367-370.

Jones TB, Sorokin Y, Bhatia R et al: Single umbilical artery: accurate diagnosis? *Am J Obstet Gynecol* 1993; 169:538-540.

Kalter CS, Williams MC, Vaughn V et al: Sonographic diagnosis of a large umbilical cord pseudocyst. *J Ultrasound Med* 1994; 13:487-489.

Middleton MA, Middleton WD, Wiele K: Case Report 2: allantoic cyst of the umbilical cord. *Am J Roentgenol* 1989; 152:1324-1325.

Morin LR: Sonography of umbilical cord hematoma. *Am J Roentgenol* 1991; 156:1115.

Nyberg DA, Mahony BS, Luthy D et al: Single umbilical artery: prenatal detection of concurrent anomalies. *J Ultrasound Med* 1991; 10:247-253.

Nyberg DA, Shepard T, Mack LA et al: Significance of a single umbilical artery in fetuses with central nervous system malformations. *J Ultrasound Med* 1988; 7:265-273.

Pollack MS, Bound LM: Hemangioma of the umbilical cord: sonographic appearance. *J Ultrasound Med* 1989; 8:163-166.

Rempen A: Sonographic first-trimester diagnosis of umbilical cord cyst. *J Clin Ultrasound* 1989; 17:53-55.

Resta RG, Luthy DA, Mahony BS: Umbilical cord hemangioma associated with extremely high alpha-fetoprotein levels. *Obstet Gynecol* 1988; 72:488-491.

Rosenberg JC, Chervenak FA, Walker BA et al: Antenatal sonographic appearance of omphalomesenteric duct cyst. *J Ultrasound Med* 1986; 5:719-720.

Ruvinsky ED, Wiley TL, Morrison JC et al: In utero diagnosis of umbilical cord hematoma by ultrasonography. *Am J Obstet Gynecol* 1981; 140:833-834.

Sachs L, Fourcroy JL, Wenzel DJ et al: Prenatal detection of umbilical cord allantoic cyst. *Radiology* 1982; 145:445-446.

Schuman AJ: How to assess single umbilical artery. *Contemp OB GYN* 1992; Oct:61-66.

Siddiqi TA, Bendon R, Schultz DM et al: Umbilical artery aneurysm: prenatal diagnosis and management. *Obstet Gynecol* 1992; 80:530-533.

Sutro WH, Tuck SM, Loesevitz A et al: Prenatal observation of umbilical cord hematoma. *Am J Roentgenol* 1984; 142:801-802.

Vesce F, Guerrini P, Perri G et al: Ultrasonographic diagnosis of ectasia of the umbilical vein. *J Clin Ultrasound* 1987; 15:346-349.

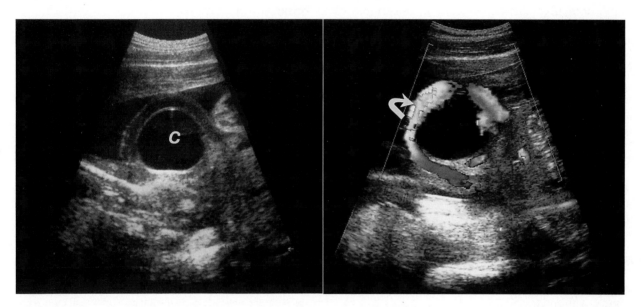

Left, Allantoic cyst associated with the cord. A cyst is completely echo-free and single. It is located quite close to the fetal abdominal wall (*C*). *Right,* View of the cord cyst with color flow used to demonstrate the cord (*arrow*).

13.3 Intrauterine Growth Retardation

EPIDEMIOLOGY/GENETICS

Definition   There is considerable variability in the definition of what constitutes a growth retarded infant. Definitions include a birth weight below 2500 g, a birth weight below the third percentile for gestational age, a birth weight below the tenth percentile for gestational age, or a birth weight more than two standard deviations below the mean for gestational age. The most commonly used definition is a birth weight below the tenth percentile for gestational age.

Epidemiology   Intrauterine growth retardation (IUGR) affects 3% to 10% of all pregnancies, depending on the definition used.

Embryology   Subnormal fetal growth may result from chronic uteroplacental insufficiency, exposure to drugs or environmental agents, congenital infections, or intrinsic genetic limitations of growth potential. Fetuses with growth restriction due to nutritional compromise tend to have sparing of head growth (asymmetric growth retardation).

Inheritance Patterns   Recurrent IUGR most commonly represents an underlying maternal medical condition. There is no genetic basis for true IUGR. Healthy, but small for gestational age infants may be the result of as yet unknown genetic factors.

Prognosis   Perinatal mortality is four to eight times higher for the growth retarded fetus and significant morbidity is noted in up to 50% of the survivors.

SONOGRAPHY

Findings
1. **Fetus:** Diminished soft tissue mass.
2. **Amniotic Fluid:** Usually diminished. If the fluid is increased, consider the possibility of a chromosomal anomaly.
3. **Placenta**
   a. Usually thin and small.
   b. If enlarged and thickened or "molar" in appearance, consider triploidy.
   c. Grade 3 placenta occurring prior to 34 to 36 weeks often heralds or accompanies IUGR of vascular origin, as with maternal hypertension or placental infarcts.
4. **Measurement Data:** Estimated fetal weight is based on ultrasonic measurement of:
   a. Abdominal circumference;
   b. Biparietal diameter and head circumference;
   c. Femur length.
   Various formulas use the abdominal circumference in combination with other parameters to determine weight. Three different growth patterns are seen:

   a. Symmetrical—All measurement data are small compared with known dates (early sonogram, known conception date, early exam = regular menstrual dating);
   b. Asymmetrical—head measurements are consistent with dates or not far behind, whereas abdomen measurements are at least 2 weeks less and below the tenth percentile;
   c. Femur sparing—head and abdomen measurements are small, whereas the femur and cerebellar measurements are consistent with dates. If dates are unclear and all other measurements are 3 to 4 weeks less than the femur, IUGR is likely.
5. **When Detectable:** Very early, for example, 15 weeks, in association with karyotypic abnormalities; or 28 to 32 weeks with preeclampsia and hypertension.

Pitfalls
1. Distinction from wrong dates is difficult when a patient presents late with uncertain dates. Oligohydramnios and an abnormal Doppler and biophysical profile favor true IUGR.
2. Distinction from the small for gestational age (SGA) baby is difficult. A family history of small children, normal fluid, biophysical profile, and Doppler suggest a normal fetus.
3. Quality views of the abdominal circumference are crucial because weight estimates are so dependent on this measurement. Weight estimation errors are less with small fetuses but are, in the best of hands, +/- 1 to 200 g per 1000 g.
4. The long, thin fetus is easily overlooked with ultrasonographic measurements.

Differential Diagnosis
1. Wrong dates and normal fetus.
2. Normal small fetus.

Where Else to Look
1. Do tests of fetal well being:
   a. Biophysical profile including the nonstress test.
   b. Umbilical artery doppler.
   c. Amniotic fluid index.
2. With early IUGR look for:
   a. Stigmata of chromosomal anomalies
      i. Trisomy 18—choroid plexus cyst, clenched hands and club feet, neural crest anomaly, and congenital heart defects.
      ii. Stigmata of triploidy—large placenta with molar aspects, asymmetrical IUGR, micrognathia, cleft palate, hand and feet deformities, hydrocephalus, and neural crest anomalies.
      iii. Trisomy 13—holoprosencephaly, facial deformities, omphalocele, renal cystic dysplasia, hand and feet abnormalities, and congenital heart defects.

b. Nonchromosomal syndromes
  i. Cytomegalovirus infection—hepatospleno-megaly, microcephaly with lateral ventricular dilation with echogenic borders, and hydrops.
  ii. Neu-Laxova syndrome—microcephaly, micrognathia, protruding eyeballs, joint contractures, edematous skin, heart defects, cleft lip, and polyhydramnios.
  iii. Cornelia de Lange syndrome—micrognathia, clinodactyly, micromelia, hypospadias, and undescended testes.
  iv. Fetal alcohol syndrome—cardiac abnormalities, microcephaly, micrognathia, and cleft lip and palate.

PREGNANCY MANAGEMENT

Investigations and Consultations Required   Chromosome evaluation of the fetus and maternal toxoplasmosis, other, rubella, cytomegalovirus, and herpes simplex virus (TORCH) titers should be performed with otherwise unaccounted for IUGR.

Fetal Intervention   Experimental work evaluating methods of increasing fetal "nutrition" by instillation of amino acids into the amniotic fluid or by direct intravascular injections have been attempted. However, at present these methods are not appropriate for clinical management.

Monitoring   The management of the fetus with IUGR should be in the hands of a perinatologist. The timing of fetal assessment methods such as nonstress testing and biophysical profile must be individualized, depending on the clinical circumstances.

Early delivery is often the treatment of choice when fetal lung maturity has been attained.

Pregnancy Course   Intrauterine growth retardation places the fetus at significant risk for stillbirth or hypoxic damage to the central nervous system (CNS). Oligohydramnios is a later manifestation of severe IUGR.

Pregnancy Termination Issues   Not applicable to this clinical circumstance.

Delivery   The site for delivery must be one with the capabilities to manage premature or compromised infants.

NEONATOLOGY

Resuscitation   Growth retarded fetuses, in general, are less tolerant of the stress of labor and are more prone to experience asphyxia than normally grown fetuses. They are, therefore, more likely to require immediate resuscitation, particularly if delivery is either preterm or postterm. The more severe the growth retardation, the greater the risk for severe asphyxia. Any special techniques required relate to the etiology of the growth retardation.

Transport   Indications for referral to a tertiary perinatal center are very low birth weight (less than 1.5 kg), very early gestation (less than 32 weeks), concomitant illness or life-threatening complications or associated organ malformations. Care during transport will be determined by the indication for referral.

Testing and Confirmation   Establishing an etiologic diagnosis, if such was not completed prior to delivery, is important and difficult, as there are myriad causes, many of which cannot be excluded definitively. In some large series of IUGR, a definite etiology cannot be determined in more than half of instances. A careful physical examination and review of the maternal social, medical, and obstetrical history are the first and most important diagnostic steps. Further evaluations—serologic testing, radiographic imaging, chemical analysis, karyotyping, and so on—will be determined by the information from the history and physical assessment.

Nursery Management   Care following birth is directed toward stabilization of cardiorespiratory function and recovery from perinatal asphyxia. As a group, IUGR infants are more prone to postasphyxial cardiovascular and CNS syndromes, hypoglycemia, polycythemia, and coagulopathies. Other neonatal problems are dependent upon the etiology of the growth retardation and therefore, care requirements will vary with the specific diagnoses.

BIBLIOGRAPHY

Barros FC, Huttly SR, Victoria CG et al: Comparison of the causes and consequences of prematurity and intruterine growth retardation: a longitudinal study in southern Brazil. *Pediatrics* 1992; 90:238-244

Benson CB, Boswell SB, Brown DL et al: Improved prediction of intrauterine growth retardation with use of multiple parameters. *Radiology* 1988; 168:7-12.

Brown HL, Miller JM Jr, Gabert HA et al: Ultrasonic recognition of the small-for-gestational-age fetus. *Obstet Gynecol* 1987; 69:631-635.

Davies BR, Casanueva E, Arroyo P: Placentas of small-for-dates infants: a small controlled series from Mexico City, Mexico. *Am J Obstet Gynecol* 1984; 149:731-736.

Gulmezoglu AM, Ekici E: Sonographic diagnosis of Neu-Laxova syndrome. *J Clin Ultrasound* 1994; 22:48-51.

Khoury MJ, Erickson JD, Cordero JF et al: Congenital malformations and intrauterine growth retardation: a population study. *Pediatrics* 1988; 82:83-90.

Kramer MS, Olivier M, McLean FH et al: Impact of intrauterine growth retardation and body proportionality on fetal and neonatal outcome. *Pediatrics* 1990; 86:707-713.

Medchill MT, Peterson CM, Kreinick C et al: Prediction of estimated fetal weight in extremely low birth weight neonates (500-1000 g). *Obstet Gynecol* 1991; 78:286-290.

Ott WJ: Defining altered fetal growth by second-trimester sonography. *Obstet Gynecol* 1990; 75:1053-1059.

Villar J, de Onis M, Kestler E et al: The differential neonatal morbidity of the intrauterine growth retardation syndrome. *Am J Obstet Gynecol* 1990; 163:151-157.

Warshaw JB: Intrauterine growth retardation. *Pediatr Rev* 1986; 8:107-114.

Yogman MW, Kraemer HC, Kindlon D et al: Identification of intrauterine growth retardation among low birth weight preterm infants. *J Pediatr* 1989; 115:799-807.

13.4 MACROSOMIA

EPIDEMIOLOGY/GENETICS

Definition   Macrosomia is defined as a birth weight of 4500 g or greater (4000 g or greater in diabetics) or as a weight that is over the 90th percentile for gestational age.

Epidemiology   Macrosomic infants account for 1% to 2% of all deliveries. Significant risk factors are advanced maternal age, multiparity, obesity, maternal diabetes, and gestational age greater than 42 weeks.

Embryology   The mechanisms that result in excessive fetal growth are unknown. Patients with glucose intolerance (gestational diabetes or overt diabetes) are at significant risk for this complication.

Inheritance Patterns   Although no precise genetic mechanism has been elucidated, a previous delivery of a macrosomic infant is associated with a markedly increased risk in subsequent pregnancies.

Prognosis   Providing delivery problems, such as birth trauma, do not occur, the long-term prognosis is good.

SONOGRAPHY

Findings
1. **Fetus:** Skin thickening, without a central echopenic component as is seen in hydrops, is usually present.
2. **Amniotic Fluid:** Mild polyhydramnios is usually present and may be the presenting finding.
3. **Placenta:** The placenta is usually unaffected.
4. **Measurement Data:** All measurement data, especially the abdominal circumference, are larger than usual (above the 90th percentile). The cheek to cheek ratio is helpful; babies with fat cheeks are usually macrosomic. A study at 35 weeks may be valuable in deciding on early induction at 38 weeks.
5. **When Detectable:** Increased fetal size first becomes apparent at about 28 weeks. Polyhydramnios may be seen earlier when it is subsequently shown to be related to macrosomia.

Pitfalls   Measurement data for large babies is often inaccurate in weight estimation by as much as 700 gms.

Differential Diagnosis   Hydropic skin thickening—there will be an echopenic subdermal area with hydrops. Pleural effusion and ascites will be seen. Although several of the genetic syndromes with excessive fetal growth (Beckwith-Wiedemann syndrome, Weaver syndrome, Sotos' syndrome) may be confused with "benign" macrosomia, the obstetric management would not be modified in most circumstances. A prospective diagnosis is possi-

ble for Beckwith-Wiedemann syndrome if an omphalocele is present, but unlikely for the other overgrowth syndromes.

Where Else to Look
1. Some fetuses with macrosomia have mothers who have diabetes mellitus known to be associated with the vertebral abnormalities, anal atresia, cardiac abnormalities, tracheoesophageal fistula and esophageal atresia, renal agenesis and dysplasia, and limb defects (VACTERL) syndrome. A detailed look at the heart, spine, gut, and kidneys is required.
2. Look for large tongue, enlarged liver and kidneys, the features of Beckwith-Wiedemann syndrome.

PREGNANCY MANAGEMENT

Investigations and Consultations Required   Fetal echocardiography should be performed to exclude cardiac malformations. Consultation with a neonatologist to plan perinatal management is appropriate. Assessment of maternal glucose tolerance should be done to exclude diabetes.

Fetal Intervention   None is indicated.

Monitoring   If the patient is found to have gestational diabetes, maternal dietary control may slow the rate of fetal growth. However, by definition this diagnosis will not be made until late in pregnancy at which time management options are limited.

Pregnancy Course   There is a significant risk of birth trauma, and shoulder dystocia, long-term neurologic complications, and perinatal death.

Pregnancy Termination Issues   Not applicable.

Delivery   Some authors have recommended pursuing cesarean section if estimated fetal weight is 4700 g or more. If vaginal delivery is attempted, a physician experienced in the management of shoulder dystocia should be present and appropriate anesthesia and pediatric support should be available. Delivery should occur in a tertiary center.

NEONATOLOGY

Resuscitation   The risk for fetal distress is higher than for infants of normal birth weight and is related both to pregnancy complications resulting in fetal overgrowth and to the size of the infant. A resuscitation team should be present for the delivery of any infant anticipated to weigh 4.5 kg or more. No special techniques are required. Tension on the neck and upper extremities should be avoided until brachial plexus injury has been excluded by careful physical examination.

Transport   Referral to a tertiary perinatal center is indicated only if neonatal complications develop or congenital malformations are suspected.

Nursery Management   Admission to a special care nursery for observation during the early transition period is advisable and mandatory if maternal diabetes or postterm delivery (after 42 completed weeks) are etiological factors. Soft tissue injury—bruising, brachial plexus injury, respiratory distress, hypoglycemia, polycythemia, and hyperbilirubinemia are the more common neonatal problems irrespective of the maternal factors present. In addition, postasphyxial organ injury syndromes are more likely with postmaturity. Cyanosis unrelieved by oxygen in a macrosomic infant should be considered a neonatal emergency requiring immediate evaluation for cardiac defects. In the absence of pregnancy or intrapartum complications the nursery course is usually benign.

BIBLIOGRAPHY

Abramowicz JS, Sherer DM, Woods JR Jr: Ultrasonographic measurement of cheek-to-cheek diameter in fetal growth disturbances. *Am J Obstet Gynecol* 1993; 169:405-408.

Ballard JL, Rosenn B, Khoury JC, et al: Diabetic fetal macrosomia: Significance of disproportionate growth. *J Pediatr* 1993; 122:115-119.

Benson CB, Doubilet PM, Saltzman DH: Sonographic determination of fetal weights in diabetic pregnancies. *Am J Obstet Gynecol* 1987; 156:441-444.

Chervenak JL, Divon MY, Hirsch J, et al: Macrosomia in the postdate pregnancy: is routine ultrasonographic screening indicated? *Am J Obstet Gynecol* 1989; 161:753-756.

Jovanovic-Peterson L, Peterson CM, Reed GF, et al: Maternal postprandial glucose levels and infant birth weight: National Institute of Child Health and Human Development—diabetes in early pregnancy study. *Am J Obstet Gynecol* 1991; 164:103-111.

Leikin EL, Jenkins JH, Pomerantz GA, et al: Abnormal glucose screening tests in pregnancy: a risk factor for fetal macrosomia. *Obstet Gynecol* 1987; 69:570-573.

Lubchenco LO: The high risk infant. In: *The infant who is large for gestational age.* Philadelphia. WB Saunders, 1976.

Sacks DA: Fetal macrosomia and gestational diabetes: What's the problem? *Obstet Gynecol* 1993; 81:775-781.

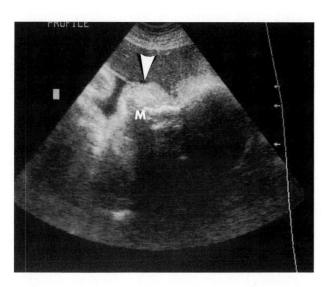

Macrosomia. The fetal skin is thick and the cheeks are prominent (*arrow*). M, mouth.

13.5 Oligohydramnios

EPIDEMIOLOGY/GENETICS

Definition Diminished amniotic fluid volume for a given gestational age.

Epidemiology Common.

Teratogens Indomethacin, used to inhibit labor, can induce oligohydramnios.

Screening Increased alpha-fetoprotein (AFP) may be due to oligohydramnios.

Prognosis Poor with first and second trimester oligohydramnios. Oligohydramnios in a normally grown fetus, occurring for the first time in the third trimester, usually carries a good prognosis.

SONOGRAPHY

Findings
1. **Fetus:** Check for renal problems such as infantile polycystic kidney disease, bilateral renal obstruction, multicystic dysplastic disease, or renal agenesis.
2. **Amniotic Fluid:** The severity of the oligohydramnios depends on the underlying process. Normal standards for amniotic fluid exist, based on the amniotic fluid index. The amniotic fluid index is measured in the following fashion: the pregnant uterus is arbitrarily divided into four quadrants, a vertical measurement is made of the deepest uninterrupted fluid pocket in each quadrant, and the four measurements are added together.
3. **Placenta:** Appearance varies, depending on the underlying cause.
4. **Measurement Data:** If the oligohydramnios is associated with IUGR, all measurements, particularly the abdominal circumference, will be decreased. Often the fetal head is dolichocephalic—the head shape is long and thin.
5. **When Detectable:** Maternal control of amniotic fluid volume exists until somewhere between 14 and 20 weeks, so oligohydramnios of fetal origin may not be evident until 20 weeks. Oligohydramnios related to premature rupture of membranes (PROM), chorionic villus sampling (CVS), or severe IUGR can present early in the second trimester.

Pitfalls
1. Amniotic fluid volume normally decreases markedly in the late third trimester.
2. The amniotic fluid index is a very subjective method of measuring the amount of fluid. Two examiners can come up with different results, depending on the fetal alignment, within a short interval.

Where Else to Look
1. Renal causes—Look for absence of the kidneys, obstructed or dysplastic kidneys, and abnormally large kidneys, as with infantile polycystic kidney or adult polycystic kidney disease.
2. All measurement data may be decreased if there is IUGR.
3. Check the cervix for cervical incompetence. The bladder should be empty. A translabial or endovaginal approach should be used, so the whole length of the cervix can be seen. If there is PROM, the cervix will be short (less than 2.7 cm) and the internal os will have some fluid within it.
4. The presence of fetal breathing is reported to decrease the likelihood of pulmonary hypoplasia.
5. Due to the decreased amniotic fluid, club feet and deviated hands develop. Limb changes are hard to see because they only develop when there is almost no fluid.

PREGNANCY MANAGEMENT

Investigations and Consultation Required Amnioinfusion—If the cause of the decreased fluid is not apparent with sonography and there is little or no fluid present, instillation of a mixture of ringer solution, dextrose, and indigo carmine may be helpful. About 150 to 250 ml are instilled. The increased "amniotic fluid" will allow better visualization of the fetus. If there is an amniotic fluid leak, the indigo carmine will stain a tampon left in the vagina. Additionally, the fetus will drink the fluid and the stomach and bladder will fill, if the kidneys are functioning. A false-positive diagnosis of ruptured membranes may occur if fluid is instilled in the extraamniotic space.

Monitoring
1. Renal—If fluid disappears altogether, lung development is impaired or absent. If there is severe bilateral obstructive renal disease, sonograms every 2 to 3 weeks are required to check fluid volume.
2. PROM—The prognosis is very poor and the likelihood of hypoplastic lungs and limb contractures is high. However, in rare cases of PROM, resealing of membranes has been reported. Sonograms every 2 weeks will show if there is increased fluid accumulation.
3. IUGR—Severe IUGR and oligohydramnios at an early stage, that is 23 weeks, have a poor prognosis and usually fetal death ensues. Sonograms every 2 weeks, accompanied by twice-weekly biophysical profiles are recommended. Timing for delivery will depend on the findings of the parameters of fetal well-being such as biophysical profile, nonstress test, and Doppler (see Chapter 13).

Delivery Delivery should occur in a tertiary center.

BIBLIOGRAPHY

Barss VA, Benacerraf BR, Frigoletto FD Jr: Second trimester oligo-hydramnios, a predictor of poor fetal outcome. *Obstet Gynecol* 1984; 64:608-610.

Blott M, Greenough A, Nicolaides KH et al: The ultrasonographic assessment of the fetal thorax and fetal breathing movements in the prediction of pulmonary hypoplasia. *Early Human Devel* 1990; 21:143-151.

Bronshtein M, Blumenfeld Z: First- and early second-trimester oligohydramnios—a predictor of poor fetal outcome except in iatrogenic oligohydramnios post chorionic villus biopsy. *Ultrasound Obstet Gynecol* 1991; 1:245-249.

Fisk NM, Ronderos-Dumit D, Soliani A et al: Diagnostic and therapeutic transabdominal amnioinfusion in oligohydramnios. *Obstet Gynecol* 1991; 78:270-278.

Hill LM, Breckle R, Gehrking WC: The variable effects of oligohy-dramnios on the biparietal diameter and the cephalic index. *J Ultrasound Med* 1984; 3:93-95.

Horsager R, Nathan L, Leveno KJ: Correlation of measured amni-otic fluid volume and sonographic preductions of oligohy-dramnios. *Obstet Gynecol* 1994; 83:955-958.

Mandell J, Peters CA, Estroff JA et al: Late onset severe oligohy-dramnios associated with genitourinary abnormalities. *J Urol* 1992; 148:515-518.

Mercer LJ, Brown LG: Fetal outcome with oligohydramnios in the second trimester. *Obstet Gynecol* 1986; 67:840-842.

13.6 Polyhydramnios

EPIDEMIOLOGY/GENETICS

Definition   Excess amniotic fluid for the stage of pregnancy.

Epidemiology   Polyhydramnos is present in about 1% of pregnancies. It is particularly common in diabetes mellitus and in obese women. In about 20% of cases, it is associated with a serious fetal anomaly.

Embryology   In many instances, it is due to defective or obstructed fetal ingestion of amniotic fluid.

Prognosis   Dependent upon underlying cause.

SONOGRAPHY

Findings
1. **Fetus:** With polyhydramnios related to maternal obesity or diabetes mellitus, the fetus is enlarged (macrosomic). Polyhydramnios may precede the macrosomia.
2. **Amniotic Fluid:**   The amniotic fluid volume is increased and there will be an amniotic fluid index of over 20. In the late third trimester, an amniotic fluid index of 15 or more is suggestive of polyhydramnios, because the fluid volume normally decreases.
3. **Placenta:** Often appears thin as it is spread over a wider area.
4. **Measurement Data:** Depends on the underlying cause, but often increased.
5. **When Detectable:** Polyhydramnios may be seen at about 16 weeks, but is rare before 25 weeks gestation.

Pitfalls
1. The amniotic fluid normally decreases in the third trimester, so polyhydramnios may be present with indices of under 20 in the late third trimester.
2. A single large pocket may give a spuriously low amniotic fluid index because only one or two vertical fluid measurements will be counted in the amniotic fluid index.

Where Else to Look:
1. Look in the gastrointestinal tract for obstruction—There will be dilated loops of bowel at most levels with obstruction. The most severe polyhydramnios occurs with proximal obstruction, as with tracheoesophageal atresia when the stomach may not be seen.
2. Look in the chest or abdomen for a compressing mass as with congenital adenatoid malformation, diaphragmatic hernia, or severe ureteropelvic junction obstruction.
3. Look for intracranial malformations that result in defective swallowing, for example, holoprosencephaly or anencephaly.
4. Look for short-limbed dwarfism—The limbs will be very short and the chest will be small, so there will be secondary esophageal compression. Look for limb contractures in congenital arthrogryposis syndromes.
5. All measurement data may be increased as in macrosomia. This is the most common association of polyhydramnios.

PREGNANCY MANAGEMENT

Investigations and Consultation Required   Many of the entities that cause polyhydramnios, such as duodenal atresia or tracheoesophageal fistula are associated with karyotypic abnormalities. There is debate as to whether isolated polyhydramnios warrants amniocentesis, with most feeling that karyotypic analysis is not necessary if there is no sonographic fetal abnormality or growth deficiency.

Fetal Intervention   Very severe polyhydramnios, with resultant maternal respiratory inhibition may warrant repeated withdrawal of amniotic fluid in quantities of several liters at a time. Indomethacin will reduce fetal urine output, and secondarily, amniotic fluid volume, and may delay delivery in severe cases. Three fetal side effects have been reported: 1. premature closure of the ductus arteriosus; 2. necrotizing enterocolitis; and 3. neonatal oliguria.

Monitoring   Sonograms every 2 to 3 weeks are desirable to monitor the amount of amniotic fluid and to institute early treatment of preterm labor.

Delivery   The site of delivery should be a tertiary center in all cases with severe polyhydramnios. In the absence of structural malformation, mild polyhydramnios should not alter obstetric management.

BIBLIOGRAPHY

Carlson DE, Platt LD, Medearis AL et al: Quantifiable polyhydramnios: diagnosis and management. *Obstet Gynecol* 1990; 75:989-992.

Hill LM, Breckle R, Thomas ML et al: Polyhydramnios: ultrasonically detected prevalence and neonatal outcome. *Obstet Gynecol* 1987; 69:21-25.

Sivit CJ, Hill MC, Larsen JW et al: Second-trimester polyhydramnios: evaluation with US. *Radiology* 1987; 165:467-469.

Stoll CG, Alembik Y, Dott B: Study of 156 cases of polyhydramnios and congenital malformations in a series of 118,265 consecutive births. *J Obstet Gynecol* 1991; 165:586-590.

Appendices

APPENDIX 1 DIFFERENTIAL DIAGNOSES OF ABNORMAL IN UTERO SONOGRAPHIC FINDINGS

ABDOMINAL WALL PROCESS

Omphalocele
Gastroschisis
Physiological gut herniation (8 to 12 weeks)
Amniotic band syndrome
Umbilical hernia

Amyloplasia congenita
Beckwith-Wiedemann syndrome
Bladder exstrophy
Limb-body wall complex
Pentalogy of Cantrell
Vesicoallantoic cyst

ABSENT BLADDER

Following voiding
Renal agenesis (bilateral)
Technical—obese patient and prone fetus

Bladder exstrophy
Infantile polycystic kidney disease
Severe intrauterine growth retardation

STOMACH NONVISUALIZATION

Diaphragmatic hernia (left sided)
Normal variant
Tracheoesophageal atresia or fistula/esophageal atresia

CNS problems that prevent swallowing
Facial cleft
Micrognathia

ASCITES (ISOLATED)

Renal obstruction

Lymphatic—Turner's
Meconium peritonitis
Midgut volvulus
Small-bowel atresia

DILATED STOMACH AND DUODENUM

Duodenal atresia
Normal variant

Annular pancreas
Antral web
Diabetic embryopathy
Fetal anticonvulsant syndrome
Focal femoral deficiency
Fryns syndrome
Gut malrotation
Townes-Brock syndrome

ECHOGENIC AREA IN ABDOMEN

Echogenic Mass
Adrenal hemorrhage
Dysplastic second collecting system
Extralobar sequestration
Hepatic tumor
Intragut or intraabdominal bleed
Neuroblastoma
Ovarian cyst with hemorrhage

Echogenic Bowel
Cystic fibrosis
Intragut or intraabdominal bleed
Meconium in the third trimester
Normal variant
Trisomy 21

Fetal infections (cytomegalovirus)
Meconium peritonitis
Other chromosomal abnormality

Calcification
Normal variant

Fetal infections (cytomegalovirus, toxoplasmosis)
Gallstones
Idiopathic arterial calcification
Teratoma (intrapelvic or in adrenal region)

HYDRONEPHROSIS

Ectopic ureter
Multicystic dysplastic kidney (hydronephrotic form)
Posterior urethral valves
Reflux
Ureterocele and ectopic ureter
Ureteropelvic junction obstruction
Ureterovesicle junction obstruction

Apert syndrome
Bladder exstrophy
Chromosome—trisomy 13 and 21
Cloacal extrophy
Ectrodactyly–ectodermal dysplasia–clefting syndrome
Fraser syndrome (cryptophthalmos)
Hemifacial microsomia (Goldenhar's syndrome)
McKusik-Kaufman syndrome
Megacystis megaureter
Megacystis microcolon
Sacrococcygeal teratoma

INTRAABDOMINAL CYST

Dilated bladder
Dilated bowel
Hydroureter
Ovarian cyst (in females)
Renal cystic lesions particularly UPJ with anterior pelvis or pelvic dysplastic kidney (see separate differential)

Choledochal cyst
Duodenal atresia, anal atresia, gut atresia
Enteric duplication cyst
Hepatic arterioventricular malformation
Hydrometrocolpos
Liver cyst
Lymphangioma
McKusik-Kaufman syndrome
Meckels diverticulum
Meconium pseudocyst
Mesenteric cyst
Rectal dilation
Sacrococcygeal (cystic) teratoma
Splenic cyst
Umbilical vein varix
Urachal cyst

ABNORMAL KIDNEY

Horseshoe kidney
Pelvic kidney

Adrenal hemorrhage
Baller-Gerold syndrome
Beckwith-Wiedemann syndrome—large kidneys
Chromosome—trisomy 13–horseshoe

Continued
Chromosome—trisomy 18–horseshoe
Chromosome—45,X (Turner's syndrome)–horseshoe
Diabetic embryopathy
Pancake kidney
Wilms' tumor

POSSIBLE SUPRARENAL MASS

Adrenal hematoma
Duplex collecting system

Hepatoblastoma
Liver cyst
Neuroblastoma
Extrapulmonary sequestration

OMPHALOCELE

Amniotic band syndrome
Chromosome—trisomy 13
Isolated
Umbilical hernia

Beckwith-Wiedemann syndrome
CHARGE association
Chromosome—triploidy
Chromosome—trisomy 18
Meckel-Gruber syndrome
Pentalogy of Cantrell
Short-rib–polydactyly syndromes—various types

RENAL AGENESIS

Isolated
VACTERL association

Chromosome—trisomy 21 (Down syndrome)
Diabetic embryopathy
Fraser syndrome (cryptophthalmos)
Hemifacial microsomia (Goldenhar syndrome)
Limb-body wall complex
Smith-Lemli-Opitz syndrome
Townes-Brock syndrome
Turner's syndrome
Twin-twin transfusion syndrome

CYSTIC KIDNEY DISEASE

Multicystic dysplastic kidney
Severe hydronephrosis in single or double systems

Adult polycystic kidney
Apert syndrome
Chromosome—trisomy 13
Chromosome—trisomy 18

Continued
Ellis van Creveld syndrome (chondroectodermal dysplasia)
Fryns syndrome
Infantile polycystic kidney disease
Jeune asphyxiating thoracic dystrophy
McKusik-Kaufman syndrome
Meckel-Gruber syndrome
Oralfacial-digital syndrome—various types (microcysts)
Roberts' syndrome
Short-rib–polydactyly syndromes—various types
Smith-Lemli-Opitz syndrome
Tuberous sclerosis
Zellweger syndrome

CARDIAC ABNORMALITY

Chromosome—trisomy 18
Chromosome—trisomy 21 (Down syndrome)
Noonan syndrome
VACTERL association

CHARGE Association
Chromosome—triploidy
Chromosome—trisomy 13
Chromosome—4p- (Wolf-Hirschhorn)
Chromosome—45,X (Turner's syndrome)
Cornelia de Lange syndrome
Diabetic embryopathy
DiGeorge syndrome (includes velocardiofacial syndrome)
Ellis-van Creveld syndrome (chondroectodermal dysplasia)
Fanconi's syndrome
Fetal alcohol syndrome
Fetal infections
Hemifacial microsomia (Goldenhar's syndrome)
Holt-Oram syndrome
Ivemark's—situs inversus
McKusik-Kaufman syndrome
Maternal phenylketonuria
Meckel-Gruber syndrome
Retinoic acid embryopathy
Roberts' syndrome
Short-rib–polydactyly syndromes
Smith-Lemli-Opitz syndrome
Thrombocytopenia-absent radius syndrome
Tuberous sclerosis
Velocardiofacial syndrome

CARDIAC MASS

Papillary muscles/echogenicity
Rhabdomyoma (Tuberous sclerosis)

Continued
Basal cell nevus syndrome (Gorlin syndrome)
Fibroma
Hypertrophic cardiomyopathy
Valve prolapse

CHEST MASS

Cystic Masses
Cystadenomatoid malformation of lung
Diaphragmatic hernia

Alimentary duplications
Enlarged cardiac chamber
Klippel-Trenaunay-Weber syndrome
Mediastinal teratoma
Neurenteric cyst
Pericardial cyst
Tracheal atresia

Solid Masses
Cystadenomatoid malformation of lung

Cardiac tumor—rhabdomyoma
Chest-wall hematoma
Diaphragmatic hernia
Klippel-Trenaunay-Weber syndrome
Mediastinal teratoma
Pulmonary sequestration

PERICARDIAL EFFUSION

Cardiac malformation
Dysrhythmia
Early sign of anemia—Rh, parvovirus, and alpha thalassemia
Early sign of hydrops
Normal echopenic rim

Cardiac tumor
Chromosome—45,X (Turner's syndrome)
Confusion with pleural effusion

PLEURAL EFFUSION

Chylothorax
Earliest sign of hydrops (secondary to hydrops)

Chromosome—Trisomy 21 (Down syndrome) (secondary to hydrops)
Chromosome—45,X (Turner's syndrome) (secondary to hydrops)
Hemothorax
Pulmonary sequestration

SMALL CHEST

Osteogenesis Imperfecta—type II
Thanatophoric dysplasia

Achondrogenesis—all types
Achondroplasia
Atelosteogenesis—all types
Campomelic dysplasia
Chondrodysplasia punctata
Ellis-van Creveld syndrome (chondroectodermal dysplasia)
Fibrochondrogenesis
Hypophosphatasia
Jeune asphyxiating thoracic dystrophy
Multiple pterygium syndrome—lethal
Short-rib–polydactyly syndromes—all type
Spondyloepiphyseal dysplasia congenita (SED congenita)

AGENESIS OF THE CORPUS CALLOSUM

Dandy-Walker cyst
Isolated

Acrocallosal syndrome
Apert syndrome
Basal cell nevus syndrome (Gorlin syndrome)
Cleft lip/palate—ectrodactyly
Chromosome—trisomy 13
Chromosome—trisomy 18
Chromosome—trisomy 21 (Down syndrome)
Encephalocele
Fetal alcohol syndrome
Fetal infections
Hydrolethalus
Meckel-Gruber syndrome
Neu-Laxova syndrome
Smith-Lemli-Opitz syndrome
Thanatophoric dysplasia
Tuberous sclerosis
Warburg syndrome

BRAIN TOO EASILY SEEN

Osteogenesis imperfecta, type II

Achondrogenesis—some types
Acrania
Hypophosphatasia

CEREBELLAR HYPOPLASIA

Dandy-Walker cyst
Spinal dysraphism

Continued
Chromosome—trisomy 13
Chromosome—trisomy 18
Chromosome—trisomy 21 (Down syndrome)
Fetal infections
Fetal vitamin A syndrome
Joubert syndrome
Meckel-Gruber syndrome
Neu-Laxova syndrome
Smith-Lemli-Opitz syndrome
Warburg syndrome

DANDY-WALKER CYST

Aicardi's syndrome
Alcohol
Chromosome—triploidy
Chromosome—trisomy 13
Chromosome—trisomy 18
Cytomegalovirus
Cornelia de Lange syndrome
Diabetes
Ellis-van Creveld
Fetal infections (cytomegalovirus)
Meckel-Gruber syndrome
Neural tube defect
Rubella
Toxoplasmosis
Warburg syndrome

ECHOGENIC BRAIN FOCUS OR FOCI

Cerebellar vermis
Choroid plexus

Fetal infections (cytomegalovirus [wall of lateral ventricles] and toxoplasmosis)
Gyri in third trimester
Intrabrain hemorrhage when fresh
Intracranial tumor (teratoma)
Neu-Laxova syndrome
Tuberous sclerosis

ENCEPHALOCELE

Amniotic band syndrome—asymmetrical top of the head lesions
Isolated

Apert syndrome
Chemtel syndrome
Chromosome—trisomy 13
Chromosome—trisomy 18
Crytophthalmos syndrome
Dandy-Walker cyst

Continued
Dysegmental dysplasia
Knoblock
Meckel-Gruber syndrome
Roberts' syndrome (pseudothalidomide)
Von Vos
Warburg syndrome

HOLOPROSENCEPHALY

Chromosome—trisomy 13
Isolated

Aicardi syndrome
Campomelic dysplasia
CHARGE association
Chromosome—triploidy
Chromosome—trisomy 18
Chromosome—18p-
Diabetic embryopathy
DiGeorge syndrome (includes velocardiofacial syndrome)
Focal femoral deficiency
Frontonasal dysplasia
Fryns syndrome
Hemifacial microsomia (Goldenhar syndrome)
Meckel-Gruber syndrome
Short-rib–polydactyly syndromes
Smith-Lemli-Opitz syndrome

HYDRANENCEPHALY

Fetal infections
Isolated
Stuck twin (death of co-twin)

Cocaine embryopathy
Familial hydranencephaly (autosomal recessive)

INTRACRANIAL CYST

Arachnoid cyst
Cavum vergi
Choroid plexus cyst
Cisterna magna
Dandy-Walker cyst
Large cavum septum pelucidum
Quadrigeminal cistern

Cyst associated with agenesis of corpus callosum
Cystic encephalomalacia
Intracranial teratoma
Periventricular leukomalacia
Porencephalic cyst
Posterior fossa extraaxial cyst
Schizencephaly

Continued
Subdural hygroma
Unilateral hydrocephalus
Vein of Galen aneurysm

KLEEBLATTSCHÄDEL DEFORMITY OF SKULL (CLOVERLEAF SKULL)

Apert syndrome
Pfeiffer syndrome
Thanatophoric dysplasia

Amniotic band syndrome
Campomelic dysplasia
Crouzon syndrome

MACROCEPHALY

Familial macrocephaly
Ventriculomegaly

Achondrogenesis—all types
Achondroplasia
Basal-cell-nevus syndrome (Gorlin syndrome)
Beckwith-Wiedemann syndrome
Chromosome—triploidy (relative enlargement)
Greig's cephalopolysyndactyly syndrome
Intracranial tumor
Sotos syndrome
Thanatophoric dysplasia
Vein of Galen aneurysm

MICROCEPHALY

Drugs (alcohol, hydantoin, aminopterin)
Fetal infections (cytomegalovirus, toxoplasmosis, rubella)
Isolated
Spina bifida

Atrophy
Chromosome—triploidy
Chromosome—trisomy 13
Chromosome—trisomy 18
Chromosome—trisomy 21
Cornelia de Lange syndrome
Craniosynostosis—asymmetric head or cloverleaf skull
Encephalocele
Holoprosencephaly
Hydranencephaly
Maternal phenylketonuria
Meckel-Gruber syndrome
Neu-Laxova syndrome
Seckel syndrome
Smith-Lemli-Opitz syndrome
X-linked microcephaly

MILD VENTRICULOMEGALY (LATERAL VENTRICLE WIDTH > 10 MM)

Arnold Chiari malformation (neural tube defect)
Dandy-Walker malformation
Encephalocele
Normal variant

Agenesis of the corpus callosum (colpocephaly)
Amniotic band syndrome
Apert syndrome
Aqueductal stenosis (X-linked hydrocephalus)
Arachnoid cysts
Baller-Gerold syndrome
Camptomelic dysplasia
Chromosome—triploidy
Chromosome—trisomy 13
Chromosome—trisomy 18
Chromosome—trisomy 21 (Down syndrome)
Fetal alcohol syndrome
Fetal infections (cytomegalovirus and toxoplasmosis)
Fragile X
Holoprosencephaly
Hydrolethalis
Intracranial bleed
Jeune asphyxiating thoracic dystrophy
Meckel-Gruber syndrome
Neoplasms
Osteogenesis imperfecta, type II
Roberts' syndrome (pseudothalidomide)
Short-rib–polydactyly syndromes
Smith-Lemli-Opitz
Thanatophoric dysplasia
Vein of Galen aneurysm
Warburg syndrome

POSTERIOR FOSSA CYST

Arachnoid cyst (extraaxial cyst)
Dandy-Walker cyst
Dilated cisterna magna

Porencephalic cyst
Quadrigeminal cyst
Vein of Galen aneurysm

SPINAL DYSRAPHISM

Chromosome—triploidy
Chromosome—trisomy 18
Diabetic embryopathy
Isolated

Aminopterin
Amniotic band syndrome
Anencephaly
Chromosome—trisomy 13
Chromosome—trisomy 21 (Down syndrome)
Cloacal exstrophy

Continued
Diastematomyelia
Encephalocele
Fetal anticonvulsant syndrome (valproic acid)
Fetal vitamin A syndrome
Iniencephaly
Jarcho-Levin
Meckel-Gruber syndrome
Rachischisis
Roberts' syndrome (pseudothalidomide)
Sacrococcygeal teratoma
Warburg syndrome

CATARACT

Fetal infections (rubella, varicella, toxoplasmosis)

Neu-Laxova syndrome
Osteogenesis imperfecta—various types
Roberts' syndrome
Smith-Lemli-Opitz syndrome
Warburg syndrome
Zellweger syndrome

EXOPHTHALMUS/PROPTOSIS/PROMINENT EYES

Apert syndrome (acrocephalosyndactyly—type I)
Carpenter syndrome
Crouzon syndrome
Jackson-Weiss syndrome
Neu-Laxova syndrome
Pfeiffer syndrome
Saethre-Chotzen syndrome

HYPERTELORISM

Aarskog syndrome
Acrocallosal syndrome
Apert syndrome and other types of craniosynostosis
Atelosteogenesis
Chromosome—4p- (Wolf-Hirschhorn syndrome)
Crouzon syndrome
Frontal encephalocele
Frontonasal dysplasia
Greig's cephalopolysyndactyly syndrome
Noonan syndrome
Opitz hypertelorism hypospadias syndrome
Otopalatodigital syndrome
Pfeiffer syndrome
Robinow's syndrome (fetal face syndrome)

HYPOTELORISM

Holoprosencephaly

Baller-Gerold syndrome
Chromosome—trisomy 13

Continued
Chromosome—trisomy 18
Chromosome—18p-
Chromosome—duplication 20p
Hemifacial microsomia (Goldenhar's syndrome)
Meckel-Gruber syndrome
Trigonocephaly

MICROPHTHALMIA OR ANOPHTHALMIA

Chromosome—trisomy 13
Isolated

Chromosome—18q-
Fetal infections (rubella, varicella, toxoplasmosis)
Fraser syndrome
Goldenhar's syndrome (hemifacial microsomia)
Hydrolethalus
Hypoplasia of one side of the face
Meckel-Gruber syndrome
Neu-Laxova syndrome
Oculodentodigital syndrome
Warburg syndrome

FACIAL ASYMMETRY

Amniotic band syndrome with facial cleft
Craniosynostosis

Apert syndrome
Carpenter syndrome
Crouzon syndrome
Greig's cephalopolysyndactyly syndrome
Goldenhar's syndrome (hemifacial microsomia)
Jackson-Weiss syndrome
Pfeiffer syndrome
Saethre-Chotzen syndrome
Townes-Brock syndrome

CLEFT LIP AND PALATE

Amniotic band syndrome (L)
Chromosome—trisomy 13 (M,L,P)
Holoprosencephaly (M,L)
Isolated
Stickler syndrome (P)

Apert syndrome (acrocephalosyndactyly)—various types (P)
Atelosteogenesis (P)
Camptomelic dysplasia (P)
CHARGE association (P)
Chromosome—triploidy (L,P)
Chromosome—trisomy 18 (L,P)
Crouzon syndrome (acrocephalosyndactyly) (P)
Diastrophic dysplasia (P)

M, midline cleft lip; L, lateral cleft lip; P, cleft palate only.

Continued
Ectrodactyly-ectodermal dysplasia-clefting syndrome (L,P)
Fetal anticonvulsant syndrome (L)
Fetal vitamin A syndrome (L,P)
Fryns syndrome (L,P)
Hemifacial microsomia (Goldenhar syndrome) (L,P)
Maternal phenylketonuria (P)
Meckel-Gruber syndrome (M,L,P)
Multiple pterygium syndrome—lethal (P)
Orofacial-digital syndrome—various types (M,L,P)
Roberts' syndrome (L,P)
Robinow's syndrome (L,P)
Short-rib–polydactyly syndromes—various types (L,P)
Spondyloepiphyseal dysplasia congenita (SED congenita) (P)
Treacher Collins syndrome (P)
Velocardiofacial syndrome/DiGeorge sequence (P)

MACROGLOSSIA

Beckwith-Wiedemann syndrome
Chromosome—trisomy 21 (Down syndrome)
Oral teratoma

MALFORMED EARS

Chromosome—trisomy 18

Acrofacial dysostoses (microtia)
Branchiootorenal syndrome
CHARGE association
Chromosome—4p- (tags) (Wolf-Hirschhorn)
Fetal vitamin A syndrome
Hemifacial microsomia (Goldenhar syndrome) (tags, microtia)
Oligohydramnios sequence with large ears
Townes-Brock syndrome (tags)
Treacher Collins syndrome (tags)(microtia)

MICROGNATHIA

Chromosome—trisomy 18
Pierre Robin sequence
Stickler syndrome

Acrofacial dysostoses—various types
Arthrogryposis
Atelosteogenesis
Camptomelic dysplasia
CHARGE association
Chromosome—trisomy 13
Diastrophic dysplasia
DiGeorge syndrome (includes velocardiofacial syndrome)
Fetal alcohol syndrome

Continued
Fetal anticonvulsant syndrome (valproic acid)
Fetal vitamin A syndrome
Focal femoral deficiency—unusual facies
Freeman-Sheldon syndrome (whistling facies)
Fryns syndrome
Harlequin syndrome
Hemifacial microsomia (Goldenhar syndrome)
Hypoglossia—hypodactyly
Multiple pterygium syndrome
Orofacial-digital syndrome—various types
Otocephaly
Pena-Shokeir syndrome
Seckel syndrome
Short-rib–polydactyly syndromes—various types
Smith-Lemli-Opitz syndrome
Treacher Collins syndrome

SHORT NOSE

Chromosome—trisomy 18
Chromosome—trisomy 21 (Down syndrome)
Holoprosencephaly
Stickler syndrome

Aarskog syndrome
Apert syndrome
Cornelia de Lange syndrome
Fetal alcohol syndrome
Fetal anticonvulsant syndrome
Fetal warfarin syndrome
Miller-Dieker syndrome
Osteogenesis imperfecta, type II
Pfeiffer syndrome
Robinow's syndrome
Smith-Lemli-Opitz syndrome

ABNORMAL THUMB

Diabetic embryopathy
Holt-Oram syndrome
VACTERL association

Acrofacial dysostoses—various types
Apert syndrome (acrocephalosyndactyly, type I)
Baller-Gerold syndrome
Carpenter syndrome (acrocephalopolysyndactyly, type II)
Chromosome—trisomy 13
Chromosome—trisomy 18
Cornelia de Lange syndrome
Diastrophic dysplasia
Ectrodactyly-tibial aplasia syndrome
Fanconi's syndrome
Greig's cephalopolysyndactyly syndrome
Hemifacial microsomia (Goldenhar's syndrome)
Orofacial-digital syndrome—various types
Pfeiffer syndrome (acrocephalosyndactyly, type V)
Poland anomaly

Continued
Rubinstein-Taybi syndrome
Smith-Lemli-Opitz syndrome
Townes-Brock syndrome

ABSENT DIGITS

Amniotic band syndrome
Poland anomaly
Terminal transverse limb defect

Acrofacial dysostoses—various types
Atelosteogenesis
Baller-Gerold syndrome
Carpenter syndrome (acrocephalopolysyndactyly, type II)
Chromosome—triploidy
Chromosome—trisomy 18
Cornelia de Lange syndrome
Ectrodactyly-ectodermal dysplasia-clefting syndrome
Ectrodactyly-tibial aplasia syndrome
Fanconi's syndrome
Fryn's syndrome
Holt-Oram syndrome
Oromandibular limb hypogenesis
Pfeiffer syndrome (acrocephalosyndactyly, type V)
Roberts' syndrome (pseudothalidomide)
Smith-Lemli-Opitz syndrome
Townes-Brock syndrome
VACTERL association

ABSENT LIMBS

Amniotic band syndrome
Diabetic embryopathy
Limb body wall complex

Acrofacial dysostoses—various types
Atelosteogenesis
Cornelia de Lange syndrome
Ectrodactyly-ectodermal dysplasia-clefting syndrome
Fetal alcohol syndrome
Grebe syndrome
Holt-Oram syndrome
Oromandibular limb hypogenesis
Poland anomaly
Roberts' syndrome (pseudothalidomide)
Sirenomelia
Thalidomide embryopathy
Thrombocytopenia-absent radius syndrome

BOWING

Camptomelic dysplasia—particularly tibia and femur
Osteogenesis Imperfecta—type II, particularly tibia and femur
Thanatophoric dysplasia

Continued
Achondrogenesis
Boomerang dysplasia
Chondroectoterminal dysplasia
Diabetic embryopathy
Diastrophic dysplasia
Dyssegmental dysplasia
Fibrochondrogenesis
Focal femoral deficiency—only involves tibia and femur
Hypophosphatasia
Normal (if femur scanned from medial aspect)
Oligohydramnios sequence
Roberts' syndrome
Spondyloepiphyseal dysplasia

CLENCHED HANDS

Arthrogryposis—various types
Chromosome—trisomy 18

Apert syndrome
Chromosome—trisomy 13
Congenital muscular dystrophy—various types
Fetal alcohol syndrome
Freeman-Sheldon syndrome
Multiple pterygium syndrome
Neu-Laxova syndrome
Pena-Shokeir syndrome

CLINODACTYLY

Chromosome—trisomy 18
Chromosome—trisomy 21 (Down syndrome)

Aarskog syndrome
Amniotic band syndrome
Camptomelic dysplasia
Carpenter syndrome (acrocephalopolysyndactyly, type II)
Chromosome—triploidy
Chromosome—trisomy 13
Cornelia de Lange syndrome
Ectrodactyly-ectodermal dysplasia-clefting syndrome
Fetal alcohol syndrome
Holt-Oram syndrome
Miller-Dieker syndrome
Orofacial-digital syndrome—various types
Pfeiffer syndrome (acrocephalosyndactyly, type V)
Poland anomaly
Roberts' syndrome
Saethre-Chotzen syndrome (acrocephalosyndactyly, type III)
Seckel syndrome
Townes-Brock syndrome
Treacher Collins syndrome

CLUB FOOT

Arthrogryposis—various types
Chromosome—trisomy 18
Isolated
Neural tube defect

Amniotic band syndrome
Amyloplasia congenita
Atelosteogenesis
Camptomelic dysplasia
Carpenter syndrome (acrocephalopolysyndactyly, type II)
Chondrodysplasia punctata (rhizomelic type) lethal
Chromosome—triploidy
Chromosome—18p-
Diabetic embryopathy
Diastrophic dysplasia
Distal arthrogryposis syndrome
Ellis-van Creveld syndrome (chondroectodermal dysplasia)
Focal femoral deficiency
Freeman-Sheldon syndrome (whistling face)
Fryns syndrome
Larsen syndrome
Meckel-Gruber syndrome
Multiple pterygium syndrome
Pena-Shokeir syndrome
Seckel syndrome
Short-rib–polydactyly syndromes—various types
Smith-Lemli-Opitz syndrome
Thrombocytopenia-absent radius syndrome (TAR)
Zellweger syndrome

FRACTURES

Osteogenesis imperfecta, all types

Achondrogenesis
Hypophosphatasia

JOINT CONTRACTURES

Arthrogryposis—various types
Caudal dysplasia sequence
Chromosome—trisomy 18

Amyloplasia congenita
Apert syndrome (acrocephalosyndactyly, type I)
Beals' syndrome (contractual arachnodactyly)
Chromosome—Triploidy
Chromosome—trisomy 13
Diabetic embryopathy
Diastrophic dysplasia
Distal arthrogryposis syndrome
Fetal alcohol syndrome
Focal femoral deficiency
Freeman-Sheldon syndrome

Continued
Multiple pterygium syndrome—various types
Neu-Laxova syndrome
Oligohydramnios sequence
Pena-Shokeir syndrome
Seckel syndrome
X-linked hydrocephalus (thumb)
Zellweger syndrome

MESOMELIC SHORTNESS

Acromesomelic dysplasia
Camptomelic dysplasia
Fetal aminopterin/methotrexate syndrome

MUSCLE WASTING

Arthrogryposis—various types
Congenital muscular dystrophy—various types
Neural tube defect—various types (lower limbs only)

Freeman-Sheldon syndrome (whistling facies)
Multiple pterygium syndrome (lethal)
Pena-Shokeir syndrome

POLYDACTYLY

Preaxial
Atelosteogenesis
Carpenter syndrome
Diabetic embryopathy
Greig's cephalopolysyndactyly syndrome
Pfeiffer syndrome
Townes-Brock syndrome

Postaxial
Chromosome—trisomy 13
Familial in blacks

Acrocallosal syndrome
Atelosteogenesis
Ellis-van Creveld syndrome (chondroectodermal dysplasia)
Grebe syndrome
Greig's cephalopolysyndactyly syndrome
Hydrolethalus
Jeune asphyxiating thoracic dystrophy
McKusik-Kaufman syndrome
Meckel-Gruber syndrome
Orofacial-digital syndrome
Pallister-Hall syndrome
Short-rib–polydactyly syndromes
Smith-Lemli-Opitz syndrome

RADIAL HYPOPLASIA

Chromosome—trisomy 18
Cornelia de Lange syndrome
Holt-Oram syndrome
VACTERL association

Aase syndrome
Acrofacial dysostoses—various types
Baller-Gerold syndrome
Chromosome—triploidy
Chromosome—trisomy 13
Fanconi's syndrome
Hemifacial microsomia (Goldenhar syndrome)
Roberts' syndrome (pseudothalidomide)
Thrombocytopenia-absent radius syndrome
Townes-Brock syndrome

RHIZOMELIC SHORTENING

Achondroplasia
Thanatophoric dysplasia

Atelosteogenesis
Diabetic embryopathy
Familial
Focal femoral deficiency
Fetal warfarin syndrome
Fibrochondrogenesis
Short-rib–polydactyly syndromes

ROCKER-BOTTOM FEET

Arthrogryposis—various types
Chromosome—trisomy 18

Fryns syndrome
Multiple pterygium syndrome—various types
Neu-Laxova syndrome
Neural tube defect
Pena-Shokeir syndrome

SHORT LIMBS

Generalized
Achondroplasia
Thanatophoric dysplasia

Achondrogenesis
Ellis-van Creveld syndrome (chondroectodermal dysplasia)
Jeune asphyxiating thoracic dystrophy
Kniest syndrome

Continued
Osteogenesis imperfecta—all types
Roberts' syndrome
Short-rib–polydactyly syndromes
Spondyloepiphyseal dysplasia congenita

Not all limbs
Focal femoral deficiency
Osteogenesis imperfecta—all types
Camptomelic dysplasia
Cornelia deLange syndrome
Diastrophic dysplasia

CYSTIC HYGROMA

Chromosome—45,X (Turner's syndrome)
Chromosome—trisomy 21 (Down syndrome)
Regression to normal (common)

Acardiac acephalic twin
Achondrogenesis
Chromosome—trisomy 13
Chromosome—trisomy 18
Chromosome—47,XXY (Klinefelter syndrome)
Multiple pterygium syndrome
Noonan syndrome
Pena-Shokeir syndrome
Roberts' syndrome

HYPEREXTENDED NECK

Anterior lymphangioma
Cervical neural tube defect (iniencephaly)
Cervical teratoma
Goiter
Neuromuscular disorder
Normal variant

NECK MASS

Anterior lymphangioma
Cervical meningocele
Cystic hygroma—bilateral
Cystic hygroma—unilateral
Encephalocele
Goiter
Hemangioma
Nuchal thickening
Teratoma of neck

VERTEBRAL DEFECTS

Diabetic embryopathy
Neural tube defect
VACTERL association

Continued
Cloacal extrophy
Diastomatomyelia
Hemifacial microsomia (Goldenhar syndrome)
Klippel-Feil syndrome
Kniest syndrome
Multiple pterygium syndrome
Osteogenesis imperfecta
Skeletal dysplasia—many types

AMNIOTIC BAND

Amniotic band syndrome
Amniotic sheet
Subamniotic or chorionic bleed
Twin membrane
Unfused amniotic membrane

Amniotic displacement following amniocentesis
Limb-body wall complex (amniotic disruption sequence)
Placental cyst

CORD MASS

Allantoic cyst

Angiomyxoma
Cord cyst
Cord knot
Hemangioma
Hematoma
Mucoid degeneration of the cord
Thrombosis of umbilical vessels
Umbilical vein varix
Wharton's jelly

HYDROPS

Alpha thalassemia (anemias)
Cardiac malformation (congenital heart disease)
Chromosome—trisomy 21 (Down syndrome)
Chromosome—45,X (Turner's syndrome)
Fetal infections (cytomegalovirus, parvovirus, syphilis, toxoplasmosis)
Rh incompatibility and other blood antibody syndromes
Twin-twin transfusion syndrome
Urinary-tract obstruction

Achondrogenesis
Cardiac tumor—rhabdomyoma—tuberous sclerosis
Chondrodysplasia punctata
Chromosome—triploidy
Chromosome—trisomy 18 (rare)
Congenital nephrotic syndrome—Finnish type

Continued
Cornelia de Lange syndrome
Cystadenomatoid malformation of lung
Diabetic embryopathy/meconium peritonitis
Diaphragmatic hernia
Dysrhythmia
Extralobar pulmonary sequestration
Fetomaternal transfusion
Fibrochondrogenesis
Hypophosphatasia
Multiple pterygium syndrome—lethal
Osteogenesis imperfecta—various types
Pena-Shokeir syndrome
Placental mass—chorioangioma
Sacrococcygeal teratoma
Short-rib–polydactyly syndromes—various types
Thanatophoric dysplasia
Tracheal atresia

INTRAUTERINE GROWTH RETARDATION

Chromosome—triploidy
Chromosome—trisomy 18
Poor-quality measurements
Small normal fetus

Achondroplasia
Achondrogenesis, various types
Atelosteogenesis
Camptomelic dysplasia
Chromosome—trisomy 13
Cornelia de Lange syndrome
Diabetic embryopathy—severe
Diastrophic dysplasia
Ellis-van Creveld syndrome (chondroectodermal dysplasia)
Fetal infections (cytomegalovirus, varicella, rubella)
Fetal alcohol syndrome
Fetal aminopterin/methotrexate syndrome
Fetal anticonvulsant syndrome
Fetal warfarin syndrome
Fibrochondrogenesis
Focal femoral deficiency
Fryn's syndrome
Hypophosphatasia
Meckel-Gruber syndrome
Neu-Laxova syndrome
Osteogenesis imperfecta, various types
Pena-Shokeir syndrome
Roberts' syndrome (pseudothalidomide)
Seckel syndrome
Short-rib–polydactyly syndromes—various types
Spondyloepiphyseal dysplasia congenita
Thanatophoric dysplasia

MACROSOMIA

Diabetic embryopathy
Large mother

Continued
Poor-quality measurements
Wrong dates

Beckwith-Wiedemann syndrome
Simpson-Golabi-Behnel syndrome

OLIGOHYDRAMNIOS

Bilateral dysplastic kidney
Bilateral renal agenesis (see Renal Agenesis)
Bilateral ureteral obstruction
Infantile polycystic kidney disease
Intrauterine growth retardation
Late third trimester
Posterior urethral valves
Postmaturity
Premature rupture of membranes
Stuck twin

Amniotic band syndrome
Caudal regression
Congenital infection
Neural tube defect
Sirenomelia
Triploidy

PLACENTAL MASS

Chorioangioma
Venous lake
Wharton's jelly deposition

Fetal lobulation
Partial molar changes
Mole and normal fetus
Placental cyst
Placental infarct

POLYHYDRAMNIOS

Associated with fetal hydrops including: Turner's syndrome, fetal infections—parvovirus, trisomy 13
Duodenal atresia
Gut atresia
Macrosomia
Tracheoesophageal fistula (esophageal atresia)
Twins

Achondrogenesis—various types
Achondroplasia
Anemias
Camptomelic dysplasia
Cardiac malformation—heart failure: various types—tuberous sclerosis
Chorioangioma
Chromosome—triploidy
Chromosome—trisomy 18

Continued
Cleft palate
Congenital nephrotic syndrome—Finnish type
Cystadenomatoid malformation of lung
Diabetic embryopathy
Diaphragmatic hernia
Epignathus
Fetal goiter
Fryns syndrome
Holoprosencephaly
Idiopathic
Intraabdominal mass (e.g., mesoblastic nephroma)
Intracranial abnormality
Jeune asphyxiating thoracic dystrophy
Large ovarian cysts
Megacystis microcolon
Micrognathia
Multiple pterygium syndrome
Neck teratoma
Omphalocele
Osteogenesis imperfecta—various types
Pena-Shokeir syndrome
Sacrococcygeal teratoma
Short-rib–polydactyly syndromes
Thanatophoric dysplasia
Twin-twin transfusion syndrome

THICK PLACENTA

Normal variant

Chorioangioma
Chromosome—triploidy
Diabetic embryopathy
Fetal infections (cytomegalovirus, rubella, syphilis, toxoplasmosis)
Hydrops
Rh incompatibility
Beckwith-Wiedemann syndrome
Sacrococcygeal teratoma

BONE HYPOMINERALIZATION

Achondrogenesis
Hypophosphatasia
Osteogenesis imperfecta

ENLARGED HEART

Cardiomyopathy
Hydrops
Small chest

LEFT HEART ENLARGEMENT

Anomalous left coronary artery
Aortic stenosis—some
Cardiomyopathy

RIGHT HEART ENLARGEMENT

Aortic stenosis—some
Coarctation of the aorta
Hypoplastic left heart syndrome
Pulmonary stenosis
Tetralogy of Fallot

RIGHT ATRIAL ENLARGEMENT

Complete arterioventricular canal
Ebstein's syndrome
Total anomalous pulmonary venous return
Tricuspid regurgitation
Tricuspid stenosis

BRIGHT ECHOES IN THE HEART

Angioma
Chordae tendineae (normal variant)
Papillary muscle (normal variant)
Rhabdomyoma (usually large)

PERICARDIAL EFFUSION

Cytomegalovirus (parvovirus)
Fifth disease
Hydrops

SMALL BOWEL DILATATION

Jejunoileal atresia
Volvulus
Meconium ileus
Meconium peritonitis
Hirschsprung's disease
Enteric duplications
Congenital choridorrhea
Gastroschisis
Hydronephrosis

LARGE BOWEL DILATATION

Anorectal atresia
Meconium plug syndrome
Hirschsprung's disease

ECHOGENIC FOCI IN THE ABDOMEN

Cytomegalovirus
Echogenic bowel
Idiopathic
Liver infarction
Meconium peritonitis

Hepatic tumors
Kidney tumor
Neuroblastoma
Renal vein thrombosis
Retroperitoneal tumors
Toxoplasmosis
Vascular calcification—intravascular thrombus

LIMB SHORTENING

Diffuse Shortening
Achondrogenesis
Osteogenesis imperfecta—types II, III
Thanatophoric dysplasia

Camptomelic dysplasia
Diastrophic dysplasia
Homozygous achondroplasia
Hypophosphatasia
Metatropic dysplasia
Short-rib–polydactyly syndrome
Other rare dysplasias

Rhizomelia
Asphyxiating thoracic dysplasia
Heterozygous achondroplasia

Chondrodysplasia punctata, rhizomelic type
Chondroectodermal dysplasia
Spondyloepiphyseal dysplasia

Mesomelia
Acromesomelic dysplasias
Mesomelic dysplasias

CHROMOSOMAL ANOMALY SONOGRAPHIC FINDINGS

Central nervous system anomalies
    Holoprosencephaly
    Dandy-Walker malformation, cerebellar hypoplasia
    Hydrocephalus
    Spina bifida
    Agenesis of the corpus callosum
Choroid plexus cysts—large or associated with other abnormalities
Hypotelorism, cleft lip and palate, single nostril, absent nose
Cystic hygroma
Nuchal thickening
Cardiac malformations
Duodenal atresia
Gut atresia
Omphalocele
Hydrothorax
Genitourinary anomalies
    Obstructive uropathy (obstruction at or distal to the urethrovesical junction)
    Renal cystic dysplasia with other abnormalities
Clubfoot, rocker bottom foot
Clubhand
Severe early intrauterine growth retardation
Polyhydramnios or oligohydramnios
Single umbilical artery
Multiple cord cysts

Appendix II Sonographic Features of Less Common Fetal Abnormalities

AARSKOG SYNDROME

Hypertelorism
Short nose
Clinodactyly

AASE SYNDROME

Radial hypoplasia

ACROCALLOSAL SYNDROME

Agenesis of corpus callosum
Hypertelorism
Polydactyly—postaxial

ACROFACIAL DYSOSTOSIS

Malformed ears
Micrognathia
Abnormal thumb
Absent digits
Radial hypoplasia

ACROMESOMELIC DYSPLASIA

Mesomelic shortness

AICARDI SYNDROME

Agenesis of corpus callosum
Dandy-Walker syndrome
Holoprosencephaly

ALPHA-THALASSEMIA

Hydrops

AMYLOPLASIA CONGENITA

Abdominal-wall process
Club foot
Joint contractures

APERT SYNDROME

Hydronephrosis
Coronal craniosynostosis
Renal cystic structure

Continued
Agenesis of the corpus callosum
Encephalocele
Mild ventriculomegaly
Exophthalmus
Short nose
Abnormal thumb
Clenched hands
Joint contractures
Hypertelorism

ATELOSTEOGENESIS

Small chest
Hypertelorism
Cleft lip and palate
Micrognathia
Absent limbs
Club foot
Polydactyly—postaxial
Rhizomelic shortening
Intrauterine growth retardation

BALLER-GEROLD SYNDROME

Malformed kidney
Mild ventriculomegaly
Hypotelorism
Absent digits
Abnormal thumb
Radial hypoplasia

BASAL CELL NEVUS SYNDROME

Macrocephaly
Cardiac mass

BEALS' SYNDROME

Joint contractures

BECKWITH-WIEDEMANN SYNDROME

Omphalocele or umbilical hernia
Malformed kidney
Visceromegaly
Macroglossia

BOOMERANG DYSPLASIA

Bowing

BRANCHIOOTORENAL SYNDROME

Malformed ears

CARPENTER'S SYNDROME

Abnormal thumb
Absent digits
Clinodactyly
Club foot
Polydactyly—preaxial

CHARGE ASSOCIATION

Omphalocele
Cardiac abnormality
Holoprosencephaly
Cleft palate
Micrognathia
Intrauterine growth retardation

CHONDRODYSPLASIA PUNCTATA

Small chest
Club foot
Rhizomelic shortening
Hydrops
Stippled epiphyses

CHROMOSOME—18P-

Holoprosencephaly
Hypotelorism
Club foot

CHROMOSOME—18Q-

Microphthalmia/anophthalmia

CHROMOSOME—47,XXY

Cystic hygroma

CHROMOSOME—4P-

Hypertelorism
Cardiac abnormality
Malformed ears (tags)

CHROMOSOME—DUPLICATION 20P

Hypertelorism

CLEIDOCRANIAL DYSPLASIA

Partial or total asplasia of the clavicles
Brachycephaly

CONGENITAL MUSCULAR DYSTROPHY

Clenched hands
Muscle wasting

CONGENITAL NEPHROTIC SYNDROME

Polyhydramnios
Hydrops

CORNELIA DE LANGE SYNDROME

Cardiac abnormality
Dandy-Walker cyst
Microcephaly
Short nose
Abnormal thumb
Absent digits
Absent limbs
Clinodactyly
Radial hypoplasia
Short limbs
Hydrops
Intrauterine growth retardation

CROUZON SYNDROME

Brachycephaly—prominent forehead
Hypertelorism
Exophthalmos/proptosis
Midface hypoplasia—beaked nose

DIABETIC EMBRYOPATHY

Duodenal atresia
Malformed kidney
Renal agenesis
Cardiac abnormality
Holoprosencephaly
Spinal dysraphism
Abnormal thumb
Absent limbs
Thick placenta
Bowing
Club foot
Joint contractures
Polydactyly—preaxial
Rhizomelic shortening
Vertebral defects
Hydrops

Continued
Macrosomia
Polyhydramnios

DIGEORGE SYNDROME

Cardiac abnormality—defects of the aortic arch
Holoprosencephaly
Micrognathia

DYSSEGMENTAL DYSPLASIA

Bowing

ECTRODACTYLY-ECTODERMAL DYSPLASIA-CLEFTING SYNDROME

Hydronephrosis
Cleft lip and palate (L,P)
Absent digits
Absent limbs
Clinodactyly

ECTRODACTYLY-TIBIAL APLASIA SYNDROME

Abnormal thumbs
Absent digits

ELLIS-VAN CREVELD SYNDROME

Renal cystic structure
Cardiac abnormality
Small chest
Club foot
Polydactyly—postaxial
Short limbs
Intrauterine growth retardation

ENLARGED KIDNEYS

Evenly echogenic or with variably sized cysts

FANCONI'S SYNDROME

Cardiac abnormality
Abnormal thumb
Absent digits
Radial hypoplasia

FETAL AMINOPTERIN/METHOTREXATE SYNDROME

Mesomelic shortness
Intrauterine growth retardation

FETAL INFECTIONS

Echogenic area in abdomen (cytomegalovirus)
Cardiac mass
Agenesis of the corpus callosum
Cerebellar hypoplasia
Dandy-Walker cyst
Echogenic brain foci
Microcephaly
Mild ventriculomegaly
Cataract
Microphthalmia or anophthalmia
Hydrops
Intrauterine growth retardation
Thick placenta

FETAL VITAMIN A SYNDROME

Cerebellar hypoplasia
Spinal dysraphism
Lateral cleft lip
Cleft palate
Malformed ears
Micrognathia

FETAL WARFARIN SYNDROME

Short nose
Rhizomelic shortening
Intrauterine growth retardation

FIBROCHONDROGENESIS

Small chest
Rhizomelic shortening
Hydrops
Intrauterine growth retardation

FRASER SYNDROME

Microphthalmia or anophthalmia

FREEMAN-SHELDON SYNDROME

Micrognathia
Clenched hands

Continued
Club foot
Joint contractures
Muscle wasting

FRONTONASAL DYSPLASIA

Holoprosencephaly
Hypertelorism

FRYN'S SYNDROME

Duodenal atresia
Renal cystic structure
Diaphragmatic hernia
Chest mass—pulmonary hypoplasia/abnormal lobulation
Holoprosencephaly
Lateral cleft lip
Cleft palate
Micrognathia
Absent digits
Club foot
Rocker bottom feet
Intrauterine growth retardation
Polyhydramnios

GOLDENHAR'S SYNDROME (SEE CHAPTER 13.4)

GREBE SYNDROME

Absent limbs
Polydactyly—preaxial

GREIG'S CEPHALOPOLYSYNDACTYLY SYNDROME

Macrocephaly
Hypertelorism
Facial asymmetry
Abnormal thumb
Polydactyly—preaxial/postaxial

HEMIFACIAL MICROSOMIA (GOLDENHARS SYNDROME)

Hydronephrosis
Renal agenesis
Cardiac abnormality
Holoprosencephaly
Hypotelorism
Microphthalmia or anophthalmia
Facial asymmetry

Continued
Lateral cleft lip
Cleft palate
Malformed ears
Micrognathia
Abnormal thumb
Radial hypoplasia
Vertebral defects

HOLT-ORAM SYNDROME

Cardiac abnormality
Abnormal thumb
Absent digits
Absent limbs
Clinodactyly
Radial hypoplasia

HYDROLETHALUS

Agenesis of the corpus callosum
Microphthalmia or anophthalmia
Polydactyly—postaxial
Hydrocephalus
Polyhydramnios
Macrognathia
Cleft palate
Heart defect
Club foot

HYPOPHOSPHATASIA

Small chest
Exposed brain
Bowing
Continued
Moderate to severe bone shortening
Hydrops
Intrauterine growth retardation
Diffuse hypomineralization

IVEMARK SYNDROME

Situs inversus
Complex heart defect
Polysplenia

JACKSON-WEISS SYNDROME

Exophthalmos/proptosis/prominent eyes
Facial asymmetry

ASPHYXIATING THORACIC DYSTROPHY—JEUNE

Renal dysplasia
Small chest
Mild ventriculomegaly
Polydactyly—postaxial (14%)
Short limbs
Polyhydramnios

JOUBERT SYNDROME

Cerebellar hypoplasia

KLIPPEL-FEIL SYNDROME

Vertebral defects

KNIEST SYNDROME

Short limbs
Kyphoscoliosis
Platyspondyly
Epiphyseal splaying

LARSEN SYNDROME

Club foot
Abnormal vertebral segmentation with kyphoscoliosis
Hypertelorism
Depressed nasal bridge
Micrognathia
Prominent forehead
Joint dislocation

LENZ SYNDROME

Microcephaly
Renal dysgenesis
Microphthalmia

MARDEN-WALKER SYNDROME

Micrognathia
Hypertelorism
Joint contractures
Renal cysts

MARFAN SYNDROME

Aortic widening
Unduly long bones

MATERNAL PHENYLKETONURIA

Cardiac abnormality
Microcephaly
Cleft palate

MCKUSIK-KAUFMAN SYNDROME

Hydronephrosis
Cardiac abnormality
Polydactyly—postaxial
Vaginal atresia or duplication
Hydrometrocolpos
Other genitourinary anomalies
Anorectal atresia

MECKEL-GRUBER SYNDROME

Omphalocele
Renal cystic structures
Cardiac abnormality
Agenesis of the corpus callosum
Cerebellar hypoplasia
Dandy-Walker cyst
Encephalocele
Holoprosencephaly
Microcephaly
Mild ventriculomegaly
Spinal dysraphism
Hypotelorism
Microphthalmia or anophthalmia
Cleft lip and palate
Club foot
Polydactyly—postaxial
Intrauterine growth retardation

MEGACYSTIS MEGAURETER

Hydronephrosis
Large bladder

MEGACYSTIS MICROCOLON

Large bladder
Polyhydramnios
Dilated small bowel
Mostly female

MILLER-DIEKER SYNDROME

Short nose
Clinodactyly

NARGER ACROFACIAL DYSOSTOSIS

Micrognathia
Deformed ears
Absent digits

NEU-LAXOVA SYNDROME

Agenesis of the corpus callosum
Cerebellar hypoplasia
Lissencephaly
Microcephaly with sloping forehead
Cataract
Exophthalmus/proptosis/prominent eyes with hyper-
  telorism
Microphthalmia or anophthalmia
Clenched hands
Joint contractures
Rocker-bottom feet
Micrognathia with flat nose

NOONAN SYNDROME

Cardiac abnormality—pulmonary stenosis
Hypertelorism
Cystic hygroma

OCULODENTODIGITAL SYNDROME

Microphthalmia or anophthalmia

OPITZ HYPERTELORISM HYPOSPADIAS SYNDROME

Hypertelorism

OROFACIAL-DIGITAL SYNDROME

Renal cystic structure
Cleft lip and palate
Micrognathia

Continued
Abnormal thumb
Clinodactyly
Polydactyly—postaxial
Males only

OROMANDIBULAR LIMB HYPOGENESIS

Absent digits
Absent limbs

OTOPALATODIGITAL SYNDROME

Hypertelorism
Cleft lip and palate

PALLISTER-HALL SYNDROME

Intracranial tumor—hypothalamic mass
Polydactyly—postaxial

PENA-SHOKEIR SYNDROME

Clenched hands
Club foot
Joint contractures
Rocker-bottom feet
Hydrops
Intrauterine growth retardation
Polyhydramnios
Micrognathia
Cleft palate
Hypertelorism

PFEIFFER SYNDROME

Kleeblattschädel deformity of skull
Exophthalmus/proptosis/prominent eyes
Hypertelorism
Facial asymmetry
Short nose
Abnormal thumb
Absent digits
Clinodactyly
Polydactyly—preaxial

POLAND ANOMALY

Absent digits
Absent limbs
Clinodactyly

RETINOIC ACID EMBRYOPATHY

Absent limbs
Cardiac abnormality
Micrognathia

ROBERTS' SYNDROME

Cardiac abnormality
Encephalocele
Mild ventriculomegaly
Spinal dysraphism
Cataract
Lateral cleft lip and cleft palate
Absent digits
Absent limbs
Clinodactyly
Short limbs
Intrauterine growth retardation
Phocomelia
Genitourinary anomaly

ROBIN SEQUENCE (PIERRE ROBIN)

Micrognathia
Cleft palate

ROBINOW SYNDROME

Hypertelorism
Lateral cleft lip and cleft palate
Short nose

RUBINSTEIN-TAYBI SYNDROME

Abnormal thumb
Microcephaly
Beaked nose
Cardiac defects

SAETHRE-CHOTZEN SYNDROME

Exophthalmus/proptosis/prominent eyes
Facial asymmetry
Clinodactyly

SECKEL SYNDROME

Microcephaly
Micrognathia
Clinodactyly
Club foot
Joint contractures
Intrauterine growth retardation

SHORT-RIB–POLYDACTYLY SYNDROMES

Omphalocele
Renal dysplasia
Cardiac abnormality
Holoprosencephaly
Mild ventriculomegaly
Lateral cleft lip and cleft palate
Micrognathia
Club foot
Polydactyly—postaxial
Rhizomelic shortening
Short limbs
Hydrops
Intrauterine growth retardation
Polyhydramnios

SIMPSON-GOLABI-BEHNEL SYNDROME

Macrosomia

SMITH-LEMLI-OPITZ SYNDROME

Renal agenesis
Renal cystic structure
Cardiac abnormality
Agenesis of the corpus callosum
Cerebellar hypoplasia
Holoprosencephaly
Microcephaly
Cataract
Micrognathia
Short nose
Abnormal thumb
Absent digits
Club foot
Polydactyly—postaxial
Microcephaly
Hydrocephalus
Cleft palate

SOTOS' SYNDROME

Macrocephaly

SPONDYLOEPIPHYSEAL DYSPLASIA CONGENITA

Small chest
Cleft palate
Short limbs
Intrauterine growth retardation
Short, mildly bowed femurs

STICKLER SYNDROME

Cleft palate
Micrognathia
Short nose
Cataracts
Scoliosis

THALIDOMIDE EMBRYOPATHY

Absent limbs
Phocomelia

THROMBOCYTOPENIA–ABSENT RADIUS SYNDROME

Cardiac abnormality
Absent limbs
Club foot
Radial hypoplasia

TOWNES-BROCK SYNDROME

Duodenal atresia
Renal agenesis
Facial asymmetry
Malformed ears
Abnormal thumb
Absent digits
Clinodactyly
Polydactyly—preaxial/radial hypoplasia

TREACHER COLLINS SYNDROME

Cleft palate
Malformed ears
Clinodactyly
Micrognathia

TUBEROUS SCLEROSIS

Renal cystic structure
Cardiac abnormality
Cardiac mass
Agenesis of the corpus callosum
Echogenic brain foci
Intracranial cyst/tumor
Renal cysts

VELOCARDIOFACIAL SYNDROME

Cardiac abnormality
Cleft palate

WARBURG SYNDROME (WALKER-WARBURG)

Agenesis of the corpus callosum
Dandy-Walker cyst
Encephalocele
Mild ventriculomegaly
Cataract
Microphthalmia or anophthalmia

WILLIAMS SYNDROME

Cardiac defects—supravalvular aortic stenosis

ZELLWEGER SYNDROME

Renal cystic structure
Cataract
Club foot
Joint contractures

Index

Note: "f" following page numbers indicates figures.

A

Aarskog syndrome, 269
Aase syndrome, 199, 269
Abdomen
 calcifications, 144
 cyst in, 256
 echogenicity, 255, 268
Abdominal wall process, 255
Acardiac twin, 221-222, 222f
Achondrogenesis, 163-164, 164-165f
 osteogenesis imperfecta versus, 193
 thanatophoric dwarfism versus, 201
Achondroplasia, 166-167, 168f, 201
Acrocallosal syndrome, 269
Acrofacial dysostosis, 269
Acromesomelic dysplasia, 269
Adrenal gland
 hematoma, 89-90, 90f
 renal agenesis and, 110f
Agenesis
 corpus callosum, 14-15, 15-16f, 27, 34, 258
 renal, 109-110, 110-111f
Aicardi syndrome, 14, 27, 269
Alcohol, fetal alcohol syndrome, 215-216, 249
Allantoic cysts, 149, 246, 247f
Alobar holoprosencephaly, 34, 35f
Alphathalassemia, 269
Aminopterin/methotrexate syndrome, 271
Amniotic bands, 244, 245f, 265
Amniotic band syndrome, 169-170, 171f
 anencephaly and, 17
 cystic hygroma and, 158
 encephalocele and, 30
 Klippel-Trenaunay-Weber syndrome versus, 185
Amniotic fluid; see Oligohydramnios; Polyhydramnios
Amniotic membranes, 158, 244-245, 245f
Amniotic sac, unfused, 244
Amniotic sheet, 244, 245f
Amputations, in focal femoral hypoplasia, 183
Amyloplasia congenita, 269
Anal atresia, 132-133, 133f, 243
Anencephaly, 17-18, 18-19f
Aneurysms
 umbilical artery, 246
 vein of Galen, 23, 51-52, 53f
Angiomyxomas, 246
Annular pancreas, 134
Anophthalmia, 261
Antiseizure drugs, 217-218
Aorta
 coarctation, 59-60, 61f
 in tetralogy of Fallot, 81, 83f
Apert syndrome, 269
Aqueductal stenosis, 20-22, 22f, 34
Arachnoid cysts, 23-24, 24f
 corpus callosum agenesis versus, 14
 Dandy-Walker cysts versus, 27
Arms; see Limb entries
Arnold-Chiari malformation

Arnold-Chiari malformation—cont'd
 aqueductal stenosis versus, 20
 cranial changes, 49f
 microcephaly and, 45
 myelomeningocele and, 47
Arrhythmias
 bradycardias, 54-56, 56f
 premature atrial contractions, 76, 77f
 tachycardias, 78-79, 80f
Arterial switch procedure, 85
Arteries, great, transposition of, 84-85, 86f
Arthrogryposis, 172-173, 173f
 club and rocker-bottom feet versus, 176
 multiple pterygium syndrome versus, 191
Ascites, 239f
 in cystic hygroma, 159f
 differential diagnosis, 255
 in meconium peritonitis, 144
 parvovirus and, 207f
 posterior urethral valves and, 106, 108f
 in varicella-zoster infection, 214f
Asphyxiating thoracic dystrophy—Jeune, 273
Atelosteogenesis, 269
Atrial bigeminy, 54, 55
Atrial contractions, premature, 76, 77f
Atrial enlargement, right, 267
Atrial flutter, 78, 79, 80f
Atrial septal defects, 71, 72
Atrioventricular valve defect, 72f

B

Baller-Gerold syndrome, 269
Banana sign, in spinal dysraphism, 48, 49f
Basal-cell nevus syndrome, 269
Beals' syndrome, 269
Beckwith-Wiedemann syndrome
 macrosomia and, 250
 omphalocele and, 149, 150
 sonographic fetures, 269
Bladder
 absence, 255
 exstrophy, 91-92, 92f, 149
 ureterocele and, 116, 117f
Bleeding
 adrenal, 89-90
 arachnoid cyst and, 23, 24
 intracranial, 41-42, 42f
Body-stalk anomaly, 149, 150, 188
Bone grafting for cleft lip and palate, 155
Bone hypomineralization, 267
Boomerang dysplasia, 269
Bowel atresias
 duodenal, 134-136, 136f
 gastroschisis and, 141
 nonduodenal, 137-139, 139f
Bowel echogenicity, 9, 144, 147
Bowing
 camptomelic dysplasia, 174-175, 175f
 differential diagnosis, 262-263

Bradycardias, 54-56, 56f
Brain
    in anencephaly, 17
    echogenic focus, 258
    in holoprosencephaly, 34
    in hydranencephaly, 37
    too easily seen, 258
Branchiootorenal syndrome, 270
Bronchogenic cysts, 118

C

Caffey's cortical hyperostosis, 130
Calcifications
    abdominal, 144
    in cytomegalic inclusion disease, 203, 205f
    in toxoplasmosis, 212f
    in varicella-zoster infection, 214f
Camptomelic dwarfism, 193
Camptomelic dysplasia, 174-175, 175f
Cantrell's pentalogy, 68, 69
    omphalocele versus, 149, 150
Carbamazepine, 217, 218
Cardiac abnormalities, 54-88; *see also* Heart disease
    from antiseizure drugs, 217
    differential diagnoses, 257, 267
    in fetal alcohol syndrome, 215
    hydrops and, 237
Cardiac rhabdomyoma, 57-58, 58f
Cardiac transplant, neonatal, 74
Carpenter's syndrome, 270
Casting, for club foot or vertical talus, 177
Cataracts, 260
Caudal regression, 25-26, 26f
    in limb body wall complex, 188, 189f
Cauliflower ear, 181f
Central nervous system abnormalities, 14-53
    from antiseizure drugs, 217
    in fetal alcohol syndrome, 215
    in hypoplastic left heart syndrome, 73
    from illegal drugs, 219
Cephalohematomas, 30
Cerebellar hypoplasia, 258
Cervical incompetence, 252
Cervical spine, in iniencephaly, 37
Cervical teratomas, 161
CHARGE association, 270
Cheeks, in macrosomia, 250, 251f
Chest
    abnormalities, 118-131
    mass, 257
    small, 257-258
Choledochal cysts, 103
Chondrodysplasia punctata, 270
Chorangiomas, 235-236, 236f
Choroid plexus cysts, 6, 7f
Chromosomal abnormalities, 1-13
    differential diagnoses, 268
    growth retardation and, 248
    sonographic features, 270
Cisterna magna, large, 7f, 205f
Cleft lip, 155f, 156f
Cleft lip and palate, 153-155, 155-157f
    care of, 154-155, 218
    differential diagnosis, 154, 261
Cleft palate, 4f, 155f
Cleft sternum, 69
Cleidocranial dysplasia, 270
Clinodactyly, 263
Cloacal exstrophy, 149
Cloverleaf skull, 259
Club foot, 176-177, 177-178f
    in diastrophic dysplasia, 179, 180

Club foot—cont'd
    differential diagnosis, 176, 263
    in limb body wall complex, 190f
Coarctation of aorta, 59-60, 61f
Cocaine, 219, 220
Colon dilation, 133f
Colpocephaly, 16
Congenital heart disease; see Heart disease
Conjoined twins, 223-225, 226-227f
Cord cysts, 150, 246-247, 247f
Cord hematomas, 246
Cord mass, 265
Cord pseudocysts, 246
Cord tumors, 246
Cornelia de Lange syndrome, 249, 270
Corpus callosum agenesis, 14-15, 15-16f
    Dandy-Walker malformation and, 27
    differential diagnosis, 14, 258
    holoprosencephaly versus, 34
Craniofacial abnormalities
    in amniotic band syndrome, 169
    aqueductal stenosis, 20
    Dandy-Walker malformation, 27
    differential diagnoses, 258-262
    encephalocele, 30
    holoprosencephaly, 34, 35, 36f
    hydranencephaly, 37, 38f
    from intracranial teratoma, 43
    microcephaly, 45, 46f
    in spinal dysraphism, 47
    in trisomy 18, 6
    in trisomy 21, 9, 11f
Craniopagus twins, 224, 225, 227f
Cranium, cyst in, 259
Crouzon syndrome, 270
Cyanosis, in tetralogy of Fallot, 82
Cyllosomas, 188
Cystic adenomatoid malformation of lung, 118-120, 120-121f, 122
Cystic fibrosis
    gastrointestinal atresia and, 137
    meconium ileus and, 144, 145, 147
Cystic hygromas, 158-159, 159-160f
    differential diagnosis, 158, 265
    hydrops and, 237
    multiple pterygium syndrome and, 191
    in Turner syndrome, 12, 13f
Cystic kidneys
    differential diagnosis, 256-257
    in trisomy 13, 3, 4f
Cysts
    allantoic, 149, 246, 247f
    arachnoid, 14, 23-24, 24f, 27
    bronchogenic, 118
    choledochal, 103
    choroid plexus, 6, 7f
    cord, 150, 246-247, 247f
    in corpus callosum agenesis, 14, 15, 16f
    Dandy-Walker, 27, 29f, 34, 258
    duplication, 103, 144
    infantile polycystic kidney disease, 97-98, 98-99f
    intraabdominal, 256
    intracranial, 259
    liver, 103, 144
    meconium, 144-145, 146f
    mesenteric, 103, 144
    multicystic dysplastic kidney, 100-101, 102f
    neurogenic, 118
    ovarian, 103-104, 104-105f, 144
    placental, 235, 244
    posterior fossa, 260
    urachal, 246
    ureteroceles, 116-117, 117f

Cytomegalovirus, 203-205, 205f
    growth retardation and, 249
    meconium cysts and, 144
    meconium ileus and, 147
    microcephaly and, 45
    toxoplasmosis versus, 210

D

Dandy-Walker cyst, 258
Dandy-Walker malformations, 27-29, 29f, 34
Dandy-Walker syndrome, 14
Depakote (valproic acid), 199, 217
Dextrocardia, 122
Diabetes, maternal, in caudal regression, 25
Diabetic embryopathy, 271
Diagnosis
    differential, 255-268
    sonographic features of less common abnormalities, 269-276
Diaphragmatic hernia, 118, 122-124, 125f
Diastrophic dysplasia, 179-180, 180-181f
Differential diagnoses, 255-268
DiGeorge syndrome, 59, 271
Digits
    absent, 262
    polydactyly, 5f, 197, 198f, 264
    syndactyly, 2f
Dilantin (phenytoin), 217
Distal arthrogryposis syndrome, 271
Double bubble sign, 134, 135
Double-outlet right ventricle, 62-63, 64f
Down syndrome, 9-11, 11f
    duodenal atresia and, 134, 135
    endocardial cushion defect in, 9, 71
    pleural effusion and, 130
Drug-induced abnormalities, 215-220
Duodenum
    atresia, 134-136, 136f
        in Down syndrome, 9
        polyhydramnios and, 254
    dilated, 255
    stenosis, 134
Duplication cysts, 103, 144
Dwarfism
    camptomelic, 175f, 193
    diastrophic, 180f
    polyhydramnios and, 254
    thanatophoric, 201-202, 202f
        achondrogenesis versus, 163
        achondroplasia versus, 166
Dyssegmental dysplasia, 271

E

Eagle-Barrett syndrome, 106
Ear cartilage hematomas, 181f
Ear malformations, 261
Ebstein's anomaly, 65-66, 67f
ECMO, 119, 123-124
Ectopia cordis, 68-69, 70f
Ectrodactyly-ectodermal dysplasia-clefting syndrome, 271
Electrodactyly-tibial aplasia syndrome, 271
Ellis-van Creveld syndrome, 271
Encephaloceles, 30-32, 32-33f
    anencephaly versus, 17
    corpus callosum agenesis and, 14
    cystic hygromas versus, 158
    Dandy-Walker malformation and, 27
    differential diagnosis, 30, 258
    iniencephaly versus, 37
Endocardial cushion defects, 9, 71-72, 72f
Epignathus, 154
Epilepsy drugs, 217-218

Epispadias repair, 92
Esophageal atresia, 126-128, 128-129f
Exophthalmos, 260
Exstrophy of bladder, 91-92, 92f
Extracorporeal membrane oxygenation, 119, 123-124
Extremities; *see* Limb *entries*
Eyes
    hypertelorism, 260
    hypotelorism, 4f, 36f, 260-261
    prominent, 260

F

Facial abnormalities, 153-157; *see also* Craniofacial abnormalities
    from antiseizure drugs, 217
    asymmetry, 261
    differential diagnoses, 261-262
    in fetal alcohol syndrome, 215
Facial cleft
    cleft lip and palate, 153-155, 155-157f
    in trisomy 13, 5f
Fallot's tetralogy, 26f, 62, 81-83, 83f
Fanconi's anemia, 199, 200
Fanconi syndrome, 271
Femur
    in achondrogenesis, 165f
    in achondroplasia, 168f
    bowing, 174, 175f
    in Down syndrome, 9
    focal hypoplasia, 182-183, 183-184f
    lengthening, 167, 183
    in osteogenesis imperfecta, 195f
Fetal alcohol syndrome, 215-216, 249
Fetal hydrops; *see* Hydrops
Fibrochondrogenesis, 272
Fibromas, 57
Fingers; *see also* Digits
    hitchhiker thumb, 179, 180f, 181f
Focal femoral hypoplasia, 182-183, 183-184f
Fontan procedure, 74
Foot deformities, 176-178, 197; *see also* Digits
    differential diagnoses, 263, 264
Fractures, 194, 195f, 263
Fraser syndrome, 272
Freeman-Sheldon syndrome, 272
Frontonasal dysplasia, 272
Fryns syndrome, 272

G

Galen's vein malformation, 23, 51-52, 53f
Gallbladder dilation, 144
Gastrointestinal abnormalities, 132-152
Gastrointestinal atresia or stenosis, 137-139, 139f
Gastrointestinal obstruction, 254
Gastroschisis, 140-142, 142-143f
    amniotic bands and, 169
    omphalocele versus, 149
Genitourinary malformations
    from antiseizure drugs, 217
    in fetal alcohol syndrome, 215
Genitourinary tract abnormalities, 89-117
Genu varum, 167
Glomerulosclerosis, 97
Goiter, 161-162, 162f
Goldenhar's syndrome, 272
Graves' disease, 161
Great arteries, transposition of, 84-85, 86f
Grebe syndrome, 272
Greig's cephalopolysyndactyly syndrome, 272
Growth retardation, 248-249
    achondroplasia versus, 166

Growth retardation—cont'd
    in cytomegalic inclusion disease, 204
    differential diagnosis, 266
    in fetal alcohol syndrome, 215, 249
    from illegal drugs, 219
    oligohydramnios and, 252
    triploidy and, 1
    twins and, 230-231, 232

H

Hand abnormalities, 197-200, 198f, 200f; *see also* Digits
    clenched hands, 263
    in triploidy, 2f
    in trisomy 18, 8f
Hanging choroid sign, 20, 22f
Heart
    displaced, 68-69, 70f
    enlarged, 267
    neonatal transplant, 74
Heart block, 54, 55
Heart disease, 54-88; *see also* Cardiac abnormalities
    in Down syndrome, 9
    in trisomy 13, 3
    in trisomy 18, 6
    in Turner syndrome, 12, 13
Hemangioma of umbilial cord, 246
Hematomas
    adrenal, 89-90, 90f
    cord, 246
    ear cartilage, 181f
    preplacental, 235
Hemifacial microsomia, 272
Hemorrhage
    adrenal, 89-90
    arachnoid cyst and, 23, 24
    intracranial, 41-42, 42f
Hepatomegaly, 205f, 212f
Hepatosplenomegaly, 208
Hernia
    diaphragmatic, 118, 122-124, 125f
    umbilical, 149
Heroin, 219
Hitchhiker thumb, 179, 180f, 181f
Holoprosencephaly, 34-35, 35-36f
    aqueductal stenosis versus, 20
    corpus callosum agenesis versus, 14
    differential diagnosis, 34, 259
    in trisomy 13, 4f
Holt-Oram syndrome, 199, 242, 272
Humerus
    in Down syndrome, 9
    in osteogenesis imperfecta, 195f
Hydantoin, 217-218
Hydranencephaly, 37-38, 38f
    differential diagnosis, 37, 259
    holoprosencephaly versus, 34
Hydrocephalus
    from aqueductal stenosis, 20
    in cytomegalic inclusion disease, 204
    in Dandy-Walker malformation, 28
    in intracranial hemorrhage, 41
    toxoplasmosis and, 210, 211
Hydrolethalus, 272
Hydronephrosis, 93-95, 96f
    differential diagnosis, 256
    multicystic dysplastic kidney versus, 100
    posterior urethral valves and, 108f
Hydrops
    bradycardia and, 54, 55
    cystic adenomatoid malformation of lung versus, 118, 119
    in cystic hygroma, 158, 159, 159f
    differential diagnosis, 265-266
    endocardial cusion defect and, 71

Hydrops—cont'd
    hypoplastic left heart syndrome and, 73
    Klippel-Trenaunay-Weber syndrome versus, 185
    macrosomia and, 250
    nonimmune hydrops fetalis, 237-238, 239f
    from parvovirus, 206, 207, 207f
    pleural effusion and, 130
    Rh disease and, 240, 241
    stuck twin and, 228
    tachycardias and, 78, 79
    vein of Galen aneurysm and, 51
Hypertelorism, 260
Hyperthyroidism, 161
Hypophosphatasia, 193, 272-273
Hypoplastic left heart syndrome, 73-74, 75f
Hypotelorism
    differential diagnosis, 260-261
    in holoprosencepahly, 36f
    in trisomy 13, 4f
Hypothyroidism, 161

I

Ileal atresia, 137
Ileus, meconium, 144, 145, 147-148
Ilizarov method, 167
Illegal drugs, 219-220
Imperforate anus, 132-133, 133f
Indomethacin, 252, 254
Infantile polycystic kidney disease, 97-98, 98-99f, 100
Infections, 203-214
    sonographic features, 271
Iniencephaly, 17, 39-40, 40f
Intestinal atresias
    duodenal, 134-136, 136f
    gastroschisis and, 141
    nonduodenal, 137-139, 139f
Intestinal duplications, proximal, 134
Intraabdominal cysts, 256
Intracranial cysts, 259
Intracranial hemorrhage, 41-42, 42f
Intracranial teratoma, 43-44, 44f
Intrauterine growth retardation; *see* Growth retardation
Ischiopagus twins, 224-225, 226-227f
Ivemark syndrome, 71, 273

J

Jacho-Levin syndrome, 243
Jackson-Weiss syndrome, 273
Jejunal atresia, 134, 137, 139f
Joint contractures, 263-264
Joubert syndrome, 273

K

Kidneys; *see also* Renal *entries*
    agenesis, 109-110, 110-111f, 256
    cystic, 3, 4f, 256-257
        infantile polycystic kidney disease, 97-98, 98-99f
        multicystic dysplastic kidney, 100-101, 103f
    enlarged, 271
    ureterocele and, 116
Kleeblattschädel deformity of skull, 259
Klippel-Feil syndrome, 273
Klippel-Trenaunay-Weber syndrome, 169, 185-186, 186-187f
Kniest syndrome, 273
Kyphoscoliosis, 179, 180
Kyphosis, thoracolumbar, 167

L

Ladd's bands, 134
Large bowel dilatation, 267

Larsen syndrome, 273
Left ventricle hypoplasia, 73-74, 75f
Legs; see Limb entries
Lemon sign, in spinal dysraphism, 48, 49f
Lenz syndrome, 273
Limb abnormalities, 163-202
    differential diagnoses, 262-265, 268
    oligohydramnios and, 252
    polyhydramnios and, 254
    in spinal dysraphism, 47
    in trisomy 18, 6
    in trisomy 21, 9
Limb-body wall complex, 188-189, 189f
    amniotic bands in, 169
    gastroschisis versus, 140
Limb lengthening, 167, 183
Lipomas, 43
Lips
    cleft lip, 155f, 156f
    cleft lip and palate, 153-155, 155-157f, 261
Liver
    cysts, 103, 144
    enlarged, 205f, 208, 212f
    omphalocele and, 149
Lobar holoprosencephaly, 34
    corpus callosum agenesis versus, 14
    hydranencephaly versus, 37
Lungs
    cystic adenomatoid malformation, 118-120, 120-121f
    stenosis in tetralogy of Fallot, 81, 82
    tumors, 122
Lymphangioma of neck, 160f
Lymphedema, in Turner syndrome, 12, 13f

M

Macrocephaly
    differential diagnosis, 259
    in thanatophoric dwarfism, 202f
    in triploidy, 2f
Macroglossia, 261
Macrosomia, 250-251, 251f, 266
Marden-Walker syndrome, 273
Marfan syndrome, 273
McKusick-Kaufman syndrome, 103, 273
Meckel-Gruber syndrome
    Dandy-Walker malformation and, 27
    encephalocele and, 30
    infantile polycystic kidney disease versus, 97
    kidney cysts in, 33f
    multicystic dysplastic kidney versus, 100
    polydactyly and, 197
    sonographic features, 273-274
Meconium cysts, 144-145, 146f
Meconium ileus, 147-148
    cystic fibrosis and, 144, 145, 147
Meconium peritonitis, 137, 144, 147
Meconium pseudocysts, 144
Megacystis megaureter syndrome, 106, 274
Megacystis microcolon syndrome, 106, 274
Meningoceles, 47, 158
Mental retardation, in fetal alcohol syndrome, 215
Mesenteric cysts, 103, 144
Mesomelic shortness, 264
Microcephaly, 45-46, 46f
    anencephaly versus, 17
    from cytomegalovirus, 205f
    differential diagnosis, 45, 259
Micrognathia, 8f, 261-262
Microphthalmia, 261
Midgut volvulus, 134
Miller-Dieker syndrome, 274
Multicystic dysplastic kidney, 100-101, 102f
Multiple pterygium syndrome, 191-192, 192f

Multiple pterygium syndrome—cont'd
    arthrogryposis versus, 172
    cystic hygroma and, 158
    Turner's syndrome versus, 12
Muscle wasting, 264
Muscular dystrophy, 270
Myelomeningoceles, 47-49, 49-50f
    corpus callosum agenesis and, 14
    in limb-body wall complex, 188
    microcephaly and, 45
    sacrococcygeal teratomas versus, 112
    valproic acid and, 217
Myeloschisis, 47, 50f

N

Narger acrofacial dysostosis, 274
Neck abnormalities, 158-162
    hyperextension, 265
    lymphangioma, 160f
    mass, 265
Nephrotic syndrome, 270
Neu-Laxova syndrome
    growth retardation and, 249
    microcephaly and, 45
    sonographic features, 274
Neuroblastomas, 89
Neurogenic cysts, 118
Nonimmune hydrops fetalis, 237-238, 239f
Noonan syndrome
    cystic hygroma and, 158
    sonographic features, 274
    Turner's syndrome versus, 12
Norwood procedure, 74
Nose, short, 262
Nuchal fold thickening, 9, 11f
Nuchal translucency, 158

O

Oculodentodigital syndrome, 274
Oligohydramnios, 252-253
    amniotic band syndrome and, 170
    differential diagnosis, 266
    in infantile polycystic kidney disease, 97
    in renal agenesis, 111f
    stuck twin and, 228
Omphaloceles, 149-151, 151-152f
    bladder exstrophy versus, 91
    differential diagnosis, 149, 256
    iniencephaly and, 40f
    ruptured, gastroschisis versus, 140
    in trisomy 13, 5f
Omphalomesenteric cyst, 246
Omphalopagus twins, 224, 226f
Opitz-Frias hypertelorism hypospadias syndrome, 130
Opitz hypertelorism hypospadias syndrome, 274
Orofacial-digital syndrome, 198f, 274
Oromandibular limb hypogenesis, 274
Osteogenesis imperfecta, 193-194, 195-196f
    camptomelic dysplasia versus, 174
    focal femoral hypoplasia versus, 182
    radial ray problems versus, 199
Otopalatodigital syndrome, 274
Ovarian cysts, 103-104, 104-105f, 144

P

Pacemaker insertion, 56
Palate
    cleft lip and palate, 153-155, 155-157f, 261
    cleft palate, 4f, 155f
Pallister-Hall syndrome, 274
Pancreas, annular, 134

Parvovirus, 206-207, 207f
Pena-Shokeir syndrome
 arthrogryposis versus, 172
 cystic hygroma and, 158
 sonographic features, 274
Pendred's syndrome, 161
Pentalogy of Cantrell, 68, 69
 omphalocele versus, 149, 150
Pericardial effusion, 257, 267
Peritonitis, meconium, 137, 144
Pfeiffer syndrome, 274-275
Phenobarbital, 217
Phenylketonuria, maternal, 45, 273
Phenytoin, 217
Pierre Robin sequence, 275
Placenta
 cysts, 235, 244
 mass, 266
 thick, 267
Plastic surgery for cleft lip and palate, 154-155
Platyspondyly, 202f
Pleural effusion, 130-131, 131f, 239f, 257
Poland anomaly, 275
Polycystic kidney disease, 97-98, 98-99f
 adult, 97, 100
 multicystic dysplastic kidney versus, 100
Polydactyly, 197, 198f
 differential diagnosis, 264
 in trisomy 13, 5f
Polyhydramnios, 254
 acardiac twin and, 221
 in anencephaly, 17
 cystic adenomatoid malformation of lung versus, 118, 119
 diaphragmatic hernia versus, 123
 diastrophic dysplasia and, 179
 differential diagnosis, 266-267
 esophageal atresia and, 127
 ovarian cysts and, 103
 stuck twin and, 228
Porencephalic cyst, 23
Porencephaly, 37
Posterior fossa cyst, 260
Posterior urethral valves, 106-108, 108f
 in trisomy 21, 9
 ureterocele versus, 116
Preeclampsia, vein of Galen aneurysm and, 51
Premature atrial contractions, 76, 77f
Premature rupture of membranes, 252
Proptosis, 260
Proteus syndrome, 185
Prune-belly syndrome, 106, 107
Pseudoascites, 237
Pseudocysts, cord, 246
Pseudoomphalocele, 152f
Pseudopericardial effusion, 237
Pterygia, multiple pterygium syndrome, 191-192, 192f
 differential diagnosis, 12, 158, 172, 191
Pulmonary stenosis, 81, 82
Pygopagus twins, 224, 225, 227f

R

Radial hypoplasia, 264
Radial ray problems, 199-200, 200f
Reconstructive surgery for cleft lip and palate, 154-155
Rectal dilation, 133f
Reflux, vesicoureteric, 93, 96f, 116
Renal abnormalities
 agenesis, 109-110, 110-111f, 256
 differential diagnoses, 256-257
 enlargement, 271
 hydronephrosis, 93-95, 96f
 infantile polycystic kidney disease, 97-98, 98-99f

Renal abnormalities—cont'd
 multicystic dysplastic kidney, 100-101, 102f, 256
 oligohydramnios and, 252
 in Turner syndrome, 12
Renal pelvic dilatation, 9, 93-95, 96f
Renal vein thrombosis, 89
Retardation; see Growth retardation; Mental retardation
Retinoic acid embryopathy, 275
Rhabdomyomas, cardiac, 57-58, 58f
Rhesus incompatibility, 240-241
Rhizomelic shortening, 264
Right ventricle, double-outlet, 62-63, 64f
Roberts' syndrome, 199, 275
Robin sequence, 275
Robinow syndrome, 275
Rocker-bottom foot, 176-177, 187f, 264
Rubinstein-Taybi syndrome, 275

S

Sacrococcygeal teratoma, 112-114, 114-115f
 bladder exstrophy versus, 91
 spinal dysraphism versus, 48
Saethre-Chotzen syndrome, 275
Schizencephaly, 23, 34
Scoliosis
 in arthrogryposis, 173
 in diastrophic dysplasia, 179, 180
 in osteogenesis imperfecta, 194
Seckel syndrome, 275
Seizures, drugs for, 217-218
Semilobar holoprosencephaly, 34, 36f
Short bowel syndrome, 141
Short-gut syndrome, 138, 145
Short-rib polydactyly syndrome, 197, 275
Shunts, in aqueductal stenosis, 21
Sigmoid colon dilation, 133f
Sillence classification of osteogenesis imperfecta, 193
Simpson-Golabi-Behnel syndrome, 275
Sinus bradycardia, 54, 55
Sinus tachycardia, 78, 79
Sirenomelia, 25, 109
Skeletal malformations
 from antiseizure drugs, 217
 diastrophic dysplasia, 179-180, 180-181f
 in fetal alcohol syndrome, 215
 osteogenesis imperfecta, 193-194, 195-196f
Skin thickening
 in acardiac acephalic twin, 222f
 in cystic hygroma, 158
 macrosomia and, 250, 251f
 in varicella-zoster infection, 214f
Small bowel
 dilatation, 144, 267
 echogenicity, 144
Smith-Lemli-Opitz syndrome, 275
Soft-tissue release, in arthrogryposis, 173
Sonography
 abnormal findings, 244-254
 features of less common abnormalities, 269-276
Sotos syndrome, 275
Spinal defects
 caudal regression, 25-26, 26f
 in iniencephaly, 37
 stenosis in adults, 167
Spinal dysraphism, 47-49, 49-50f, 260
Spinal surgery for achondroplasia, 167
Splenomegaly, 205f, 212f
Spondyloepiphyseal dysplasia congenita, 276
Stenosis
 aqueductal, 20-22, 22f
 duodenal, 134
 gastrointestinal, 137-139, 139f

Stenosis—cont'd
    pulmonary, 81, 82
    spinal, in adults, 167
Sternopagus twins, 224
Sternum, cleft, 69
Stickler syndrome, 276
Stomach
    dilated, differential diagnoses, 255
    nonvisualization, 126, 129f, 255
Stuck twin, 228-229, 229f
Subchorionic lucent space, 244
Supraventricular tachycardia, 78, 79
Surgery for conjoined twins, 224-225
Sylvian aqueduct stenosis, 20-22, 22f
Syndactyly, 2f
Syphilis, 208-209

T

Tachycardias, 78-79, 80f
Talectomy, 180
Talus, vertical, 176, 177
TAR syndrome, 199, 200
Tegretol (carbamazepine), 217
Teratomas
    cardiac rhabdomyomas versus, 57
    cleft lip and palate versus, 154
    intracranial, 43-44, 44f
    sacrococcygeal, 112-114, 114-115f
        bladder exstrophy versus, 91
        spinal dysraphism versus, 48
        thyroid enlargement versus, 161
Tetralogy of Fallot, 26f, 62, 81-83, 83f
Thalidomide embryopathy, 276
Thanatophoric dwarfism (dysplasia), 201-202, 202f
    achondrogenesis versus, 163
    achondroplasia versus, 166
Third ventriculostomy, 21
Thoracolumbar kyphosis, 167
Thoracopagus twins, 224, 225, 226f
Thrombocytopenia—absent radius syndrome, 242, 276
Thumb abnormalities
    differential diagnosis, 262
    hitchhiker thumb, 179, 180f, 181f
Thyroid enlargement, 161-162, 162f
Tibia
    bowing, 174, 175f
    lengthening, 167, 183
    in osteogenesis imperfecta, 195f
Toes; see Digits
Townes-Brock syndrome, 276
Toxoplasmosis, 110-111, 112f, 144
Tracheal atresia, 126, 128f
Tracheoesophageal fistula, 126, 127, 128, 243, 254
Transfusions
    parvovirus and, 207
    in Rh disease, 240
Transplantation, neonatal cardiac, 74
Transposition of great arteries, 84-85, 86f
Treacher-Collins syndrome, 276
Treponema pallidum, 208
Tricuspid valve, Ebstein anomaly of, 65-66, 67f
Triploidy, 1-2, 2f, 248
Trisomy 13, 3-4, 4-5f
    Dandy-Walker malformation and, 27
    growth retardation and, 248
    infantile polycystic kidney disease versus, 97
    multicystic dysplastic kidney versus, 100
    omphaloceles versus, 149
    polydactyly and, 197
    rocker-bottom feet in, 178f
Trisomy 18, 6-7, 7-8f
    Dandy-Walker malformation and, 27

Trisomy 18—cont'd
    growth retardation and, 248
    omphaloceles versus, 149
    radial ray problems and, 199
Trisomy 21, 9-11, 11f
Tuberous sclerosis, 276
Tumors
    cardiac rhabdomyoma, 57-58, 58f
    chorangioma, 235-236, 236f
    intracranial teratoma, 43-44, 44f
    sacrococcygeal teratoma, 112-114, 114-115f
        differential diagnosis, 48, 91, 112
Turner syndrome, 12-13, 13f
    aortic coarctation in, 59
    cystic hygroma and, 158
    pleural effusion and, 130
    trisomy 21 versus, 10
Twin gestational sac membrane, 244
Twin reversed arterial perfusion sequence, 221
Twins, 221-234
Twin-twin transfusion syndrome, 232-233, 234f
    growth retardation and, 230
    stuck twin and, 228, 229

U

Ultrasonography
    abnormal findings, 244-254
    features of less common abnormalities, 269-276
Umbilical artery aneurysm, 246
Umbilical cord hemangioma, 246
Umbilical hernia, 149
Urachal cysts, 246
Ureteroceles, 116-117, 117f
Ureteropelvic junction obstruction and reflux, 93-95, 96f
Urethral valves, posterior, 106-108, 108f
    in trisomy 21, 9
    ureterocele versus, 116
Urinomas, 96f
Urofacial syndrome, 93
Urogenital abnormalities, 89-117

V

VACTERL association/syndrome, 242-243
    in anal atresia, 132
    in duodenal atresia, 135
    in esophageal atresia, 126, 127
    radial ray problems and, 199
Valproic acid, 199, 217
Varicella-zoster infection, 213-214, 214f
Vein of Galen malformation, 23, 51-52, 53f
Velocardiofacial syndrome, 276
Ventricle
    left, hypoplasia, 73-74, 75f
    right, double-outlet, 62-63, 64f
Ventricular contractions, 76, 77f, 80f
Ventricular septal defects, 87-88, 88f
    double-outlet right ventricle and, 62-63, 64f
    endocardial cushion defects and, 71
    in tetralogy of Fallot, 81, 82
    transposition of great arteries and, 84
Ventricular shunts, in aqueductal stenosis, 21
Ventricular tachycardia, 78, 79, 80f
Ventriculomegaly
    in aqueductal stenosis, 20, 21, 22f
    corpus callosum agenesis versus, 14
    from cytomegalovirus, 205f
    differential diagnosis, 260
    in intracranial hemorrhage, 42f
    vein of Galen aneurysm and, 53f
Vertebral defects, 265
Vertical talus, 176, 177

Vesicostomy, 107
Vesicoureteric reflux, 93, 96f, 116
Viral infections, 203-207, 205f, 207f, 213-214, 214f
Vitamin A syndrome, 271
Vitamin K, 218
Volvulus, midgut, 134

W

Walker-Warburg syndrome, 27, 276
Warburg syndrome, 276
Warfarin syndrome, 271
Webbing, multiple pterygium syndrome, 191-192, 192f
    differential diagnosis, 12, 158, 172, 191
Williams syndrome, 276
Wolff-Parkinson-White syndrome, 78

Z

Zellweger syndrome, 276